American Red Cross

First Aid
Responding to Emergencies

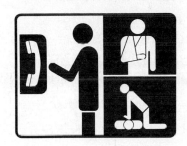

* IMPORTANT CERTIFICATION INFORMATION *

American Red Cross certificates may be issued upon successful completion of a training program, which uses this textbook as an integral part of the course. By itself, the text material does not constitute comprehensive Red Cross training. In order to issue ARC certificates, your instructor must be authorized by the American Red Cross, and must follow prescribed policies and procedures. Make certain that you have attended a course authorized by the Red Cross. Ask your instructor about receiving American Red Cross certification, or contact your local chapter for more information.

American Red Cross
First Aid
Responding to Emergencies

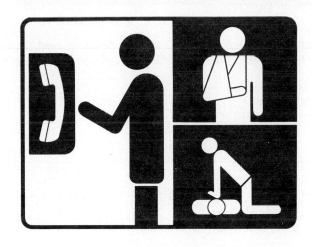

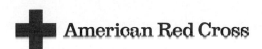 American Red Cross

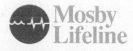 Mosby Lifeline

St. Louis Baltimore Boston Chicago London Philadelphia Sydney Toronto

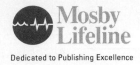

Mosby
Lifeline

Dedicated to Publishing Excellence

Printed in the United States of America

Mosby Lifeline
11830 Westline Industrial Drive
St. Louis, MO 63146

Library of Congress Cataloging in Publication Data
American Red Cross first aid responding to emergencies.
       p.   cm.
     Includes bibliographical references.
     Includes index.
     ISBN 0-8016-9009-9
     1. First aid in illness and injury.   2. Medical emergencies.
   I. American Red Cross.
     [DNLM: 1. Emergencies—programmed instructions.   2. First Aid—
   programmed instructions.   WA   18 A152]
   RC86.7.A477   1991
   616.02′52--dc20
   DNLM/DLC
   for Library of Congress   90-13642
                                                               CIP

ISBN 0-8016-9009-9

21135

94 95 96 97 CL/CD/BA 9 8 7 6 5 4

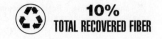

10%
TOTAL RECOVERED FIBER

This textbook is dedicated to the thousands of paid and volunteer staff of the American Red Cross who contribute their time and talents to teach lifesaving skills worldwide.

Acknowledgements

This course and textbook were developed and produced through a joint effort of the American Red Cross and the Mosby—Year Book Publishing Company. Many individuals shared in the overall process in many supportive, technical, and creative ways. This course could not have been developed without the dedication of both paid and volunteer staff. Their commitment to excellence made this course and textbook possible.

Members of the Development team at American Red Cross national headquarters responsible for designing and writing this course and textbook included: M. Elizabeth Buoy-Morrissey, M.P.H., Development Team Leader; Lawrence D. Newell, Ed.D., NREMT-P, and S. Elizabeth White, M.A.Ed., ATC, Writers/Instructional Designers; Martha F. Beshers, Elizabeth Peabody, and Joan H. Timberlake, Editors; Elaine P. McClatchey, Feature Articles Writer; Rebekah Jecker Calhoun, M.S.Ed., Application and Study Questions Writer; Marian F. H. Kirk, Artwork and Photographic Coordinator; and Ella Holloway and Jane Moore, Administrative Support.

The following American Red Cross national headquarters Health and Safety paid and volunteer staff provided guidance and review: John M. Malatak, Ph.D., Assistant Director; Frank Carroll, Manager, Development; Jean M. Wagaman, Associate, Operations; Jeanne P. Luschin, M.B.A., Associate, Marketing; Israel M. Zuñiga, Associate, Development; and Stephen Silverman, Ed.D., National Volunteer Consultant, Development.

The Mosby—Year Book Production team included: David T. Culverwell, Publisher; Richard A. Weimer, Executive Editor; Claire Merrick, Senior Editor; Patricia Gayle May, Project Manager; Mary Cusick Drone and Donna Walls, Production Editors; Kay Kramer, Art and Design Director; and Liz Fett, Senior Designer.

Special thanks go to Tom Lochhaas, Ed.D., Developmental Editor; Bruce Goldfarb, Writing Consultant; Rick Brady, Photographer; and Terry Hoff, Cover Artist.

Guidance and review were also provided by members of the American Red Cross First Aid Advisory Committee:

Sergeant Ray Cranston
Chairperson
Farmington Hills Police
  Department
Farmington Hills, Michigan

Kathleen C. Oberlin
Subcommittee Chairperson
Specialist, Health and Safety
Western Operations Headquarters
American Red Cross
Burlingame, California

Ann E. Graziadei, Ed.S., A.T.,C.
Department of Physical Education
  and Recreation
Gallaudet University
Washington, D.C.

Candace Key Gregg, M.S.
Director of Health and Safety
American Red Cross Tuscaloosa
  County Chapter
Tuscaloosa, Alabama

Stanley Henderson, M.S., E.M.T.
Assistant Professor
Department of Health and Safety
Indiana State University
Terre Haute, Indiana

Sam A. Lybarger, Ed.S.
Safety Professional III
Reynolds Electrical and
  Engineering
Las Vegas, Nevada

Mary M. Newman
Emergency Medical Services
  Consultant
Carmel, Indiana

Donna Palmieri
Manager, Safety Services
American Red Cross Southeastern
  Pennsylvania Chapter
Philadelphia, Pennsylvania

David C. Wiley, Ph.D.
Assistant Professor
Department of Health, Physical
  Education and Recreation
Southwest Texas State University
San Marcos, Texas

Peter C. Wolk, Ed.M., J.D.
Volunteer Instructor
National Capital Chapter
  and
Attorney
Dow, Lohnes and Albertson
Washington, D.C.

External review was provided by the following organizations and
individuals:

American College of Emergency
  Physicians
Dallas, Texas

National Association of Emergency
  Medical Technicians
Kansas City, Missouri

National Association of EMS
  Physicians
Pittsburgh, Pennsylvania

Jane W. Ball, RN, Dr. P.H.
Children's National Medical Center
Washington, D.C.

Judith M. Carson, M.A.
Assistant Professor and
Director of General Studies
Department of Physical Education
Northern Illinois University
DeKalb, Illinois

James W. Crowe
Associate Professor
Health, Physical Education and
  Recreation Department
Indiana University
Bloomington, Indiana

Daniel E. Della-Giustina, Ph.D.
Professor and Chairman
Department of Safety Studies
West Virginia University
Morgantown, West Virginia

Robert L. Hailey, M.Ed.
Assistant Professor
Southern Illinois University at
  Carbondale
Carbondale, Illinois

Laura Kitzmiller, EMT-P
Director, Emergency Medical Care
  Programs
Health and Kinesiology
  Department
Texas A & M University
College Station, Texas

Mark Lockhart, NREMT-P
Maryland Heights Fire Protection
  District
Maryland Heights, Missouri

Jill Moore, M.P.H.
Research Associate
Injury Prevention Research Center
The University of North Carolina
Chapel Hill, North Carolina

Lawrence Mottley, M.D.,
  F.A.C.E.P.
Senior Medical Advisor
Emergency Services
New York State Department of
  Health
Albany, New York

Terri Mulkins Manning, Ed.D.
Assistant Professor of Health
  Behavior
The University of North Carolina at
  Charlotte
Charlotte, North Carolina

James O. Page, J.D.
Publisher
Journal of Emergency Medical
  Services (JEMS)
Solana Beach, California

John W. Pappa
Supervisor V
Coordinator of Emergency Care
Department of Physical Education
University of California at Davis
Davis, California

John A. Paraskos, M.D.
Professor of Medicine
Division of Cardiovascular
  Medicine
University of Massachusetts
  Medical Center
Worcester, Massachusetts

S. Scott Polsky, M.D., F.A.C.E.P.
Department of Emergency
  Medicine
Akron City Hospital
Akron, Ohio

Charmaine R. Posten, M.A.
School Health Educator
Los Angeles Unified School District
Verdugo Hills High School
Tujunga, California

Mary Lou Smith, M. Ed.
Virginia Intermont College
Bristol, Virginia

Bernard G. Starks
Chairman, Physical Education
 Programs
University of Wisconsin at Green
 Bay
Green Bay, Wisconsin

E. V. "Lige" Turman
Assistant Professor and EMS
 Coordinator
Health, Physical Education, and
 Recreation Department
Health and Safety Division
Memphis State University
Memphis, Tennessee

Vincent P. Verdile, M.D.
Assistant Professor of Medicine
Division of Emergency Medicine
University of Pittsburgh
School of Medicine
 and
Associate Medical Director
Department of Public Safety
City of Pittsburgh
Pittsburgh, Pennsylvania

Additional assistance was provided by the Institute of Medicine of the
National Academy of Sciences. Members of a special committee, the
Committee to Advise the American National Red Cross, included:

Paul R. Meyer, Jr., M.D.
Chairperson
Director, Acute Spine Injury
 Center
Northwestern Memorial Hospital
Northwestern University Medical
 School
Chicago, Illinois

George T. Anast, M.D.
President, Northern Wisconsin
 Orthopedic Center
Woodruff, Wisconsin

Harold D. Cross, M.D.
PROMIS Health Care
Hampden, Maine

Benjamin Honigman, M.D.
Director, Emergency Medicine and
 Trauma
Assistant Professor of Surgery
University of Colorado Medical
 Center
Denver, Colorado

D. Randy Kuykendall
Operations Supervisor, Ambulance
 Department
Memorial General Hospital
Las Cruces, New Mexico

Sylvia II. Micik, M.D.
Medical Director
North County Health Services
San Marcos, California

Frederick P. Rivara, M.D., M.P.H.
Director, Harborview Injury
 Prevention and Research Center
Harborview Medical Center
Seattle, Washington

Carol W. Runyan, Ph.D.
Associate Director
Injury Prevention Research Center
 and
Research Assistant Professor
School of Public Health
The University of North Carolina
Chapel Hill, North Carolina

John A. Sterba, M.D., Ph.D.
Wright State University School of
 Medicine
Department of Emergency
 Medicine
Dayton, Ohio

Warren Winkelstein, Jr., M.D.,
 M.P.H.
Head, Epidemiology Program
School of Public Health
University of California at Berkeley
Berkeley, California

Contents

PART VII **Healthy Lifestyles**

Detailed Table of Contents

About This Course

◆ Why You Should Take This Course

People need to know what to do in an emergency before medical help arrives. Since you, the citizen responder, are the person most likely to be first on the scene of an emergency, it is important that you know how to recognize emergencies and how to respond. This course will prepare you to make appropriate decisions regarding first aid care and to act on those decisions.

The first critical step in any emergency depends on the presence of someone who will take appropriate action. After completing this course, you should be able to—

- Recognize when an emergency has occurred.
- Follow a four-step plan of action for any emergency.
- Provide care for injuries or sudden illnesses until professional medical help arrives.

The course clarifies when and how to call for emergency medical help, eliminating the confusion that is frequently a factor in any emergency.

The course also emphasizes the importance of a safe, healthy lifestyle. The Healthy Lifestyles Awareness Inventory, Appendix D in this book, provides a means for you to evaluate your lifestyle, determine how you can improve it, and help prevent lifestyle-related illness and injury.

◆ How You Will Learn

Course content is presented in various ways. The textbook, which will be assigned reading, contains the information that will be discussed in class. Videos and transparencies will support this information, as well as discussions and other class activities. These audiovisuals emphasize the key points that you will need to remember when making decisions in emergencies and will help you provide appropriate care. They also present skills that you will practice in class. Participating in all class activities will increase your confidence in your ability to respond to emergencies.

The course design allows you to frequently evaluate your progress in terms of skills competency, knowledge, and decision-making. Certain chapters in the textbook include directions for skill practice sessions that are designed to help you learn specific first aid skills. Some of the practice sessions require practice on a manikin. Others give you the opportunity to practice with another person. This will give you a sense of what it would be like to care for a real person in an emergency situation and help reduce any concerns or fears you may have about giving care. Your ability to perform specific skills competently will be checked by your instructor during the practice sessions.

Several written self-assessments are provided for you to use to evaluate your level of knowledge and understanding at particular points in the course. These assessments build on previously presented material and will help you prepare for the final written examination.

Your ability to make appropriate decisions when faced with an emergency will be enhanced as you participate in the class activities. Periodically, you will be given situations in the form of scenarios that provide you the opportunity to apply the knowledge and skills you have learned. These scenarios also provide an opportunity to discuss with your instructor the many different situations that you may encounter in any emergency.

♦ Requirements for Course Completion Certificate

When this course is taught by a currently authorized American Red Cross instructor, you will be eligible for an American Red Cross course completion certificate. In order for you to receive an American Red Cross course completion certificate, you must—

- ♦ Perform specific skills competently and demonstrate the ability to make appropriate decisions for care.
- ♦ Pass a final written examination with a score of 80 percent or higher.

The final written examination is designed to test your retention and understanding of the course material. You will take this examination at the end of the course. If you do not pass the written examination the first time, you may take a second examination.

♦ Textbook

The textbook has been designed to facilitate your learning and understanding of the material it presents. It includes the following features:

Objectives

At the beginning of each chapter is a list of objectives. Read these objectives carefully and refer back to them from time to time as you read the chapter. The objectives describe what you should be able to do after reading the chapter and participating in class activities.

Key Terms

At the beginning of each chapter is a list of defined key terms that you need to know in order to understand chapter content. Some key terms are listed in more than one chapter because they are essential to your understanding of the material presented in each. The pronunciation of certain medical and anatomical terms is provided, and a pronunciation guide is included in the glossary. In the chapter, key terms are printed in boldface the first time they appear.

For Review

This section indicates information you need to know in order to more easily understand the chapter you are about to read. For example, reviewing the information about the nervous system will help you to better understand the chapter on head and spine injuries.

Sidebars

Feature articles called sidebars enhance the information in the main body of the text. They appear in all chapters and are easily recognizable because of their lavender background. They present a variety of material ranging from historical information and accounts of actual events to everyday application of the information presented in the main body of the text. You will not be tested on any information presented in these sidebars as part of the American Red Cross course completion requirements.

Tables

Tables, on a blue background, are included in many chapters. They concisely summarize important concepts and information and may aid in studying.

Application Questions

Application questions, designated with a "Q" inside a yellow bar, challenge you to apply the information you have learned and build a solution. The answers to these application questions are at the end of each chapter.

Study Questions

Also at the end of each chapter are a series of questions designed to test your retention and understanding of the content. Completing these questions will help you evaluate how well you understand the material and also help you prepare for the final written examination. The answers are in Appendix A of the text. Sufficient space after most study questions allows you to write the answers directly in your book.

Skill Sheets

Learning specific skills that you will need to provide appropriate care for victims of sudden illness or injury is an important part of this course. Illustrated skill sheets at the end of certain chapters give step-by-step directions for performing each skill.

Appendixes

Appendixes at the end of this textbook provide not only the answers to the Study Questions but additional information on certain topics. For example, Appendix B gives detailed information on first aid and disease transmission; Appendix C discusses the relationship of Good Samaritan laws to the citizen responder.

Glossary

The glossary defines all the key terms, as well as other words in the text that may be unfamiliar. A pronunciation guide is included in the glossary.

♦ How to Use This Textbook

You should complete the following five steps for each chapter in order to gain the most from this course:

1. Read the chapter objectives before reading the chapter.
2. Review the recommended information listed under "For Review" prior to reading the chapter.
3. As you read the chapter, keep the objectives in mind. When you finish, go back and review the objectives. Check to see that you can meet them without difficulty.
4. Answer the Application Questions as you read the chapter. Check your answers with those at the end of the chapter. If you cannot answer or do not understand the answer given, ask your instructor to help you with concepts or questions with which you are having difficulty.
5. Answer the Study Questions at the end of each chapter. Mark or write your answers in the text in order to facilitate your review or study. Answer as many questions as you can without referring to the chapter. Then review the information covering any questions you were unable to answer, and try them again. Check your responses to the questions with the answers in Appendix A. If you have not answered a question appropriately, reread that part of the chapter to ensure that you understand why the answer is correct. This exercise will help you gauge how much information you are retaining and which areas you need to review. If, after rereading that part of the chapter, you still do not understand, ask your instructor to help you.

Health Precautions and Guidelines for First Aid Training

Since the beginning of citizen training in CPR (cardiopulmonary resuscitation), the American Red Cross and the American Heart Association have trained more than 50 million people in these lifesaving skills. According to the Centers for Disease Control (CDC), there has never been a documented case of any infectious disease transmitted through the use of CPR manikins.

The Red Cross follows widely accepted guidelines for the cleaning and decontamination of training manikins. **If these guidelines are consistently followed, and basic personal hygiene (for example, frequent handwashing) is practiced, the risk of any kind of disease transmission during CPR training is extremely low.**

There are also some health precautions and guidelines that you should know. You should take these precautions if you have an infection or a condition that would increase your risk or the other participants' risk of exposure to infections. You should request a separate training manikin if you—

- Have an acute condition, such as a cold, a sore throat, or breaks in the skin in or around your mouth.
- Know you are seropositive (have had a positive blood test) for hepatitis B surface antigen (HBsAg), indicating that you are currently infected with hepatitis B virus.*
- Know you have a chronic infection such as indicated by long-term seropositivity (long-term positive blood tests) for hepatitis B surface antigen (HBsAg)* or a positive

---

*A person with hepatitis B infection will test positive for the hepatitis B surface antigen (HBsAg). Most persons infected with hepatitis B will get better within a period of time. However, some hepatitis B infections will become chronic and will linger for much longer. These persons will continue to test positive for HBsAg. Their decision to participate in CPR training should be guided by their physician.

After a person has had an acute hepatitis B infection, he or she will no longer test positive for the surface antigen but will test positive for the hepatitis B antibody (anti-HBs). Persons who have been vaccinated for hepatitis B will also test positive for the hepatitis antibody. A positive test for the hepatitis B antibody (anti-HBs) should not be confused with a positive test for the hepatitis B surface antigen (HBsAg).

blood test for anti-HIV (that is, a positive test for antibodies to HIV, the virus that causes AIDS).

• Have a type of condition that makes you unusually susceptible to infection.

If, after you read and consider the above information, you decide that you should have your own manikin, ask your instructor if one can be made available for your use. You will not be required to provide details in your request. The manikin will not be used by anyone else until it has been cleaned according to the recommended end-of-class decontamination procedures. Because of limited numbers of manikins for class use, the more advance notice you provide, the more likely it is that you can be provided a separate manikin.

♦ Guidelines to Follow During Training

To protect yourself and other participants from infection, you should do the following:

• Wash your hands thoroughly before working with the manikin and repeat handwashing as often as is necessary or appropriate.
• Do not eat, drink, use tobacco products, or chew gum during classes when manikins are used.

• Before you use the manikin, dry the manikin's face with a clean gauze pad. Next, vigorously wipe the manikin's face and the inside of its mouth with a clean gauze pad soaked with either a solution of liquid chlorine bleach and water (sodium hypochlorite and water) or rubbing alcohol. Place this wet pad over the manikin's mouth and nose and wait at least 30 seconds. Then wipe the face dry with a clean gauze pad.
• When practicing what to do for an obstructed airway, simulate (pretend to do) the finger sweep.

♦ Physical Stress and Injury

CPR requires strenuous activity. If you have a medical condition or disability that will prevent you from taking part in the practice sessions, please let your instructor know.

♦ Damage to Manikins

In order to protect the manikins from damage, you should do the following before you begin to practice:

• Remove pens and pencils from your pockets.
• Remove all jewelry.
• Remove lipstick.
• Remove chewing gum and candy from your mouth.

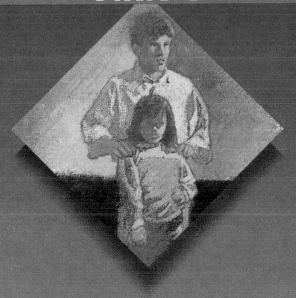

Introduction

The Citizen Responder

Objectives

After reading this chapter, you should be able to—

1. Explain how the emergency medical services (EMS) system works.

2. Describe your role as a citizen responder in the EMS system.

3. Identify the most important action you can take in a life-threatening emergency.

4. Identify four common indicators of an emergency.

5. List the five common barriers to action that may prevent people from responding to emergencies.

6. Describe the value of first aid training.

7. Explain four ways in which you can effectively prepare for emergencies.

8. Define the key terms for this chapter.

Key Terms

Citizen responder: A layperson who recognizes an emergency and decides to help.

Emergency: A situation requiring immediate action.

Emergency medical services (EMS) professionals: Trained and equipped community-based personnel dispatched through a local emergency number to provide emergency care for ill or injured victims; commonly, ambulance personnel.

Emergency medical services (EMS) system: A network of community resources and medical personnel that provides emergency care to victims of injury or sudden illness.

Emergency medical technician (EMT): Someone who has successfully completed a state-approved Emergency Medical Technician training program. There are several different levels of EMTs, including paramedics at the highest level.

First aid: Immediate care given to a victim of injury or sudden illness until more advanced care can be obtained.

First Responder: A person trained in emergency care who may be called upon to provide such care as a routine part of his or her job.

Injury: Damage that occurs when the body is subjected to an external force such as a blow, a fall, or a collision.

Medical emergency: A sudden illness requiring immediate medical attention.

Poison control center (PCC): A center staffed by medical professionals to give information about how to care for victims of poisoning.

◆ Introduction

You and several friends are driving home after a ball game. While stopped at an intersection, you see a car hit another car head-on. To your horror, one of the drivers crashes against the windshield. Glass is everywhere and the injured driver slumps over the steering wheel, motionless.

On a Saturday afternoon you enter the garage and find your father lying on the floor. He barely seems conscious and is clutching at his chest.

In each case, what would you do? What help can you give?

As a **citizen responder** trained in **first aid,** you are the first link in the **emergency medical services (EMS) system**. As this first link, you may be called upon to provide first aid to a victim of injury or sudden illness until more advanced care can be obtained. The goal of this course is to train you in the basics of first aid that will help you recognize and respond to any **emergency** appropriately. Your response may help save a life.

◆ The Citizen Responder and the EMS System

The emergency medical services (EMS) system is a network of community resources and medical personnel that provides emergency care to victims of injury or sudden illness. Think of the EMS system as a chain made up of several links. Each link depends on the others for success. Ideally, a victim will move through each link in the chain, beginning with the actions of a responsible citizen and ending with the definitive care provided to restore the victim's original health status.

The Citizen Responder

The first and most crucial link in the EMS system is the citizen responder. The citizen re-

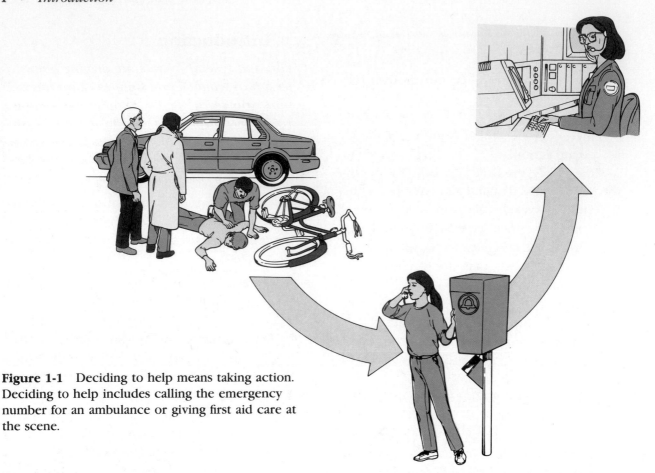

Figure 1-1 Deciding to help means taking action. Deciding to help includes calling the emergency number for an ambulance or giving first aid care at the scene.

sponder is someone like you who recognizes an emergency and decides to help (Fig. 1-1). Ideally, everyone should know what to do in an emergency. Everyone should know first aid. First aid is the immediate care given to a victim of injury or sudden illness until more advanced care can be obtained. But even if not trained in first aid, the citizen responder can provide critical help in an emergency.

The citizen responder must first recognize that the illness or injury that has occurred is an emergency. He or she must then activate the EMS system either by dialing 9-1-1 or a local seven-digit emergency number or by notifying a nearby **First Responder** such as a police officer. The sooner the EMS system is activated, the sooner more advanced medical help will arrive (Fig. 1-2).

The EMS Dispatcher

The second link in the EMS system is the dispatcher who works in a communications center. The dispatcher answers the call for help and quickly determines what help is needed. The appropriate professionals are then dispatched to the scene. The dispatcher may also give the caller instructions about how to help until EMS personnel arrive.

The First Responder

The First Responder is the third link in the EMS system. He or she is usually the first person to arrive on the scene who is trained to provide a higher level of care. First Responders are often the first people you turn to for help at the scene of an emergency. They may be firefighters, police officers, industrial safety officers, or people with similar responsibility for the safety or well-being of the community. Because of the nature of their jobs, they are often close to the scene and have the necessary supplies and equipment to provide proper care. First Responders provide a critical transition between a citizen responder's basic level of care and the care provided by advanced medical professionals.

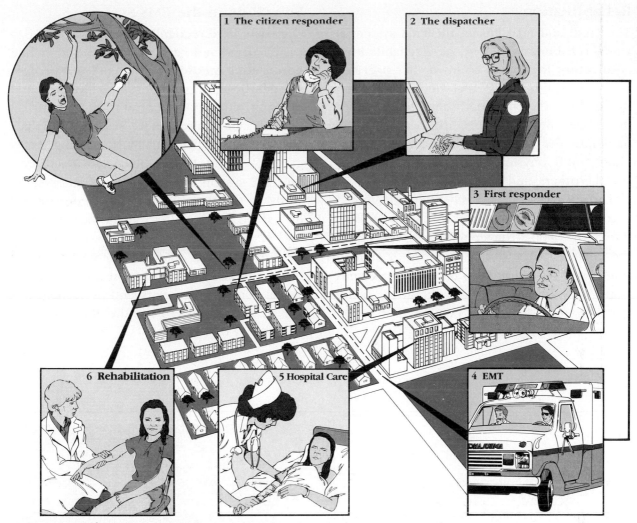

Figure 1-2 The EMS system is a network of community resources that provide emergency care.

The Emergency Medical Technician (EMT)

The **emergency medical technician (EMT)** is the fourth link in the EMS system. Depending on the level of training and certification, the EMT is capable of providing more advanced first aid and life-support techniques. In most parts of the United States, ambulance personnel are certified at least at the basic EMT level.

Paramedics are highly specialized EMTs. In addition to performing basic EMT skills, paramedics can administer medication and intravenous fluids, provide advanced airway care, and assess abnormal heart rhythms. Paramedics function at the highest level of prehospital care. They serve as the field extension of the hospital emergency physician.

Hospital Care Providers

The four links of the EMS system described in the preceding paragraphs work to give victims of injury or sudden illness the best possible prehospital medical care. The fifth link of the EMS system begins once the victim arrives at a hospital or other medical facility and the emergency department staff takes over care. Many different professionals, including emergency physicians, nurses, and other health care professionals, then become involved as needed.

Rehabilitation

The sixth and final link of the EMS system is called rehabilitation. The goal of rehabilitation is to return the victim to his or her previous state of health. After the victim has been moved from the emergency department, other health care professionals work together to rehabilitate the victim. These professionals include family physicians, consulting specialists, social workers, and physical therapists.

The six parts of the EMS system are linked together like a chain—a chain of survival for the victim. The stronger the chain, the better the chance that a victim of injury or sudden illness will be returned to his or her previous state of health. All the links should work together to provide the best possible care to victims of injury or illness.

Your Role in the EMS System

Once you have recognized that an emergency has occurred and have decided to act, calling **emergency medical services (EMS) professionals** is the most important action you and other citizen responders can take. Early arrival of EMS personnel increases the victim's chances of surviving a life-threatening emergency. Without the involvement of citizens, the EMS system would not function as effectively. In addition, a citizen responder trained in first aid can give help in the first few minutes of an emergency that can save a life. First aid *can* make the difference between life and death. Often it *does* make the difference between complete recovery and permanent disability. The citizen's role in the EMS system includes four basic steps:

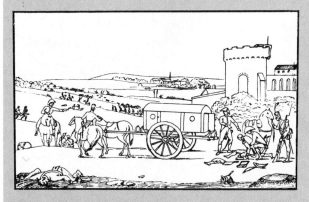

Yesterday's "Flying Ambulance." Cabanes, Chirurgiens et Blesses a travers l'Histoire, Paris, 1918.

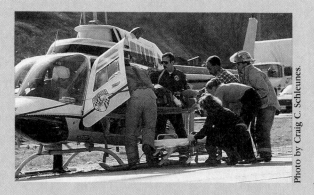

Today's "Flying Ambulance."

From Horses to Helicopters: A History of Emergency Care

Emergency care originated during the French emperor Napoleon's campaigns in the late 1700s. The surgeon-in-chief for the Grand Army, Dominique Jean Larrey, became the first doctor to try to save the wounded during battles instead of waiting until the fighting was over.[1] Using horse-drawn litters, Larrey and his men dashed onto the battlefield in what became known as "flying ambulances."

By the 1860s, the wartime principles of emergency care were applied to everyday emergencies in some American cities. In 1878, a writer for *Harper's New Monthly Magazine* explained how accidents were reported to the police, who notified the nearest hospitals by a telegraph signal. He described an early hospital ambulance ride in New York City.[2]

"A well-kept horse was quickly harnessed to the ambulance; and as the surgeon took his seat behind, having first put on a jaunty uniform cap with gold lettering, the driver sprang to the box . . . and with a sharp crack of the whip we rolled off the smooth asphalt of the courtyard and into the street. . . . As we swept around

1. Recognize that an emergency exists.
2. Decide to act.
3. Call EMS professionals.
4. Provide first aid.

By recognizing an emergency, deciding to act, and responding appropriately, you give the victim of an injury or serious illness the best chance for survival.

Q

1. If the EMS system is truly a chain of survival, explain how the adage "A chain is only as strong as its weakest link" applies to it. Also explain how the statement applies to the victim's chance of survival or recovery.

◆ Recognizing Emergencies

Recognizing an emergency is the first step in responding. What is an emergency? An emergency is a situation requiring immediate action. A **medical emergency** is a sudden illness that requires immediate medical attention, such as a heart attack. An **injury** is damage to the body, such as a broken arm, that results from a violent force. Some injuries can be serious enough to be considered emergencies. Emergencies can happen to anyone—to a friend, family member, stranger, or *you*. They can happen anywhere—on the road, at home, work, or play—*anywhere*. Recognizing an emergency may be difficult at times. You may become aware of an emergency because of certain signals. Common indicators include

corners and dashed over crossings, both doctor and driver kept up a sharp cry of warning to pedestrians."[3]

While booming industrial cities developed emergency transport systems, rural populations had only rudimentary services. In most small towns, the mortician had the only vehicle large enough to handle the litters, so emergency victims were just as likely to ride in a hearse to the hospital as in an ambulance.[4]

Cars gave Americans a faster system of transport, but over the next 50 years, car collisions also created the need for more emergency vehicles. In 1966, a major report questioned the quality of emergency services. Dismayed at the rising death toll on the nation's highways, Congress passed laws in 1966 and 1973 ordering the improved training of ambulance workers and emergency department staffs, an improved communications network, and the development of regional units with specialized care.

Today, the telegraph signal has been replaced by the 9-1-1 telephone code, which immediately connects a caller to a dispatcher who can send help. In some areas a computer connected to the enhanced 9-1-1 system displays the caller's name, address, and phone number, even if the caller cannot speak. Ambulance workers have changed from coachmen to trained medical professionals who can provide lifesaving care at the scene. Horses have been replaced by ambulances and helicopters equipped to provide the most advanced prehospital care available.

The EMS system has expanded in sheer numbers and in services. Today, New York City has 15 times as many hospitals as in the 1870s. Hospitals have also vastly improved their emergency care capabilities. If patients suffer from critical injuries such as burns, spinal cord injuries, or other traumatic injuries, the EMS system now has developed regional trauma and burn centers where specialists are always available.

In two centuries, the EMS system has gone from horses to helicopters. As technology continues to advance, it is difficult to imagine what changes the next century will bring.

REFERENCES
1. Major, Ralph, M.D. *A History of Medicine.* Springfield, Illinois. Charles C Thomas, 1954.
2. Rideing, W.H. "Hospital Life in New York." *Harper's New Monthly Magazine* 57:(1878):171.
3. Ibid.
4. Division of Medical Sciences, National Academy of Sciences—National Research Council, "Accidental Death and Disability: The Neglected Disease of Modern Society," Washington, D.C., September 1966.

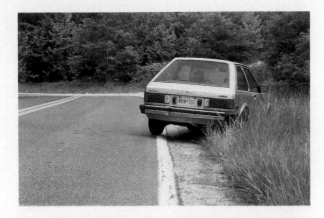
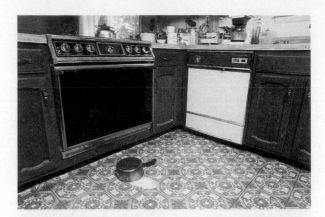
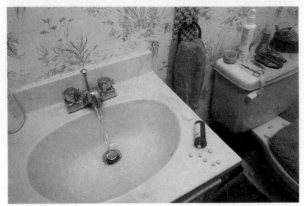
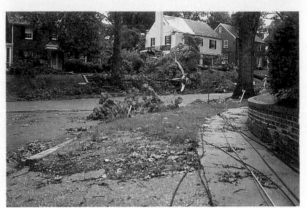

Figure 1-3 Unusual sights may indicate an emergency.

unusual noises, sights, odors, and appearance or behavior.

Unusual Noises

Noises are often the first thing that may call your attention to an emergency. Some that may signal an emergency include—
- Noises that indicate someone is in distress such as screaming, yelling, moaning, crying, and calling for help.
- Alarming, often recognizable noises such as breaking glass, crashing metal, or screeching tires.
- Abrupt or loud noises that are not identifiable such as collapsing structures or falling ladders.

Unusual Sights

Unusual sights that signal a possible emergency can go unnoticed by the unaware ob-

server (Fig. 1-3). Some examples of sights that may signal an emergency include—

- A stalled vehicle.
- An overturned pot on the kitchen floor.
- A spilled medicine container.
- Downed electrical wires.

Unusual Odors

Many odors are part of our everyday lives, for example, gasoline fumes at gas stations, the smell of chlorine at swimming pools, or smoke from a bonfire. However, when these and other odors are stronger than usual, are not easily identifiable, or otherwise seem inappropriate, they may indicate an emergency. You should always put your own safety first if you are in a situation in which there is an unusual or very strong odor, since many fumes are poisonous.

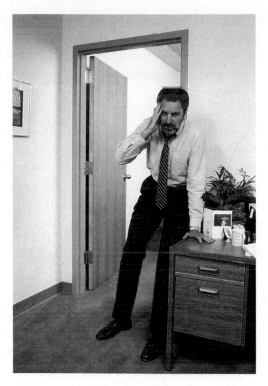

Figure 1-4 Unusual appearance may indicate an emergency.

Table 1-1	Recognizing Emergencies
Emergency indicators	**Signals**
Unusual noises	Screams, yells, moans, or calls for help
Breaking glass, crashing metal, screeching tires
Abrupt or loud unidentifiable sounds
Unusual sights	Things that look out of the ordinary—
A stalled vehicle
An overturned pot
A spilled medicine container
Broken glass
Downed electrical wires
Unusual odors	Odors that are stronger than usual
Unrecognizable odors
Unusual appearance or behavior	Unconsciousness
Difficulty breathing
Clutching the chest or throat
Slurred, confused, or hesitant speech
Unexplainable confusion or drowsiness
Sweating for no apparent reason
Uncharacteristic skin color

Unusual Appearance or Behavior

It may be difficult to tell if someone's appearance or behavior is unusual, particularly if he or she is a stranger. However, certain behaviors or appearances could indicate an emergency (Fig. 1-4). For example, if you see someone collapse to the floor, he or she obviously requires your immediate attention. However, you will not know if your help is needed until you approach the individual. He or she may merely have slipped and not be in need of any help. On the other hand, the person may be unconscious and need immediate medical assistance. Other behaviors and appearances that would indicate an emergency may be less obvious. They include—

- Breathing difficulty.
- Clutching the chest or throat.
- Slurred, confused, or hesitant speech.
- Confused behavior.
- Sweating for no apparent reason.
- Uncharacteristic skin color—pale, flushed, or bluish skin.

These and other signals may occur alone or together. For example, a heart attack may be indicated by chest pain alone, or chest pain may be accompanied by sweating and breathing difficulty.

◆ Citizen Response

You have already learned that citizen involvement is crucial in an emergency situation. Every year countless citizens recognize and respond to emergencies. Some phone for help, some comfort the victim or family members, some give first aid to victims, and still others help to keep order at the emergency scene. There are many ways citizens can help. *In order to help, you must act.*

Barriers to Action

Citizen involvement is the key to recognizing an emergency and making the EMS system work most effectively. Sometimes people simply do not recognize that an emergency has occurred. At other times, people recognize an emergency but are reluctant to act. People have various reasons for hesitating or not acting. These are called barriers to action. Some are very personal. Common reasons people give for not acting include—

* Presence of bystanders.
* Uncertainty about the victim.
* Nature of the injury or illness.
* Fear of disease transmission.
* Fear of doing something wrong.

Thinking about these things now and mentally preparing yourself to act in an emergency will enable you to respond more confidently in an actual emergency.

Presence of bystanders

The presence of bystanders can cause confusion at an emergency scene. It may not be easy to tell if anyone is providing first aid. Always ask if help is needed. Do not assume that, just because there is a crowd, someone is caring for the victim. The presence of other bystanders sometimes can make you reluctant to step forward and provide care. You may feel embarrassed about coming forward in front of strangers. This should not deter you from offering help when needed. In fact, you may be the only one at the scene who knows first aid. If someone else is already giving care, offer your assistance.

Although you might not want to become the center of attention, someone needs to take action. Ensure that the crowd does not endanger themselves or the victim unnecessarily. Sometimes you may need to ask bystanders who are not helping to back away and give the victim and rescuers ample space. But at other times, bystanders can be of great help in an emergency (Fig. 1-5). You can ask them to call for an ambulance, meet and direct the ambulance to your location, keep the area free of unnecessary traffic, or help you give care. You might send them for blankets or other supplies. Bystanders may have valuable information about what happened or the location of the nearest phone. A friend or family member who is present may know if the victim has a preexisting medical condition. Bystanders can also help comfort the victim and others at the scene.

Uncertainty about the victim

Since most emergencies happen in or near the home, you are more likely to give care to a friend or family member than to a stranger. However, this is not always the case. You may not know the victim and may feel uncomfortable with the idea of touching a stranger. Sometimes you may hesitate to act because of who the victim is. The victim may be much older or much younger than you, be of a different gender or race, have a disabling condition, or be a victim of crime. Sometimes you may have to reverse your usual role with the victim. For example, an employee may need to care for the boss, or a child may need to care for a parent or other adult (Fig. 1-6). Try to remember that, in an emergency, it is necessary to put these concerns aside and give the best care you can.

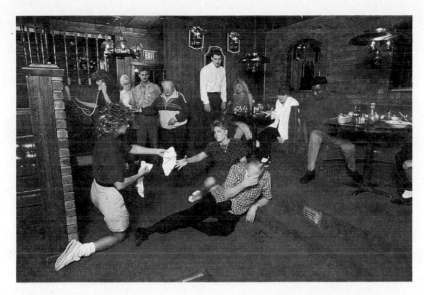

Figure 1-5 Bystanders can help you respond to emergencies.

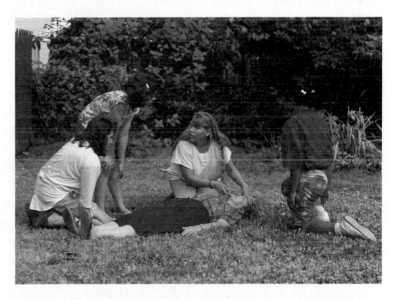

Figure 1-6 Emergencies may require that you take charge.

Sometimes victims of injury or sudden illness may act strangely or be uncooperative. The injury or illness, stress, or other factors such as the influence of alcohol or other substances may make people act offensively. Do not take such behavior personally. Remember, an emergency can cause even the nicest person to seem angry or unpleasant. If the victim's attitude or behavior keeps you from caring for him or her, you can still help. Make sure the EMS system has been activated, manage bystanders, and attempt to reassure the victim until professional help arrives. If at any time the victim's behavior becomes a threat to you, withdraw from the immediate area.

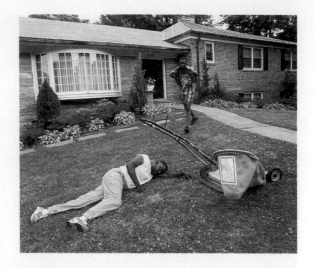

Figure 1-7 You are likely to provide care to someone you know.

Nature of the injury or illness

An injury or illness may sometimes be very unpleasant to handle. The presence of blood, vomit, unpleasant odors, or torn or burned skin is disturbing to almost everyone. You cannot predict how you will respond to these and other factors in an emergency situation. Sometimes you may need to compose yourself before acting. If you must, turn away for a moment and take a few deep breaths. Then try to provide care. Remember that this is an emergency. Your help is needed. If, however, you are still unable to provide first aid because of the appearance of the injury, you can help in other ways. You can ensure your safety, the safety of victims and bystanders, call for EMS personnel, reassure the victim, and manage bystanders.

Fear of disease transmission

A growing concern among professional rescuers and citizens alike is that of contracting a disease while giving emergency care. Spawned by the AIDS epidemic, the fear of disease transmission has become an issue to be addressed.

Having a fear of contracting a disease is understandable. Although there is a possibility of disease transmission in a first aid situation, the actual risk is far smaller than you may think.

Giving first aid in itself will not cause you to become infected with a disease. All of the conditions listed below would have to be present for it to be even possible for you to become infected:

◆ The injured or ill person who requires first aid must be infected with a disease.
◆ The rescuer providing first aid must be exposed to an infected person's body fluids such as blood, saliva, or feces.
◆ The rescuer must come in contact with infected body fluids through breaks in his or her skin or through the mucous membranes of the mouth or eyes.
◆ There must be enough body fluids that contain germs to cause infection.

Also consider that you are most likely to use your first aid skills to help someone you know personally—a family member, a friend, a co-worker (Fig. 1-7). In some instances, you may know this person's health status and be aware of risks of infection.

However, you may find yourself in an emergency situation in which you do not know what risks of infection may be present. Although you should take steps to protect yourself against the possibility of disease transmission, you should also act to reduce the risk of disease transmission from you to the victim. This can occur through any cuts or open sores on your own skin. It is safest for you to assume that all emergency situations that involve contact with body fluids have a potential for disease transmission between the victim

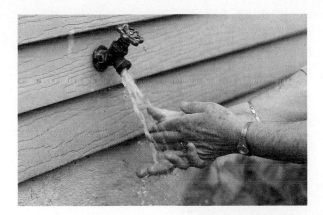
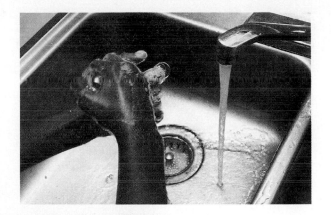
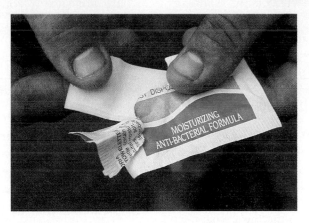

Figure 1-8 Thorough handwashing after giving care helps protect you against disease.

and rescuer. Examples of such situations are those that require bleeding control.

Disease transmission in first aid situations is rare. Your intact skin protects you as you give first aid. But if the skin is broken by a small cut or sore, germs can enter the body. Germs can also enter the body through the membranes around the eyes and mouth. For these reasons, the sensible thing to do is to always take precautions to prevent direct contact with a victim's body fluids while giving first aid. Use protective barriers that are appropriate to the emergency, and wash thoroughly as soon as possible after giving first aid (Fig. 1-8). Consult your personal physician if you come in direct contact with a victim's body fluids while giving first aid. Use caution to avoid unnecessary exposure to any hazards at the emergency scene. Appendix B contains additional information on first aid and disease transmission.

Q

2. What conditions for disease transmission must be present for it to be possible for you to become infected with HIV, the virus that causes AIDS, when you give first aid?

3. Disease transmission is a possibility when giving first aid. Who faces the greater risk of infection—you or the victim? Why?

Fear of doing something wrong

We all respond to emergencies in different ways. Whether we are trained or untrained, some of us are afraid we will do the wrong thing and make the situation worse. If you are unsure about what to do, call your emergency number for professional medical help. *The worst thing to do is nothing.*

Table 1-2 You Can Always Do Something to Help In Any Emergency

What to do	How to do it
Activate the EMS system.	Telephone your local emergency number.
Take appropriate safety precautions.	Ensure the safety of the victim, yourself, and bystanders. Be alert to possible dangers at the scene.
Communicate effectively.	Reassure the victim and others at the scene. Gather information from the victim, family, friends, bystanders. Provide necessary information to EMS personnel.
Manage bystanders.	Organize bystanders to— Call the local emergency number. Meet and direct the ambulance to the scene. Help give care. Comfort the victim and other bystanders. Help obtain supplies. Keep the area free of unnecessary traffic. Help protect the victim from possible dangers.

Sometimes people worry that they might be sued for giving first aid. Do not be overly concerned about this. Lawsuits against those who give emergency care at the scene of an accident are highly unusual and rarely successful. Most states have enacted "Good Samaritan" laws that protect people who willingly give first aid without accepting anything in return. Therefore you can provide help without worrying about lawsuits. If you want to know about Good Samaritan laws, see the additional information provided in Appendix C.

Q

4. As you approach the scene of a car crash, you see blood on the car windshield and hear people crying in pain. You begin to feel faint and nauseous and are not sure if you can proceed any farther. How can you still help?

♦ Deciding to Act

In most states, citizens have no legal duty to help victims in emergencies. Yet, obviously, each of us would want to be helped if we were the victim. People will always have feelings that make them hesitate or fail to help. Barriers to action are personal and very real to the people who experience them, as is the decision to act. The decision to act is yours and yours alone. Your decision to respond to emergencies should be guided by your own values as well as by a knowledge of the risks that may be present in various rescue situations. Ultimately, your decision to act may not involve giving first aid care. However, it should at least involve recognizing that an emergency has occurred and activating the EMS system by calling the local emergency number.

♦ Preventing Emergencies

Being a responsible citizen requires that you take reasonable precautions to prevent emergencies from occurring. Injuries remain the leading cause of death and disability in children and young adults. Thousands of Americans die each year as a result of injuries (Fig. 1-9). No one knows for sure how many of these victims die needlessly from preventable incidents.

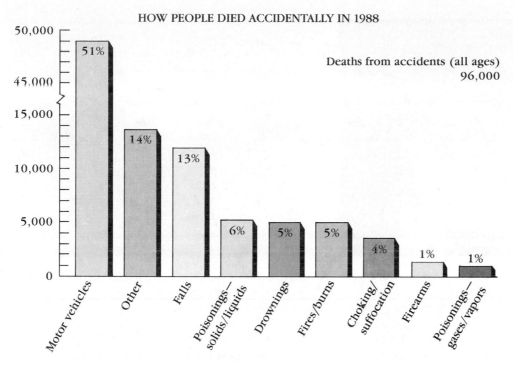

Figure 1-9 Injuries kill thousands each year. No one knows how many die needlessly from preventable injuries. Data from *Accident Facts,* 1989 edition, National Safety Council.

Emergencies also occur as a result of unhealthy lifestyles. For example, your exercise and dietary habits influence the health of your heart. Unhealthy habits, such as overeating, smoking, and lack of exercise, can increase your chances of heart attack.

In order to prevent emergencies, you must first be able to recognize potential risks in your own life. Completing the Healthy Lifestyles Awareness Inventory in Appendix D will help to identify these risks. Once you are aware of them, you can take precautions to conserve your health and safety and that of your family and friends. Later chapters will provide you with information about preventing specific emergencies.

Q
5. Knowing that most injuries can be prevented, list three things you can do to reduce the chance of being injured.

◆ Preparing for Emergencies

You will never see the emergencies you prevent. However, emergencies can and do happen, regardless of attempts to prevent them.

If you are prepared for unforeseen emergencies, you can help ensure that care begins as soon as possible—for yourself, your family, and your fellow citizens. First aid training provides you with both the knowledge and skills necessary to respond confidently to emergency situations. Your training will help you to focus on the most important aspects of care by giving you a basic plan of action that can be used in any emergency. By knowing what to do, you will be better able to manage your fears and overcome barriers to action. Your training will enable you to respond more effectively in your role as a citizen responder.

You can be ready for most emergencies if you do the following things *now*:

◆ Keep important information about you and your family in a handy place such as on the refrigerator door and in your automobile

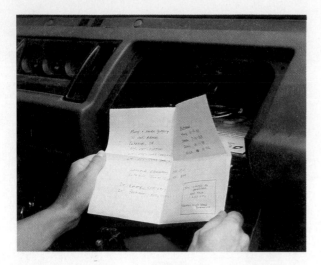

Figure 1-10 Important information should be readily available.

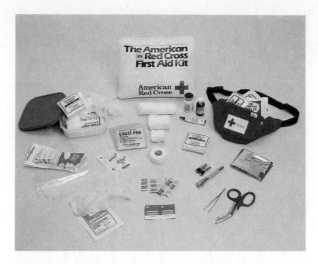

Figure 1-11 Be prepared for emergencies with a well-stocked first aid kit.

glove compartment (Fig. 1-10). Include your address, everyone's date of birth, medical conditions, allergies, and prescriptions and dosages. List physicians' names and phone numbers.

◆ Keep medical and insurance records up to date.

◆ Find out if your community is served by an emergency 9-1-1 telephone number. If it is not, look up the numbers for police, fire department, EMS, and **poison control center (PCC)**. Emergency numbers are usually listed in the front of the telephone book. Teach children how to call for help as soon as they are old enough to use the telephone.

◆ Keep emergency telephone numbers listed in a handy place such as by the telephone, and in your first aid kit. Include the home and office phone numbers of family members, friends, or neighbors who can help. Be sure to keep both the list and the telephone numbers current.

◆ Keep a first aid kit readily available in your home, automobile, workplace, and recreation area (Fig. 1-11). Store each kit in a dry place and replace used contents regularly. A first aid kit should contain the following:

a. Sterile gauze pads (dressings), 2- and 4-inch squares to place over wounds

b. Roller and triangular bandages to hold dressings in place or to make an arm sling

c. Adhesive bandages in assorted sizes

d. Scissors and tweezers

e. Ice bag or chemical ice pack

f. Disposable gloves such as surgical or examination gloves

g. Flashlight, with extra batteries in a separate bag

h. Antiseptic wipes

i. Other items as suggested by your physician

◆ Learn and stay practiced in first aid skills such as cardiopulmonary resuscitation (CPR).

◆ Make sure your house or apartment number is easy to read. Numerals are easier to read than spelled-out numbers. Report any downed or missing street signs to the proper authorities.

◆ Wear a medical alert tag if you have a potentially serious medical condition such as epilepsy, diabetes, heart disease, or allergies (Fig. 1-12). A medical alert tag, usually worn on a necklace or bracelet, provides important medical information if you cannot communicate. Family members should do the same when necessary.

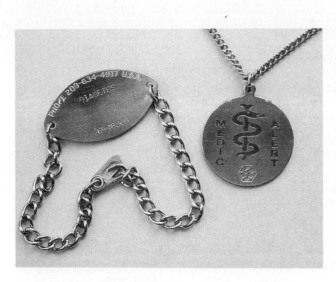

Figure 1-12   Medical alert tags can provide important medical information about the victim.

◆ Summary

You, the citizen responder trained in first aid, play a strategic role by being the first link in the chain of survival. Your actions can help save the life of a victim of injury or sudden illness. The most important things you can do are to recognize that an emergency has occurred, decide to act, and to activate the EMS system by calling your emergency number. Then give first aid until help arrives.

In the following chapters, you will learn how to manage emergencies. You will learn a plan of action that you can apply to any emergency situation and how to give first aid for both life-threatening and less serious emergencies.

Answers to Application Questions

1. The EMS system functions most effectively when its six links work together. If the chain is only as strong as its weakest link, the weakest link can determine the effectiveness of the EMS system and therefore can seriously affect the victim's chance of survival or recovery. One link can and often does make the difference between life and death or recovery and permanent disability.

2. You cannot become infected with HIV when you give first aid unless the four specific conditions for disease transmission listed on page 12 are present.

3. There is a risk of infection for both you and the victim. The degree of risk will be determined by the situation and the health status of the people involved. Disease can be transmitted as easily from you to the victim as from the victim to you. Follow the guidelines in this chapter to protect yourself and the victim.

4. Although you may feel ill and be incapacitated by the sight of blood or cries of pain, you can still help. If possible, turn away for a moment and try to control your feelings. If you are still unable to proceed, make sure EMS personnel have been called. Then find other ways to help, such as asking bystanders to assist you or helping keep the area safe.

5. You can do many things to reduce your chance of injury. Do not drive under the influence of alcohol or other substances. Do not ride with people under the influence of alcohol or other substances. Always wear a safety belt. Know the possible dangers in and around your home, neighborhood, and workplace. Know your own limitations when you do something that is physically demanding.

Study Questions

1. Match each term with the correct definition. Not all of the terms listed are defined here.

   a. Citizen responder
   b. First Responder
   c. EMT-paramedic

   d. Rehabilitation
   e. Hospital care providers
   f. EMS dispatcher

   _B_ Often the first person on the scene trained to provide a higher level of care, such as a policeman, fireman, or lifeguard.

   _C_ A field extension of the physician; provides the highest level of prehospital care such as administering medication or intravenous fluids.

   _f_ The person who answers the emergency call and determines what help is needed at the scene.

   _d_ The process of returning the victim to his or her previous state of health.

   _a_ Someone who recognizes an emergency and decides to act; the first link in the chain of survival.

2. Using all of the terms in question 1, organize the six EMS system components in the most effective order for the chain of survival to succeed.

   1. _Citizen responder_
   2. _EMS Dispatcher_
   3. _First Responder_
   4. _EMT_
   5. _Hospital care providers_
   6. _Rehabilitation_

3. List the four responses a citizen responder can make to enable the EMS system to function most effectively.

   1) Take safety precautions
   2) Call EMS
   3) communicate effectively
   4) manage bystanders

4. List four indicators of an emergency and give one example of each.

   1 unusal smell
   2 noises
   3 actions
   4 sights

5. List the five barriers to action.

   1) preascence of bystanders
   2) not sure about victum
   3) nature of illness or injury
   4) fear of disease transmittion
   5) not doing it right

6. List three ways bystanders can help in an emergency.

7. List four ways to prepare for an emergency.

1) list of #
2) list of insurance & records
3) Keep 1st Aid kit
4) teach children to call

8. Match each term with the correct definition.

a. First aid
b. Calling EMS personnel immediately
c. Medical emergency
d. Barriers to action
e. Indicator of an emergency
f. Citizen involvement
g. Emergency
h. EMS system

___G___ A situation that requires immediate action.
___H___ A network of community resources and medical personnel that provides emergency care to victims of injury or sudden illness.
___A___ The immediate care given to a victim of injury or sudden illness until more advanced care can be obtained.
___b___ The most important action you can take in a life-threatening emergency.
___C___ A sudden illness requiring immediate medical attention.
___E___ An unidentifiable odor.
___f___ Recognizing an emergency and deciding to act.
___D___ Reasons for not acting or for hesitating to act.

9. On your way to the grocery store from the parking lot, you hear the loud screech of tires and the crash of metal. You turn around and head in the direction of the sound. As you reach the corner of the parking lot, you notice that across the street a car has struck a telephone pole, causing it to lean at an odd angle. Wires are hanging down from the pole. Another vehicle is stalled in the middle of the street. List five indicators of an emergency found in this scenario.

10. A recent newspaper account of a multiple vehicle highway collision reported that the approximate time of the incident was 4:50 p.m., that EMS help did not arrive until 5:25 p.m, and that the last victim did not arrive at the hospital until 6:30 p.m. What might have happened along these links in the chain of survival to cause this delay in reaching the victims and getting them to the hospital?

Answers are in Appendix A.

Body Systems

Objectives

After reading this chapter, you should be able to—

1. Identify the major structures of the respiratory, circulatory, nervous, musculoskeletal, and integumentary systems.

2. Identify the primary functions of each system.

3. Give one example of how body systems work together.

4. Describe what can happen to the body if a problem occurs in one or more of the body systems.

5. Define the key terms for this chapter.

Key Terms

Airway: The pathway for air from the mouth and nose to the lungs.

Arteries (AR ter ez): Large blood vessels that carry oxygen-rich blood from the heart to all parts of the body.

Bone: A dense, hard tissue that forms the skeleton.

Brain: The center of the nervous system that controls all body functions.

Cells: The basic units of all living tissue.

Exhale: To breathe air out of the lungs.

Heart: A fist-size muscular organ that pumps blood throughout the body.

Infection: Condition caused by disease-producing microorganisms in the body.

Inhale: To breathe air into the lungs.

Lungs: A pair of organs in the chest that provides the mechanism for taking oxygen in and removing carbon dioxide during breathing.

Muscle: A fibrous tissue that lengthens and shortens to create movement.

Nerve: A part of the nervous system that sends impulses to and from the brain and all body parts.

Pulse: The beat felt in arteries near the skin's surface with each contraction of the heart.

Respiration: The breathing process of the body that takes in oxygen and eliminates carbon dioxide.

Shock: The failure of the circulatory system to provide adequate oxygen-rich blood to all parts of the body.

Skin: The tough, supple membrane that covers the entire surface of the body.

Spinal cord: A bundle of nerves extending from the brain at the base of the skull to the lower back; protected by the spinal column.

Tissue: A collection of similar cells that act together to perform specific body functions.

Trachea (TRA ke ah): A tube leading from the upper airway to the lungs; also called the windpipe.

Veins: Blood vessels that carry oxygen-poor blood from all parts of the body to the heart.

◆ Introduction

The human body is a miraculous machine. It performs many complex functions, each of which helps us live. The body is made up of billions of **cells** that are microscopic in size. A cell is the basic unit of all living **tissue.** There are many different types of cells, each of which contributes in a specific way to keep the body functioning normally. A collection of similar cells is a tissue.

Different cells and tissues working together make up organs (see Figure 2-1 on the next page). Organs have specialized functions. For example, the **heart** is an organ. Its job is to pump blood throughout the body. Vital organs are those whose function is essential for life. They include the **brain**, heart, and **lungs.**

A body system is a group of organs and other structures that are especially adapted to perform specific body functions. They work together to carry out a function needed for life. For example, the heart, blood, and blood vessels make up the circulatory system. The circulatory system keeps all parts of the body supplied with oxygen-rich blood.

For the body to work properly, all the different systems must work well together. The following body systems are covered in this chapter:

- Respiratory
- Circulatory
- Nervous
- Musculoskeletal
- Integumentary

You do not need to be an expert about

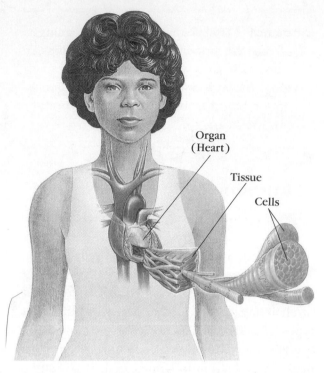

Figure 2-1 Cells and tissues make up organs.

body systems to give first aid to someone who needs it. However, knowing how the body works will help you better understand when something is wrong. You will learn that the different body systems depend on each other. Just as different body systems work together well when you are healthy, an injury or illness that affects one body system can affect others. For instance, a head injury may affect the nervous system. This in turn can affect the respiratory system and cause breathing to stop.

◆ Respiratory System

The body must have a constant supply of oxygen to stay alive. The respiratory system supplies the body with oxygen through breathing. When you **inhale,** air fills the lungs and the oxygen in the air is transferred to the blood. The blood carries oxygen to all parts of the body. This same system removes carbon dioxide. Carbon dioxide is transferred from the

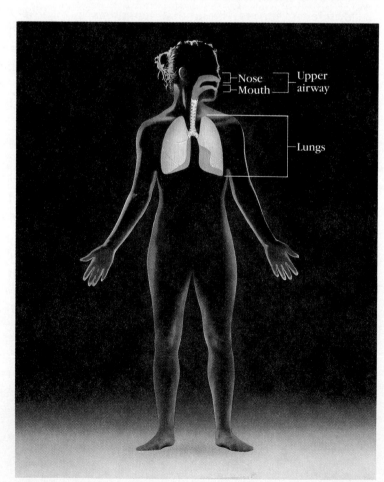

Figure 2-2 The Respiratory System

blood to the lungs. When you **exhale,** air is forced from the lungs, expelling carbon dioxide and other waste gases. This breathing process is called **respiration.**

The respiratory system includes the **airway** and lungs. Figure 2-2 shows the parts of the respiratory system in detail. The airway begins at the nose and mouth, which form the upper airway. Air passes through the mouth and nose, then through the **trachea,** on its way to the lungs (Fig. 2-3). The trachea is also called the windpipe. Behind the trachea is the esophagus. The esophagus carries food and liquids from the mouth to the stomach. A small flap of tissue, called the epiglottis, covers the trachea when you swallow to keep food and liquids out of the lungs.

Air reaches the lungs through two tubes called bronchi. The bronchi branch into increasingly smaller tubes like tree branches (Fig. 2-4, *A).* These eventually end in millions of tiny air sacs called alveoli (Fig. 2-4, *B).* Oxygen and carbon dioxide pass into and out of the blood through the thin cell walls of the alveoli and capillaries.

Air enters the lungs when you inhale and leaves the lungs when you exhale. When you inhale, the chest **muscles** and the diaphragm contract. This expands the chest and draws air

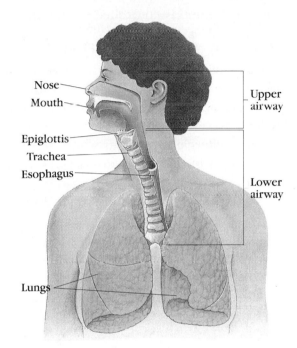

Figure 2-3 The respiratory system includes the mouth, nose, epiglottis, trachea, and lungs.

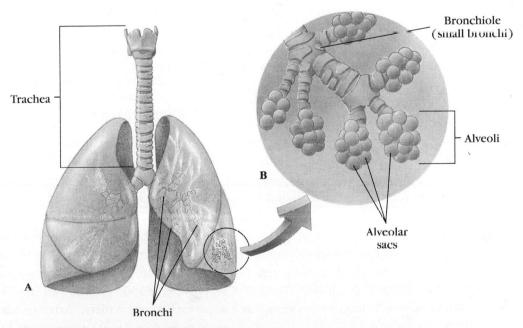

Figure 2-4 **A,** The bronchi branch into many small tubes. **B,** Oxygen and carbon dioxide pass into and out of the blood through the cell walls of alveoli.

into the lungs. When you exhale, the chest muscles and diaphragm relax, allowing air to exit the lungs (Fig. 2-5). An adult breathes about one pint of air (500 ml) per breath. The average adult breathes about 10 to 20 times per minute. This ongoing breathing process is involuntary and is controlled by the brain.

Problems That Require First Aid

Because of the body's constant need for oxygen, it is important to recognize breathing difficulties and to provide first aid immediately. Some causes of breathing difficulties are asthma, allergies, or injuries to the chest. Breathing difficulty is referred to as respiratory distress.

If a person has breathing difficulties, you may see or hear noisy breathing or gasping. The victim may be conscious or unconscious. The conscious victim may be anxious or excited or may say that he or she feels short of breath. The victim's **skin,** particularly the lips and under the nails, may have a blue tint. This is called cyanosis and occurs when the tissues do not get enough oxygen.

If a person stops breathing, it is called respiratory arrest. Respiratory arrest is a life-threatening emergency. Without the oxygen obtained from breathing, other body systems fail to function. For example, if the brain does not receive oxygen, it cannot send messages to the heart to beat. The heart will soon stop beating.

Respiratory problems require immediate attention. Making sure the airway is open and clear is an important first aid step. You may have to breathe for the nonbreathing victim or give abdominal thrusts to someone who is choking. Breathing for the victim is called rescue breathing. These first aid skills are discussed in Chapter 4.

Because it is vital for the respiratory system to keep functioning, one of your priorities is to make sure the victim is breathing. The victim must always have adequate oxygen, or other systems will fail.

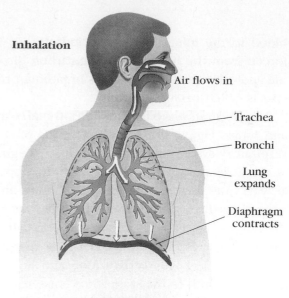

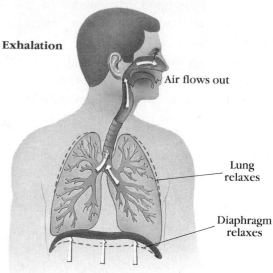

Figure 2-5   In the breathing process, the diaphragm and chest muscles contract and relax during inhalation and exhalation.

♦ Circulatory System

The circulatory system works with the respiratory system to carry oxygen to every cell in the body. It also carries other nutrients throughout the body and removes waste. The circulatory system includes the heart, blood, and blood vessels. Figure 2-6 shows this system in detail. The heart is a muscular organ behind the sternum, or breastbone. The heart pumps blood throughout the body through **arteries** and **veins.** Arteries are large blood vessels that carry oxygen-rich blood from the

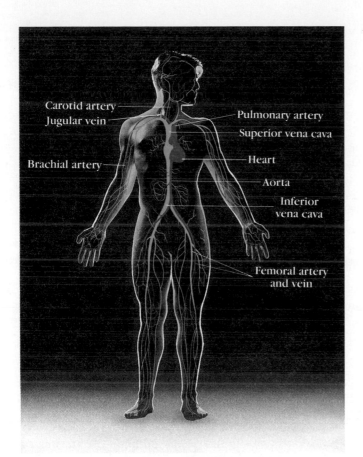

Figure 2-6 The circulatory system

heart to the rest of the body. The arteries subdivide into smaller blood vessels and ultimately become tiny capillaries. The capillaries transport blood to all the cells of the body and nourish them with oxygen. After the oxygen in the blood is given to the cells, veins carry the oxygen-poor blood back to the heart. The heart pumps this oxygen-poor blood to the lungs to pick up more oxygen, before pumping it to other parts of the body. This cycle is called the circulatory cycle. The cross section of the heart in Figure 2-7 on the next page shows how blood moves through the heart to complete the circulatory cycle.

The pumping action of the heart is called a contraction. Contractions are controlled by the heart's electrical system, which makes the heart beat regularly. You can feel the heart's contractions in the arteries that are close to the skin, for instance, at the neck or the wrist. The beat you feel with each contraction is called the **pulse.** The heart must beat regularly to deliver oxygen to body cells to keep the body functioning properly.

Problems That Require First Aid

The following problems threaten the delivery of oxygen to body cells:

1. Blood loss caused by severe bleeding (example: a severed artery)
2. Impaired circulation (example: a blood clot)
3. Failure of the heart to pump adequately (example: a heart attack)

Body tissues that do not receive oxygen die. For example, when one of the arteries supplying the brain with blood is blocked, brain tissue dies. When one of the arteries supplying the heart with blood is blocked, heart muscle tissue dies. This results in a life-threatening emergency such as a heart attack.

When someone has a heart attack, the heart functions irregularly and may stop. If the heart

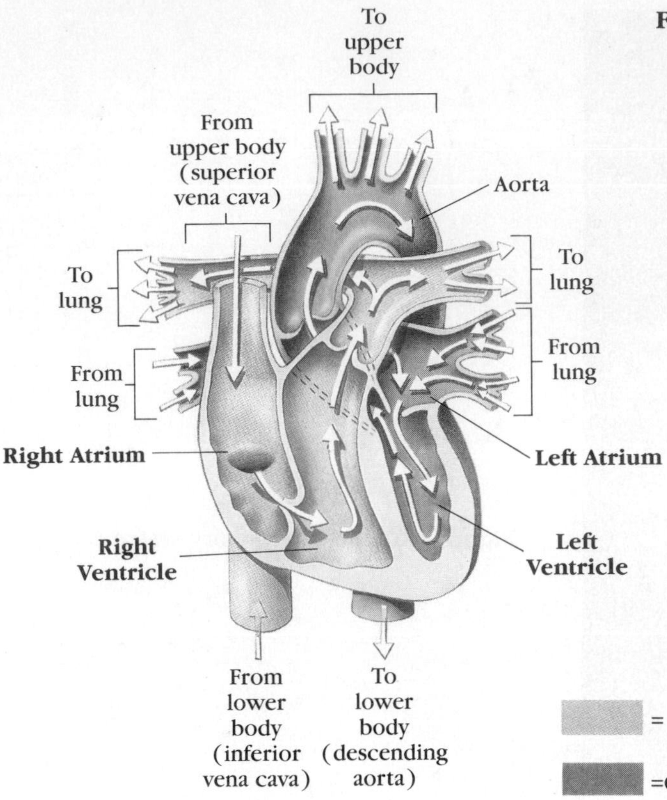

Figure 2-7 Pathway of blood through the heart.

To upper body

From upper body (superior vena cava)

Aorta

To lung

To lung

From lung

From lung

Right Atrium

Left Atrium

Right Ventricle

Left Ventricle

From lower body (inferior vena cava)

To lower body (descending aorta)

= Oxygen-poor blood pumped from the body to the lungs

= Oxygen-rich blood pumped from the lungs to the body

stops, breathing will also stop. When the heart stops beating, it is called cardiac arrest. Victims of heart attack or cardiac arrest need first aid immediately. Cardiac arrest victims need to have circulation maintained artificially by receiving chest compressions and rescue breathing. This combination of compressions and breaths is called cardiopulmonary resuscitation, or CPR. You will learn more about the heart and how to perform CPR in Chapter 5.

Q

1. If the circulatory system is functioning normally, but the body is not receiving adequate oxygen-rich blood, what might this tell you about the respiratory system?

◆ Nervous System

The nervous system is the most complex and delicate of all body systems. The brain, the center of the nervous system, is the master organ of the body. It regulates all body functions, including the respiratory and circulatory systems. The primary functions of the brain can be divided into three categories. These are the sensory, motor, and integrated functions of consciousness, memory, emotions, and use of language. The brain transmits and receives information through a network of **nerves.** Figure 2-8 shows the nervous system in detail. The **spinal cord,** a large bundle of nerves, extends from the brain through a canal in the spine, or backbone. Nerves extend from the brain and spinal cord to every part of the body.

Nerves transmit information as electrical impulses from one area of the body to another. Some nerves conduct impulses from the body to the brain. This allows you to see, hear, smell, taste, and touch. These are the sensory functions. Other nerves conduct impulses from the brain to the muscles to control the motor functions, or movement (Fig. 2-9).

The integrated functions of the brain are

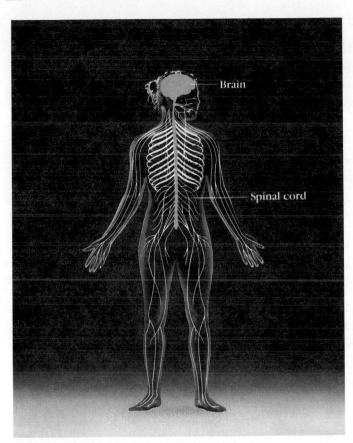

Figure 2-8 The nervous system

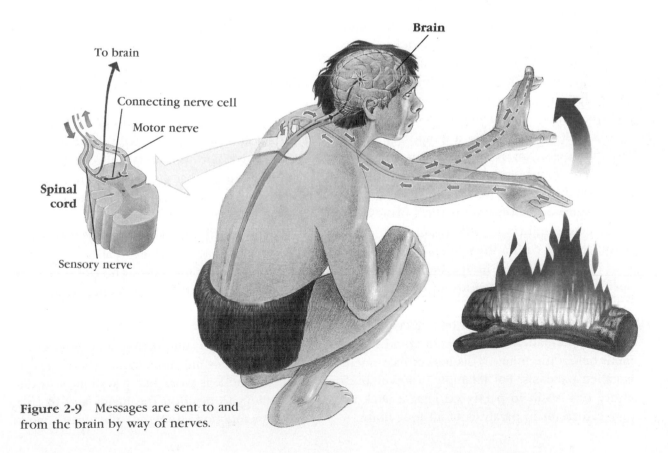

Figure 2-9 Messages are sent to and from the brain by way of nerves.

more complex. One of these functions is consciousness. Normally, when you are awake, you are conscious. Being conscious means that you know who you are, where you are, the approximate date and time, and what is happening around you. There are various degrees, or levels, of consciousness. Your level of consciousness can vary from being highly aware in certain situations to being less aware during periods of relaxation or sleep.

Problems That Require First Aid

Unlike other body cells, brain cells cannot regenerate. Once brain cells die or are damaged, they are not replaced. Brain cells may die from disease or injury. When a particular part of the brain is diseased or injured, the body functions controlled by that area of the brain may be lost forever. For example, if the part of the brain that regulates breathing is damaged, respiratory functions can be lost, and the person may stop breathing.

A person's level of consciousness may be altered as a result of illness or injury. It may be affected by emotions, in which case the victim may be intensely aware of what is going on. At other times, the victim's mind may seem to be dull, hazy, or cloudy. Illness or injury affecting the brain can also alter memory, emotions, and the ability to use language.

A head injury can cause a temporary loss of consciousness. Any head injury resulting in a loss of consciousness could cause brain injury and should be considered serious. These injuries require evaluation by medical professionals because injury to the brain can cause blood to pool within the skull. This puts pressure on the brain and limits the supply of oxygen to the brain cells. Without oxygen, brain cells die.

Injury to the spinal cord or a nerve can result in a permanent loss of feeling and movement below the injury. This loss of movement is called paralysis. For example, a lower back injury can result in paralyzed legs; a neck injury can result in paralysis of all four limbs. A broken **bone** or a deep wound can also cause nerve damage, resulting in a loss of sensation or movement. In Chapter 10, you will learn about first aid techniques for head, neck, and back injuries.

Q

2. How could a head injury cause breathing to stop?

◆ Musculoskeletal System

The musculoskeletal system consists of the bones, muscles, ligaments, and tendons. This system performs several functions:

- Supporting the body
- Protecting internal organs
- Allowing movement
- Storing minerals and producing blood cells
- Producing heat

Bones and Ligaments

The body has over 200 bones. Bone is hard, dense tissue that forms the skeleton. The skeleton forms the framework that supports the body (Fig. 2-10). Where two or more bones join, they form a joint. Figure 2-11 shows a typical joint. Bones are usually held together at joints by fibrous bands called ligaments. You will notice that bones vary in size and shape. This variation allows bones to perform specific functions.

The bones of the skull protect the brain. The spine is made of bones called vertebrae that protect the spinal cord. The ribs attach to the spine and to the breastbone, forming a protective shell for vital organs such as the heart and lungs.

In addition to supporting and protecting the body, bones aid movement. The bones of the arms and legs work like a system of levers and pulleys to position the hands and feet so they can function. Bones of the wrist, hand,

Figure 2-10 The skeleton

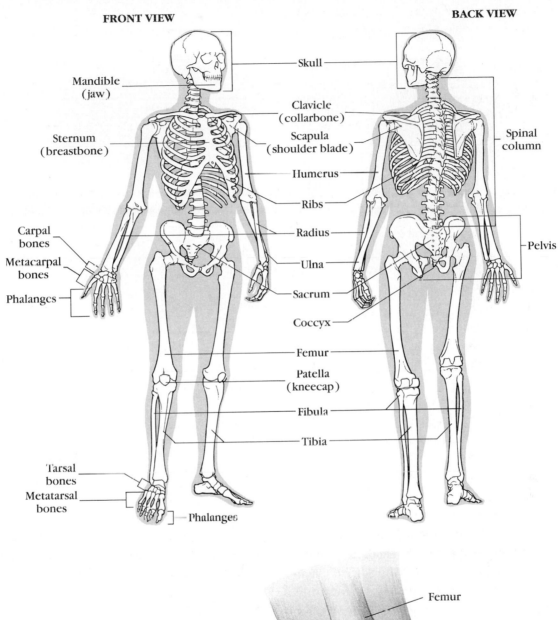

FRONT VIEW

BACK VIEW

Skull

Mandible
(jaw)

Clavicle
(collarbone)

Sternum
(breastbone)

Scapula
(shoulder blade)

Spinal
column

Humerus

Ribs

Carpal
bones

Radius

Metacarpal
bones

Ulna

Pelvis

Phalanges

Sacrum

Coccyx

Femur

Patella
(kneecap)

Fibula

Tibia

Tarsal
bones

Metatarsal
bones

Phalanges

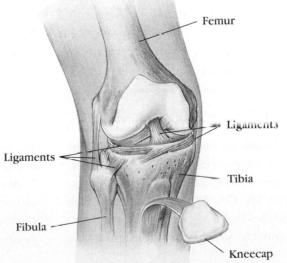

Femur

Ligaments

Ligaments

Tibia

Fibula

Kneecap

Figure 2-11 A typical joint consists of
two or more bones held together by
ligaments.

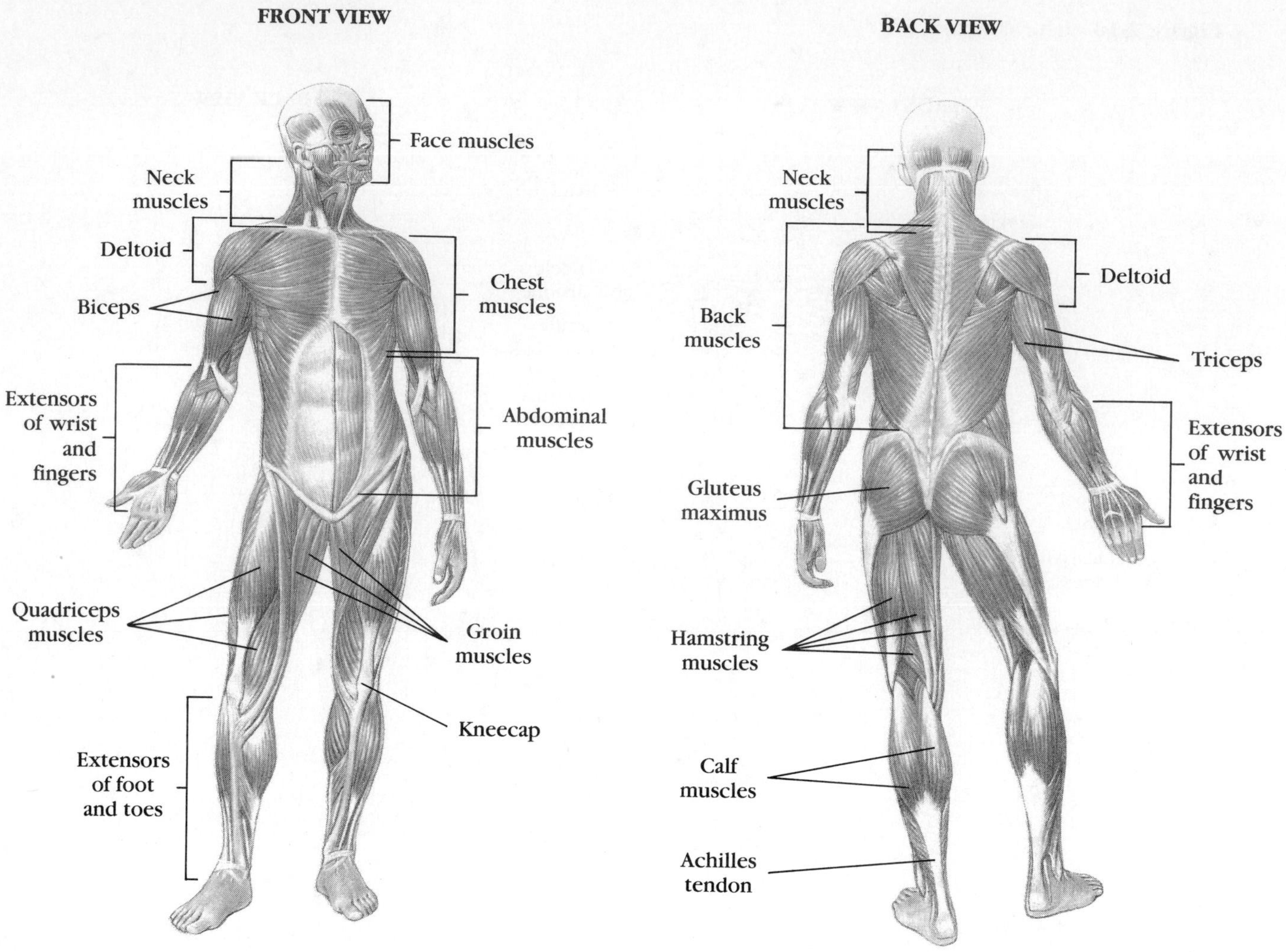

FRONT VIEW

BACK VIEW

Face muscles

Neck
muscles

Deltoid

Biceps

Chest
muscles

Extensors
of wrist
and
fingers

Abdominal
muscles

Quadriceps
muscles

Groin
muscles

Kneecap

Extensors
of foot
and toes

Neck
muscles

Back
muscles

Deltoid

Triceps

Extensors
of wrist
and
fingers

Gluteus
maximus

Hamstring
muscles

Calf
muscles

Achilles
tendon

Figure 2-12 The muscular system

and fingers are progressively smaller to allow for fine movements like writing. The small bones of the feet enable you to walk smoothly. Together they work as shock absorbers when you walk, run, or jump.

Bones also store minerals and help produce blood cells.

Muscles and Tendons

Muscles are made of special tissue that can lengthen and shorten, resulting in movement. Figure 2-12 shows the major muscles of the body. Tendons are tissues that attach muscles to bones. Muscles band together to form muscle groups. Muscle groups work together to

produce movement (Fig. 2-13). Working muscles produce heat. Muscles also protect underlying structures such as bones, nerves, and blood vessels.

Muscle action is controlled by the nervous system. Nerves carry information from the muscles to the brain. The brain processes this information and directs the muscles to move by way of the nerves. Figure 2-14 shows how the brain sends signals to muscles, directing them to move.

Muscle actions may be involuntary or voluntary. Involuntary muscles, such as the heart, diaphragm, and intestines, are automatically controlled by the brain. You don't have to

Figure 2-13 Muscles at front of thigh shorten while muscles at back of thigh lengthen, allowing lower leg to swing forward.

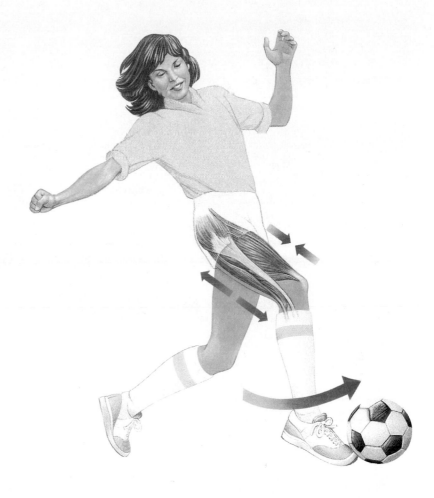

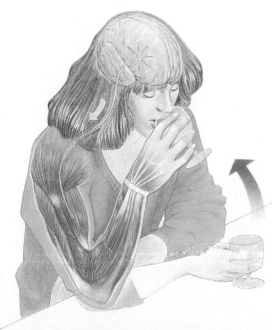

Figure 2-14 The brain controls muscle movement.

think about making them work. For example, the heart beats between 60 and 80 beats per minute without any direction from you. Voluntary muscles, such as leg and arm muscles, are under your conscious control.

Problems That Require First Aid

Injuries to bones and muscles include fractures, dislocations, strains, and sprains. A fracture is a broken bone. Dislocations occur when bones of a joint are moved out of place. Strains are injuries to muscles and tendons, whereas sprains are injuries to ligaments. Although injuries to bones and muscles may not look serious, nearby nerves, blood vessels, and other organs may be damaged. Regardless of how they appear, these injuries may cause lifelong disabilities or become life-threatening emergencies. For example, torn ligaments in the knee can limit activities, and broken ribs

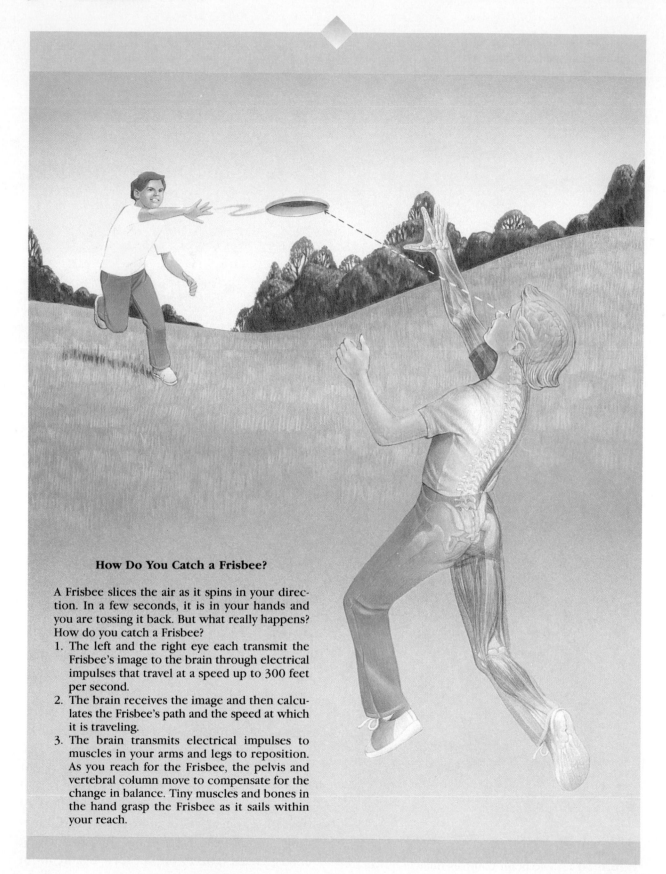

How Do You Catch a Frisbee?

A Frisbee slices the air as it spins in your direction. In a few seconds, it is in your hands and you are tossing it back. But what really happens? How do you catch a Frisbee?

1. The left and the right eye each transmit the Frisbee's image to the brain through electrical impulses that travel at a speed up to 300 feet per second.

2. The brain receives the image and then calculates the Frisbee's path and the speed at which it is traveling.

3. The brain transmits electrical impulses to muscles in your arms and legs to reposition. As you reach for the Frisbee, the pelvis and vertebral column move to compensate for the change in balance. Tiny muscles and bones in the hand grasp the Frisbee as it sails within your reach.

can puncture the lungs and threaten breathing.

When you give first aid, you should remember that injuries to muscles and bones often result in additional injuries. You will learn how to provide first aid for musculoskeletal injuries in later chapters of this book.

Q

3. Describe how a fractured leg could be a life-threatening emergency.

◆ Integumentary System

The integumentary system consists of the skin, hair, and nails (Fig. 2-15). Most important among these is the skin, because it protects the body. The skin helps keep fluids in. It prevents **infection** by keeping disease-producing microorganisms, or germs, out. The skin is made of tough, elastic fibers that stretch without easily tearing, preventing it from injury. The skin also helps make vitamin D, and it stores minerals.

The outer surface of the skin is made of dead cells that are continually rubbed away and replaced by new cells. The skin contains the hair roots, oil glands, and sweat glands. Oil glands help to keep the skin soft, supple, and waterproof. Sweat glands and pores help regulate body temperature. The nervous system monitors blood temperature and causes you to sweat if blood temperature rises even slightly. Sweat often evaporates before you even see it on the skin.

Blood supplies the skin with nutrients and helps provide skin with its color. When blood vessels dilate, the blood circulates close to the skin's surface, making the skin appear flushed, or red, and feel warm. However, you may not be able to recognize this reddening in people with darker skin. On the other hand, when the blood vessels constrict, there is not as much blood close to the skin's surface. As a result, the skin looks pale and feels cool.

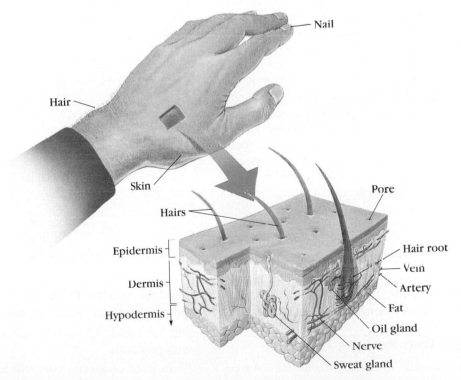

Figure 2-15 The skin, hair, and nails make up the integumentary system.

Too Much of a Good Thing

Contrary to some beliefs, tan is not in. Although brief exposure to the sun stimulates your skin to produce the vitamin D necessary for the healthy formation of bones, prolonged exposure can cause problems such as skin cancer and premature aging—a classic case of too much of a good thing being bad.

There are two kinds of ultraviolet light rays to be concerned about. Ultraviolet beta rays (UVB) are the burn-producing rays that more commonly cause skin cancer. These are the rays that damage the skin's surface and cause you to burn, blister, and perhaps peel.

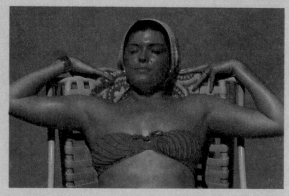

The other rays, ultraviolet alpha rays (UVA), have been heralded by tanning salons as "safe rays." Tanning salons claim to use lights that only emit UVA rays. While UVA rays may not appear as harmful as UVB rays to the skin's surface, they more readily penetrate the deeper layers of the skin. This increases the risk of skin cancer, skin aging, eye damage, and genetic changes that may alter the skin's ability to fight disease.

So, how do you get enough sun without getting too much? First, avoid exposure to the sun between 10:00 a.m. and 2:00 p.m. Ultraviolet (UV) rays are most harmful during this period. Second, wear proper clothing to prevent overexposure. Third, if you are going to be exposed to the sun at any time, take care to protect your skin and eyes.

Commercial sunscreens come in various strengths. The American Academy of Dermatology recommends year-round sun protection, including use of a high Sun Protection Factor (SPF) sunscreen, for all individuals, but particularly for those who are fair-skinned and sunburn easily. The Food and Drug Administration (FDA) has evaluated SPF readings, and recognizes values between 2 and 15. It has not been determined whether products with an SPF rating higher than 15 provide any additional protection against sun damage.

Sunscreens should be applied before exposure to the sun and should be reapplied frequently. Swimmers should use sunscreens labeled as water-resistant and reapply them as described in the labeling.

Your best bet is to use a sunscreen that claims to be broad spectrum—protecting against both UVB and UVA rays. Carefully check the label to determine the protection a product offers. Some products only offer protection against UVB rays.

It is equally important to protect your eyes from sun damage. Sunglasses are sunscreen for your eyes and provide important protection from UV rays. Be sure to wear sunglasses that are labeled with their UV-absorbing ability. Ophthalmologists recommend sunglasses that have a UV absorption of at least 90 percent.

The next time the sun beckons, put on some sunscreen, don your sunglasses, go outside, and have a great time.

Nerves in the skin make it very sensitive to sensations such as touch, pain, and temperature. Therefore, the skin is also an important part of the body's communication network.

Problems That Require First Aid

Although the skin is tough, it can be injured. Sharp objects may puncture, slice, or tear the skin. Rough objects can scrape it, and extreme heat or cold may burn or freeze it. Burns and skin injuries that cause bleeding may result in the loss of vital fluids. Germs may enter the body where there are breaks in the skin, causing infection. An infection may become a serious problem.

In later chapters, you will learn how to care for wounds, burns, and heat and cold emergencies.

◆ Interrelationships of Body Systems

Each body system plays a vital role in survival. Body systems work together to help the body maintain a constant healthy state. When the environment changes, body systems adapt to the new conditions. For example, because your musculoskeletal system works harder when you exercise, your respiratory and cir-

culatory systems must work harder to meet your body's increased oxygen demands.

None of the body systems work independently. The impact of an injury or a disease is rarely isolated to one body system, especially when the brain is affected. For example, a broken bone may result in nerve damage that will impair movement and feeling. Injuries to the ribs can make breathing difficult. If the heart

Table 2-1 Body Systems

System	Major structures	Primary functions	How the system works with other body systems
Respiratory system	Airway and lungs	Supplies the body with the oxygen it needs through breathing	Works with the circulatory system to provide oxygen to cells; is under the control of the nervous system
Circulatory system	Heart, blood vessels, and blood	Transports nutrients and oxygen to body cells and removes waste products	Works with the respiratory system to provide oxygen to cells; works in conjunction with urinary and digestive systems to remove waste products; helps give skin color; is under the control of the nervous system
Nervous system	Brain, spinal cord, and nerves	One of two primary regulatory systems in the body; transmits messages to and from the brain	The brain regulates all body systems through network of nerves
Musculoskeletal system	Bones, ligaments, muscles, and tendons	Provides body's framework; protects internal organs and other underlying structures; allows movement; produces heat; manufactures blood components	Muscles and bones provide protection to organs and structures of other body systems; muscle action is controlled by the nervous system
Integumentary system	Skin, hair, and nails	Skin is an important part of the body's communication network; prevents infection and dehydration; assists with temperature regulation; aids in production of certain vitamins	Skin helps to protect the body from disease-producing organisms; together with the circulatory system, helps to regulate body temperature under the control of the nervous system; communicates sensation to the brain by way of the nerves

stops beating for any reason, breathing will also stop.

In any significant illness or injury, body systems may be seriously affected. This may result in a progressive failure of body systems. This failure is called **shock.** Shock is caused by the inability of the circulatory system to provide adequate oxygen-rich blood to all parts of the body, especially the vital organs.

Generally, the more body systems involved in an emergency, the more serious the emergency. Body systems depend on each other for survival. In cases of serious injury or illness, the body may not be able to keep functioning. In these cases, regardless of your best efforts, the victim may die.

Q

4. You may have noticed that, after vigorous exercise, your skin is flushed, you perspire profusely, and you breathe heavily. You have learned that the musculoskeletal and respiratory systems work harder during exercise. Explain why your skin becomes flushed and why you perspire profusely. Give *specific* reasons for these conditions.

5. If someone experiences difficulty breathing, what other body systems might be affected? Why?

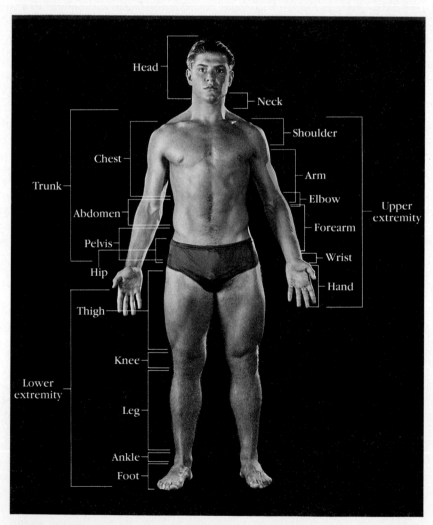

Figure 2-16 It is important to refer correctly to the parts of the body.

◆ Referencing Parts of the Body

When describing an injury or illness, it is important to understand and use standard terms for body parts in the same way. Examine Figure 2-16 to learn the exact parts of the body to which these standard terms refer.

◆ Summary

The body includes a number of systems, all of which must work together for the body to function properly. The brain, which is the center of the nervous system, controls all body functions, including those of the respiratory, circulatory, musculoskeletal, and integumentary systems.

As you have read, illness or injury that affects one body system can have a serious impact on another system. Fortunately, basic first aid is usually all that is needed to support injured body systems until more advanced care is available. By learning the basic principles of first aid described in this book, you could make the difference between life and death.

Answers to Application Questions

1. If the circulatory system is pumping blood but is still unable to deliver oxygen-rich blood to the body, there may be a problem with the respiratory system. It could be an oxygen supply problem. The airway could be blocked or injured, or an illness that affects the lungs might be preventing adequate oxygen from entering the circulatory system.

2. A head injury may result in a condition such as pooling of blood in the skull or a blood clot that would interrupt blood flow to brain cells. If oxygen flow to brain cells is interrupted, they can die from lack of oxygen, and their functions may be lost forever. If a head injury interrupts the flow of oxygen to the brain cells that control respiration, it would cause breathing to stop.

3. A fractured leg could be a life-threatening emergency if the fracture caused other injuries or conditions such as a severed artery, blood clot, internal bleeding, severe bleeding, infection, shock, or unconsciousness.

4. For working muscles to function, they require increased amounts of oxygen. Therefore, your respiratory system works harder to meet the demands of the muscles. As more oxygen is brought into the body, blood flow increases, and blood vessels dilate to accommodate and deliver it. Your skin is flushed because of the increased blood flow near the skin's surface.

   In addition to demanding more oxygen, your working muscles produce heat and cause body temperature to rise. Sweating is your body's way of cooling off and thus regulating body temperature.

5. Breathing difficulty may affect any or all other body systems because a lack of oxygen results in tissue dysfunction and eventually tissue death. Furthermore, once the oxygen supply to the brain is limited, the brain may become unable to control body functions. The functions of the nervous, musculoskeletal, and all other body systems will be severely impaired or fail.

Study Questions

1. Complete the table with the correct system, structures, or function(s).

Body Systems

System	Structures	Function(s)
a. _____	b. _____	Supplies the body with the oxygen it needs through breathing
c. _____		
Integumentary	Heart, blood, blood vessels	d. _____
	e. _____	f. _____
Musculoskeletal		
	g. _____	h. _____
i. _____	j. _____	Regulates all body functions, a communications network

2. Match each term with the correct definition.

a. Airway
b. Arteries
c. Cell
d. Bone
e. Muscle
f. Skin
g. Nerve
h. Infection

i. Pulse
j. Spinal cord
k. Lungs
l. Respiration
m. Brain
n. Shock
o. Veins

_____ Blood vessels that carry oxygen-poor blood to the heart.

_____ Dense, hard tissue that forms the skeleton.

_____ Process of breathing.

_____ Regulates all body functions.

_____ Conducts impulses between the brain and all parts of the body.

_____ Basic unit of living tissue.

_____ A pair of organs in the chest that provides the mechanism for taking oxygen in and removing carbon dioxide during breathing.

_____ Beat created by each contraction of the heart; felt in arteries near the skin's surface.

_____ Pathway for air from the mouth and nose to the lungs.

_____ A tissue that lengthens and shortens to produce movement.

_____ Condition caused by germs in the body.

_____ A tough membrane that covers the entire surface of the body.

_____ A large bundle of nerves extending from the brain through the spine.

_____ Blood vessels that carry oxygen-rich blood to all parts of the body.

_____ The failure of the circulatory system to provide adequate oxygen-rich blood to body parts, especially vital organs.

In questions 3 through 6, circle the letter of the correct answer.

3. Which of the following could result from breathing difficulty or other problems of the respiratory system?

   a. Cardiac arrest
   b. No delivery of oxygen to body parts via the circulatory system
   c. Brain cell death
   d. All of the above

4. The respiratory system works with other body systems to provide oxygen to all body cells. These systems include the—

   a. Circulatory and nervous systems.
   b. Nervous system.
   c. Musculoskeletal, nervous, and circulatory systems.
   d. Musculoskeletal and circulatory systems.

5. A blood clot in the brain could cut off all blood flow to brain cells. Which body systems would fail to function?

   a. Nervous system
   b. All body systems
   c. Circulatory and respiratory systems
   d. Nervous and respiratory systems

6. The human body rapidly adapts to new environments. For example, when you step outside of an air-conditioned building on a hot, summer day, you immediately begin to sweat. Your body adapts to its "new" environment. What systems work together to produce this specific adaptation?

   a. Nervous and musculoskeletal systems
   b. Integumentary and respiratory systems
   c. Circulatory and respiratory systems
   d. Integumentary and nervous systems

7. Why can an injury to the spinal cord or a nerve result in paralysis?

Answers are in Appendix A.

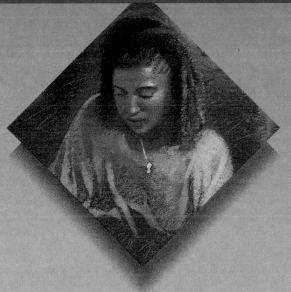

PART II

Assessment

3

Responding to Emergencies

3

Responding to Emergencies

Objectives

After reading this chapter, you should be able to—

1. List the four emergency action principles (steps to take in every emergency).

2. Explain why you should follow the emergency action principles in any emergency.

3. List four important questions to be answered when surveying the emergency scene.

4. Explain what you should do if an unsafe scene prevents you from reaching the victim.

5. List the three things you must do in order to get consent to provide care to an ill or injured person.

6. Explain why you should do a primary survey in every emergency situation.

7. Describe how to do a primary survey.

8. List at least four important facts you should give to EMS personnel when you call for help.

9. List at least six conditions that would require you to call immediately for professional help.

10. Describe when you should do a secondary survey.

11. Explain why you should do a secondary survey.

12. Explain how to do a secondary survey.

13. Explain when you should not transport a victim to the hospital yourself.

14. List two things you should do if you decide to transport the victim to the hospital yourself.

15. Define the key terms for this chapter.

After reading this chapter and completing the class activities, you should be able to—

1. Demonstrate a primary survey.

2. Demonstrate a secondary survey.

3. Make appropriate decisions for care when given an example of an emergency situation requiring you to conduct a primary and secondary survey.

Key Terms

Carotid (kah ROT id) arteries: Major blood vessels that supply blood to the head and neck.

Consent: Permission to provide care, given by the victim to the rescuer.

Emergency action principles (EAPs): Four steps to guide your actions in any emergency.

Primary survey: A check for conditions that are an immediate threat to a victim's life.

Secondary survey: A check for injuries or conditions that could become life-threatening problems if not cared for.

Vital signs: Important information about the victim's condition, obtained by checking breathing, pulse, and skin characteristics.

For Review

Before reading this chapter, you should have a basic understanding of how the respiratory and circulatory systems function (Chapter 2).

◆ Introduction

In Chapter 1, you learned that, as a citizen responder trained in first aid, you can make a difference in an emergency—you may even save a life. You learned how to recognize an emergency, ways to respond, and how to prevent and prepare for emergencies. More important, you learned that your decision to act is vital to the victim's survival. You can always do something to help.

In this chapter, you will learn a plan of action to guide you through any emergency. When an emergency occurs, you may at first feel confused. But you can train yourself to remain calm and to think before you act. Ask yourself, "What do I need to do? How can I help most effectively?" The four **emergency action principles (EAPs)** answer these questions. They are your plan of action for any emergency.

◆ Emergency Action Principles

The emergency action principles are—
1. Survey the scene.
2. Do a **primary survey** and care for life-threatening problems.

3. Call EMS personnel for help.
4. Do a **secondary survey**, when appropriate, and care for additional problems.

Having a plan of action can ensure your safety and that of the victim and other bystanders and increase the victim's chance of survival. When you call EMS for help will vary according to what you find. There is no hard, fast rule when to call your emergency number.

Survey the Scene

Once you recognize that an emergency has occurred and decide to act, you must make sure the scene of the emergency is safe for you and any bystanders. Take time to survey the scene and answer these questions:

1. Is the scene safe?
2. What happened?
3. How many victims are there?
4. Can bystanders help?

When you survey the scene, look for anything that may threaten your safety and that of the victim and bystanders. Examples of dangers that may be present are downed power lines, falling rocks, traffic, fire, smoke, dangerous fumes, extreme weather, and deep or swift-moving water (Fig. 3-1). *If any of these or other dangers are threatening, do not approach the victim. Call EMS personnel immediately for professional help.*

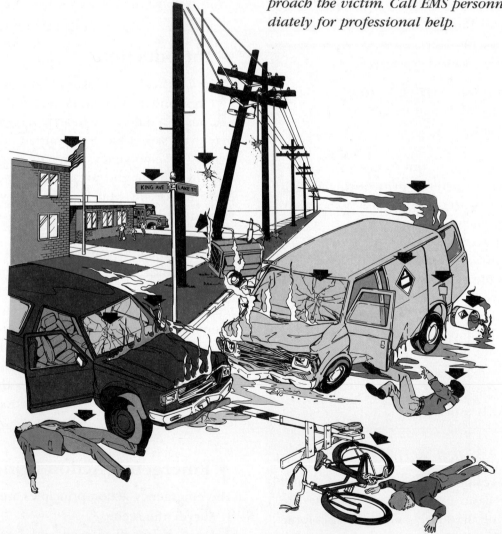

Figure 3-1 Survey the scene.

Nothing is gained by risking your own safety. An emergency that begins with one victim could end up with two if you are hurt. Leave dangerous situations for EMS professionals who have the training and proper equipment to handle them. If you suspect the scene is unsafe, wait and watch until EMS personnel arrive. If conditions change, you may then be able to approach the victim.

Find out what happened. Look around the scene for clues about what caused the emergency and the type and extent of the victim's injuries. By looking around, you may discover a situation that requires your immediate action. As you approach the victim, take in the whole picture. Nearby objects, such as shattered glass, a fallen ladder, or a spilled bottle of medicine, might tell you what happened (Fig. 3-2). If the victim is unconscious, your survey of the scene may be the only way to tell what happened.

When you survey the scene, look carefully for more than one victim. You may not spot everyone at first. For example, in a car crash, an open door may be a clue that a victim has left or was thrown from the car. If one victim is bleeding or screaming loudly, you may overlook another victim who is unconscious. It is also easy in any emergency situation to

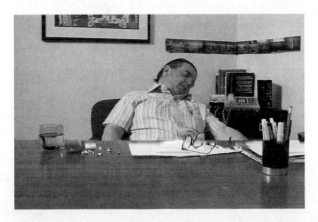

Figure 3-2 If the victim is unconscious, nearby objects may be your only clue to what has happened.

overlook an infant or small child. Ask anyone present how many people may be involved. If you find more than one victim, ask bystanders to help you care for them.

Look for bystanders who can help. Bystanders may be able to tell you what happened or help in other ways. A bystander who knows the victim may know whether he or she has any medical problems or allergies. Bystanders may call EMS professionals for help, meet and direct the ambulance to your location, keep the area free of unnecessary traffic, or help you provide care. If no bystanders are close, shout for help to summon someone who can help you.

Once you reach the victim

Once you reach the victim, quickly survey the scene again to see if it is still safe. At this point, you may see other dangers, clues to what happened, or victims and bystanders that you did not notice before.

On your way home, you notice that a car has veered off the road and landed in the ditch. You decide there may be an emergency. After surveying the scene and deciding it is safe to approach, you approach the car. As you come closer to the car, you see a woman lying on the ground, near the car. But, you also smell a strong odor of gasoline. What should you do? Is there a danger? Should you move her away from the car or try to care for her there?

As a rule, do not move a victim unless there is an immediate danger such as a fire, poisonous fumes, or an unstable structure. If this is the case, try to move the victim as quickly as possible, without making the situation worse. If there is no immediate danger, tell the victim not to move. Tell bystanders not to move the victim.

Identify yourself as a person trained in first aid. When you reach the victim, try not to alarm him or her. Try to position yourself

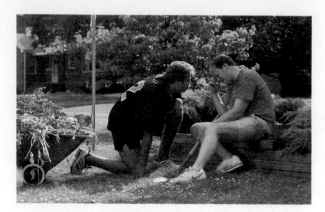

Figure 3-3 When talking to the victim, position yourself close to the victim's level and speak in a calm and positive manner.

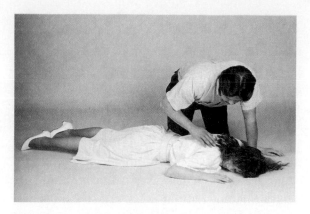

Figure 3-4 Determine if the person is conscious by gently tapping and asking, "Are you okay?"

close to the victim's eye level (Fig. 3-3). Speak in a calm and positive manner. Identify yourself to the victim and bystanders. Ask if you can help. Tell them that you have first aid training. This lets them know a caring and skilled person is giving help.

Get permission to provide care. Before giving first aid, you must get a conscious victim's permission to give care. This permission is referred to as **consent**. A conscious victim has the right to either refuse or accept care. To get consent you *must* tell the victim—

1. Who you are.
2. Your level of training.
3. What it is you would like to do.

Only then can a conscious victim give you consent, or permission to provide care. Do not give care to a conscious victim who refuses it. If the conscious victim is an infant or child, permission to provide care should be obtained from the supervising adult.

If the victim is unconscious or unable to respond because of the illness or injury, consent is implied. This means you can assume that if the person could respond, he or she would agree to be cared for. Consent is also implied for an infant or child if a supervising adult is not present.

Do a Primary Survey For Life-Threatening Conditions

In every emergency situation, you must find out if there are conditions that are an immediate threat to the victim's life. This EAP is called the primary survey. In the primary survey, you check for each of the following life-threatening conditions: unconsciousness, loss of breathing, loss of heartbeat, and severe bleeding.

First determine if the victim is conscious. Gently tap him or her and ask, "Are you okay?" (Fig. 3-4). Do not jostle or move the victim. A victim who can respond to you is conscious and breathing and has a pulse. A victim who is unable to respond may be unconscious. Unconsciousness is a life-threatening condition. When someone is unconscious, the tongue may fall to the back of the throat and block the airway. This may cause breathing to stop. Soon after, the heart will stop beating.

If the victim is unconscious, send someone to call the local emergency number for help. If you are alone, make the call yourself, then return to the victim and complete the primary survey. If you have to leave the victim, and you do not suspect a head or spine injury, position the victim on one side in case he or she vomits while you are gone. To complete the primary survey, check the unconscious victim's airway, breathing, and circulation. Remembering these steps is easy. The three steps are called the ABCs of the primary survey:

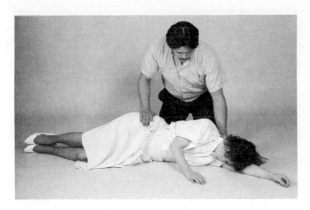

Figure 3-5 If the victim's position prevents you from checking the ABCs, roll the victim gently on to his or her back.

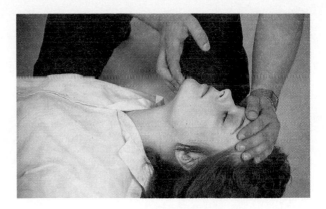

Figure 3-6 Tilt the head and lift the chin to open the airway.

```
A = Airway
B = Breathing
C = Circulation
```

If you can, attempt to check the ABCs in whatever position you find the victim. Sometimes, however, because of the victim's position, you may not be able to check the ABCs. In this case, you may roll the victim gently onto his or her back, keeping the head and spine in as straight a line as possible (Fig. 3-5).

Check the airway

Be sure the victim has an open airway. The airway is the pathway for air from the mouth and nose to the lungs. A victim who can speak, cough, or cry is conscious, has an open airway, is breathing, and has a pulse.

It is more difficult to tell if an unconscious victim has an open airway. Without an open airway, the victim cannot breathe. To open an unconscious victim's airway, tilt the head back and lift the chin (Fig. 3-6). This moves the tongue away from the back of the throat, allowing air to enter the lungs. For someone with a suspected neck injury, this technique is modified slightly, as you will read in Chapter 4.

Sometimes, opening the airway does not re-

sult in a free passage of air. This happens when a victim's airway is blocked by food, liquid, or other objects. In this case, you will need to remove what is blocking the airway. Chapter 4 describes first aid for an obstructed airway.

Check breathing

After opening the airway, check for breathing. As you learned earlier, a conscious person who can speak, cough, or cry is breathing. However, you may not know if an unconscious person is breathing until you check. An unconscious person must be watched carefully for signs of breathing. If the victim is breathing, the chest will rise and fall. However, chest movement by itself does not mean air is reaching the lungs. You must also listen and feel for signs of breathing. Position yourself so you can hear and feel air as it escapes from the nose and mouth. At the same time, watch the rise and fall of the chest. Take the time to look, listen, and feel for breathing for about 5 seconds (see Fig. 3-7 on the next page).

If the victim is not breathing, you must give 2 slow breaths. This will get air into the victim's lungs. The longer a victim goes without oxygen, the more likely he or she is to die. If the victim has a pulse but is not breathing, you will need to breathe for him or her. This process of breathing for the victim is called rescue breathing. You will learn how to give rescue breathing in Chapter 4.

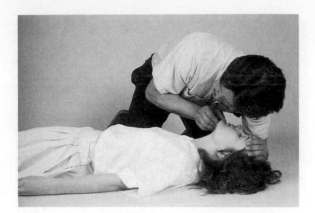

Figure 3-7 To check for breathing, look, listen, and feel for breathing for about 5 seconds.

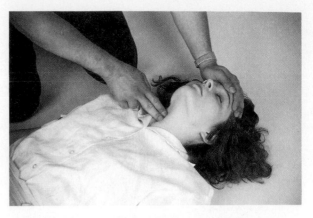

Figure 3-8 Determine if the heart is beating by feeling for a carotid pulse at either side of the neck.

1. Why is it necessary to look, listen, and feel for breathing?

Check circulation

The last step in the primary survey is checking for the circulation of blood. If the heart has stopped, blood will not circulate throughout the body. If this happens, the victim will die in just a few minutes because the brain is not getting any oxygen.

If a person is breathing, his or her heart is beating and is circulating blood. In the absence of breathing, you must determine if the victim's heart is beating. This is done by checking his or her pulse. You feel for the pulse at either of the **carotid arteries** located in the neck (Fig. 3-8). To find the pulse, feel for the Adam's apple and slide your fingers into the groove at the side of the neck. Sometimes the pulse may be difficult to find since it may be slow or weak. If at first you do not find a pulse, relocate the Adam's apple and again slide your fingers into place. When you think you are in the right spot, take about 5 to 10 seconds to feel for the pulse.

If the victim does not have a pulse, you need to give first aid to keep oxygen-rich blood circulating. This involves giving chest compressions and rescue breaths. This procedure is called cardiopulmonary resuscita-

tion (CPR). Chapter 5 describes how to do CPR.

Checking circulation also means looking for severe bleeding. Bleeding is severe when blood spurts from the wound or cannot be controlled. Check for severe bleeding by looking from head to toe for signs of external bleeding (Fig. 3-9). Severe bleeding must be controlled as soon as possible.

2. Why is it necessary to feel for a pulse?

3. Why must severe bleeding be controlled as soon as possible?

Checking infants and children

If you are alone and you find a child or an infant unconscious and not breathing, give rescue breathing for about one minute before calling the local emergency number. This will get oxygen into the child and prevent the heart from stopping.

Summary of the primary survey

The primary survey lets you know of any life-threatening conditions that need to be cared for immediately. Check for consciousness, an open airway, breathing, and circulation. Call EMS personnel or send someone else to call as soon as you determine that the victim is unconscious.

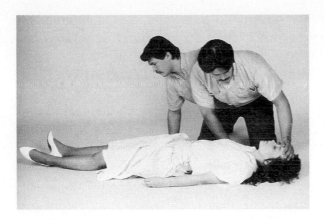

Figure 3-9 Check for severe bleeding by looking from head to toe.

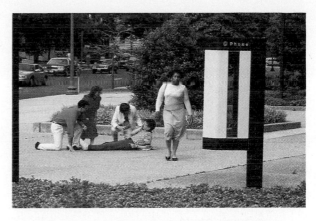

Figure 3-10 Sending someone else to call the emergency number will enable you to stay with the victim.

The skill sheets at the end of this chapter detail the steps of the primary survey.

Call EMS Personnel

Your top priority as a citizen responder is to get professional help to the victim as soon as you can. The EMS system works more effectively if you can give information about the victim's condition when the call is placed. This will help to ensure that the victim receives proper medical care as quickly as possible. By calling your local emergency number, you put into motion a response system that rushes the correct emergency care personnel to the victim.

Making the call

You may ask a bystander to call the emergency number for you. Tell him or her the victim's condition. For example, tell the bystander, "Call 9-1-1. Tell them the victim is unconscious." If you find that the victim is unconscious, do not delay calling EMS personnel. Sending someone else to make the call will enable you to stay with the victim to check breathing and circulation and to provide needed care (Fig. 3-10).

When you tell someone to call for help, you should do the following:

1. Send a bystander, or possibly two, to make the call.

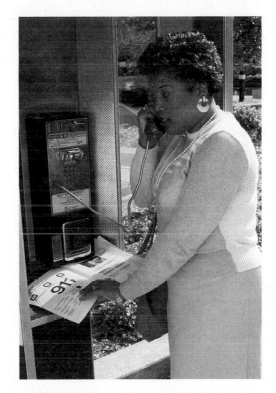

Figure 3-11 Local emergency phone numbers are easily found.

2. Give the caller(s) the EMS telephone number to call. This number is 9-1-1 in many communities. Tell the caller(s) to dial "O" (the Operator) only if you do not know the emergency number in the area. Sometimes the emergency number is on the inside front cover of telephone directories and on pay phones (Fig. 3-11).

3. Tell the caller(s) to give the dispatcher the necessary information. Most dispatchers will ask for the following important facts:

a. Where the emergency is located. Give the exact address or location and the name of the city or town. It is helpful to give the names of nearby intersecting streets (cross streets or roads), landmarks, the name of the building, the floor, and the room number.

b. Telephone number from which the call is being made.

c. Caller's name.

d. What happened—for example, a motor vehicle collision, fall, fire.

e. How many people are involved.

f. Condition of the victim(s)—for example, unconsciousness, chest pain, trouble breathing, bleeding.

g. Help (first aid) being given.

4. Tell the caller(s) not to hang up until the dispatcher hangs up. It is important to make sure the dispatcher has all the information needed to send the right help to the scene. The EMS dispatcher may also be able to give the caller instructions on how best to care for the victim until help arrives.

5. Tell the caller(s) to report to you after making the call and tell you what the dispatcher said.

If you are the only person on the scene, shout for help. If the victim is unconscious and no one comes at once to help you, you will need to get professional help fast. Find the nearest telephone as quickly as possible. Make the call and go back to the victim. Recheck the victim and give the necessary care.

If you shout and no one responds while you are giving urgent care, such as controlling severe bleeding, continue for about a minute while you think where to find the nearest telephone. Then get to that telephone as quickly as possible. After making the call, return to the victim and continue giving care.

With your first aid training, you can do two important things that can make a difference in the outcome of a seriously ill or injured person—call EMS personnel as quickly as possible and give care for life-threatening problems. If you are confused or unsure of what care to give, call your local emergency number immediately.

When to call

At times, you may be unsure if EMS personnel are needed. For example, the victim may say not to call an ambulance because he or she is embarrassed about creating a scene. Sometimes, you may be unsure if the severity of the victim's condition requires professional assistance or if the victim needs to go to the hospital. Your first aid training will help you make the decision.

As a general rule, call EMS personnel if any of the following conditions exist:

◆ Unconsciousness or altered level of consciousness

◆ Breathing problems (difficulty breathing or no breathing)

◆ Persistent chest or abdominal pain or pressure

◆ No pulse

◆ Severe bleeding

◆ Vomiting blood or passing blood

◆ Poisoning

◆ Seizures, severe headache, or slurred speech

◆ Injuries to head, neck, or back

◆ Possible broken bones

There are also special situations that warrant calling EMS personnel for assistance. These include—

◆ Fire or explosion.

◆ The presence of poisonous gas.

◆ Downed electrical wires.

◆ Swift-moving water.

◆ Motor vehicle collisions.

◆ Victims who cannot be moved easily.

These conditions and situations are by no means a complete list. It is beyond anyone's ability to provide a definitive list, since there are always exceptions. Trust your instincts. If you think there is an emergency, there probably is. Do not lose time calling untrained people such as friends or family members. Call EMS personnel for professional medical help immediately. These professionals would rather respond to a nonemergency than arrive at an emergency too late to help.

Q

4. As a citizen responder trained in first aid, your top priority is always to get professional help to the victim as soon as you can. When would you complete a primary survey before calling EMS personnel?

Do a Secondary Survey

Once you are certain that there are no life-threatening conditions needing attention, you can begin the secondary survey. If you find life-threatening conditions such as unconsciousness, call EMS personnel. Do *not* waste time with the secondary survey. Check breathing and circulation, and provide care only for the life-threatening conditions.

The secondary survey is a systematic method of finding other injuries or conditions that may need care. These are injuries or conditions that are not immediately life-threatening, but could become so if not cared for. For example, you might find possible broken bones, minor bleeding, or a specific medical condition such as epilepsy. The secondary survey has three basic steps:

1. Interview the victim and bystanders.
2. Check **vital signs**.
3. Do a head-to-toe examination.

It is a good idea to write down the information you find during the secondary survey. If possible, have someone else write down the information or help you remember it. This information can be given to EMS personnel when they arrive. It may help to decide the type of medical care the victim will get later.

When you do the secondary survey, remember not to move the victim. Most injured people will find the most comfortable position for themselves. For example, a person with a chest injury who is having trouble breathing may be supporting the injured area. Let the victim stay this way. Do not ask him or her to change positions.

Interview the victim and bystanders

Begin by asking the victim and bystanders simple questions to learn more about what happened and the victim's condition. This should not take much time.

If you have not done so already, remember to identify yourself and to get consent to help. Begin the interview by asking the victim's name. Using the victim's name will make him or her more comfortable. Ask the victim the following questions:

1. What happened?
2. Do you feel pain anywhere?
3. Do you have any allergies?
4. Do you have any medical conditions or are you taking any medication?

If the victim has pain, ask him or her to describe it. Ask when the pain started. Ask how bad the pain is. You can expect to get descriptions such as burning, throbbing, aching, or sharp pain.

Sometimes the victim will be unable to provide you with the proper information. This is often the case with an infant or child. It may also be true for an adult who momentarily lost consciousness and may not be able to recall what happened. These victims may be frightened. Be calm and patient. Speak normally and in simple terms. Offer reassurance. Ask family members, friends, or bystanders what hap-

Hundreds of Millions Served

In case of emergency, call 9-1-1. Across our country, 9-1-1 service has helped millions of people. You read a news article about a 5-year-old boy who saves his 8-year-old brother or an infant who is saved by his mother. They were instructed in lifesaving first aid over the phone by the 9-1-1 emergency dispatcher. Why 9-1-1? Why does it exist?

The 9-1-1 service was created in the United States in 1968 as a nationwide telephone number for the public to use to report emergencies and request emergency assistance. It gives the public direct access to a Public Service Answering Point that is responsible for taking the appropriate action. The numbers 9-1-1 were chosen because they best fit the needs of the public and the telephone company. They are easy to remember and dial, and they have never been used as an office, area, or service code.[1]

When should you call 9-1-1? Call 9-1-1 whenever there is a threat to life or property, or the potential for injury.[2] Fire and motor vehicle crashes are obvious emergencies that require using 9-1-1. But you should also call 9-1-1 for other situations that threaten life or property, or those that may cause injury such as a dangerous animal running loose, a downed electrical line, a burglary, or an assault.

Hundreds of millions of people call 9-1-1 each year. The majority, approximately 80 percent of 9-1-1 calls, pertain to law enforcement. Fire and EMS comprise the rest. EMS professionals alone respond to more than 19 million 9-1-1 calls each year.

What advantages does 9-1-1 offer? It was designed to save time in the overall response of a public safety agency (for example, fire, police, EMS) to a call for help.[3] This includes the time it takes a citizen to telephone the correct agency or agencies for help. For example, imagine that a house is on fire in your neighborhood and your neighbor has been seriously burned. You run to call for help. Whom should you call first—the fire department to come and put out the fire so no one else is hurt, the ambulance so EMTs can attend to your neighbor, or the police

to help secure the area? Without 9-1-1 service, you may need to place separate calls to all three agencies.

With 9-1-1 service, regardless of your needs, you make only one call. When the call comes in, a 9-1-1 dispatcher answers the call, listens to the caller, gathers needed information, and dispatches help.

Perhaps one of the most exciting lifesaving advances in computer technology in the past few years has been the development of an enhanced 9-1-1 system.

This system uses Computer-Aided Dispatch (CAD). As soon as a call comes in, CAD automatically displays the telephone number, address, and name in which the phone is listed. So, even if the caller is unable to remain on the line or unable to speak or if the call is disconnected, the dispatcher has enough information to send help.

The latest advance in 9-1-1 system development is the use of CAD units in police cars, fire engines, and ambulances. By the time these personnel start their vehicles, the built-in CAD units provide them with the location information. These CAD units are also used to send messages, establishing a vital communication link among the caller, the dispatcher, and the field unit en route.

With all of its advantages and lifesaving capabilities, 9-1-1 service today covers only approximately 50 percent of the U.S. population. While 125 cities with over 100,000 people have 9-1-1 service, other areas of the country are still without this lifesaving service.[4] As more cities establish 9-1-1 systems, response times of emergency personnel will continue to improve, resulting in more lives being saved.

REFERENCES
1. National Emergency Number Association, *Nine One One 9-1-1 (What's it all about?)*.
2. Stanton, William, Executive Director National Emergency Number Association, Interview 2/13/90.
3. National Emergency Number Association, *Nine One One 9-1-1 (What's it all about?)*.
4. Stanton, William, Executive Director National Emergency Number Association, Interview 2/13/90.

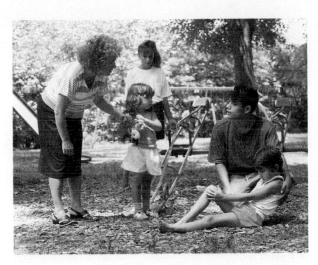

Figure 3-12 Parents or other adults may be able to provide information for a child who is sick or injured.

pened (Fig. 3-12). They may be able to give you helpful information. If a parent or adult guardian is present, ask him or her to help calm the infant or child. Parents can also tell you if the child has a medical condition that you should be aware of.

Check vital signs

A person's breathing, pulse, and skin characteristics are called vital signs. These vital signs can give you signals that tell you how the body is responding to injury or illness. Look for changes or any problems in breathing, pulse, or skin appearance and temperature. Note anything unusual. Check these vital signs about every five minutes until EMS personnel arrive.

Changes in breathing. A healthy person breathes regularly. Breathing should be effortless and quiet. In the secondary survey, watch and listen for any changes in normal breathing. Abnormal breathing may indicate a potential problem. The signals of abnormal breathing include—

◆ Gasping for air.
◆ Noisy breathing, including whistling sounds, crowing, gurgling.

◆ Excessively fast or slow breathing. (Normal breathing for adults is 10 to 20 breaths per minute. Children and infants normally breathe faster.)
◆ Painful breathing.

In later chapters, you will learn more about what changes in breathing may mean and what first aid to give.

Changes in pulse. With every heartbeat, a wave of blood moves through the blood vessels. This creates a beat called the pulse. You can feel it with your fingertips in arteries near the skin's surface.

When the heart is healthy, it beats with a steady rhythm. This creates a regular pulse. If the heartbeat changes, so does the pulse. An abnormal pulse may be a signal that indicates a potential problem. These signals include—

◆ Irregular pulse.
◆ Weak and hard-to-find pulse.
◆ Excessively fast or slow pulse. (Normal pulse for an adult is 60 to 100 beats per minute. Children and infants normally have a faster pulse.)

With a severe injury or when the heart is not healthy, the heart may beat unevenly, generating an irregular pulse. Similarly, the pulse speeds up when a person is excited, anxious, in pain, losing blood, or under stress. It slows down when a person is relaxed. Some heart conditions may also speed up or slow down the pulse rate.

These subtle changes may be difficult for a citizen responder to detect. The most important change to note is a pulse that changes from being present to no pulse at all.

Checking a pulse is a simple step. It merely involves placing two fingers on top of a major artery that is located close to the skin's surface. These include the carotid arteries in the

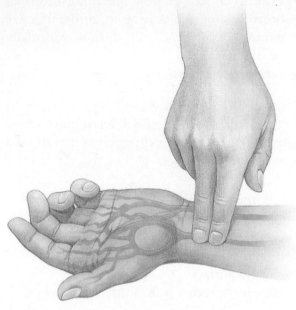

Figure 3-13 A pulse can be checked in arteries that circulate close to the surface, such as the radial artery in the wrist.

neck and radial artery in the wrist (Fig. 3-13).

A sick or injured person's pulse may be hard to find. If this happens, keep checking for a pulse periodically. Take your time. Remember, if a person is breathing, his or her heart is also beating. However, there may be a loss of pulse in the injured area. If you cannot find the pulse, check it in another major artery—in the other wrist or the neck.

In later chapters, you will learn more about what any changes in pulse may mean and what first aid to give.

Changes in skin appearance and temperature. The appearance of the skin and its temperature often indicate something about the victim's condition. For example, a victim with a breathing problem may have a flushed or pale face.

Look at the victim's face. The skin looks red when the body is forced to work harder because the heart pumps faster to get more blood to the tissues. This increased blood flow causes reddened skin and makes the skin feel warm. In contrast, the skin may look pale or bluish and feel cool and moist if the blood flow is directed

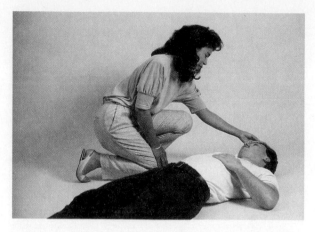

Figure 3-14 Feel the skin with your hand to determine the skin's temperature.

away from the skin's surface in order to increase the blood supply to vital organs. Determine the temperature of the skin by feeling it with your hand (Fig. 3-14). In later chapters, you will learn more about what these changes may mean and what first aid to give.

Perform a head-to-toe examination

The last step of the secondary survey is the head-to-toe examination. This examination helps gather more information about the victim's condition. When you do the head-to-toe examination, use your senses—sight, sound, and smell—to detect anything abnormal. For example, look around to determine how the incident occurred. Look for bruises, bleeding, or a deformed body part. Check for unusual odors. Listen carefully to what the victim may tell you.

Begin the head-to-toe examination by telling the victim what you are going to do. Ask the victim to remain still. A victim may move around but usually will not move a body part that is injured. Ask the victim to tell you if any areas hurt. *Avoid touching any painful areas or having the victim move any area in which there is discomfort.* Watch for facial expressions, listen for a tone of voice that may reveal pain. Look for a medical alert tag on a necklace or bracelet. This tag may tell you what might be wrong, who to call for help, and what care to give.

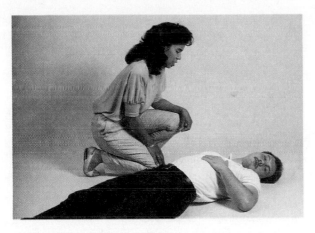

Figure 3-15 Ask the victim to gently move his head from side to side to check the neck.

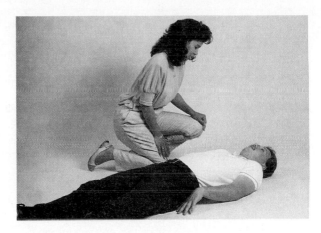

Figure 3-16 Ask the victim to shrug his shoulders to check the shoulders.

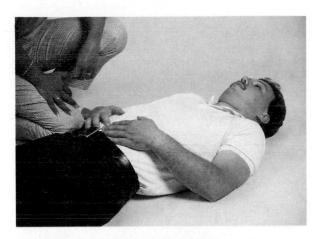

Figure 3-17 To check the chest and abdomen, ask the victim to breathe deeply and then blow the air out. Ask if he is experiencing pain.

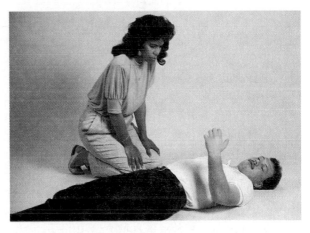

Figure 3-18 Check arms by asking the victim to bend his arms one at a time.

As you do the head-to-toe examination, think about how the body normally looks. Be alert for any sign of injuries—anything that looks or sounds unusual. If you are uncertain whether your finding is unusual, check the other side of the body.

To do a head-to-toe examination, visually inspect the entire body, starting with the head. You might see abnormal skin color from bruising, a body fluid such as blood, or an unusual position of body parts. You may notice odd bumps or depressions. The victim may seem groggy or faint. Look for signs that may indicate a serious problem. If you see or suspect a condition that requires EMS personnel, call right away and have the victim remain still.

If you do not suspect an injury to the head or spine, determine if there are any specific injuries by asking the victim to try to move each body part in which there is no pain or discomfort. To check the neck, ask if the injured person can slowly move his or her head from side to side (Fig. 3-15). Check the shoulders by asking the person to shrug them (Fig. 3-16). Check the chest and abdomen by asking the person to try to take a deep breath and then blow the air out (Fig. 3-17). Ask if he or she is experiencing pain during breathing. Check each arm by first asking the person if he or she can move the fingers and the hand. Next, ask if he or she can bend the arm (Fig. 3-18). In the same way, check the hips and legs by first asking if he or she can move the toes, foot, and

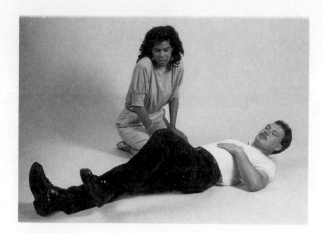

Figure 3-19 Check the legs by asking the victim to bend his legs one at a time.

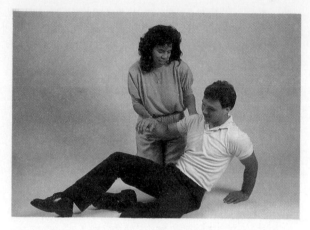

Figure 3-20 If there are no signs of obvious injuries, help the victim into a sitting position.

ankle. Then determine if he or she can bend the leg (Fig. 3-19). It is best to check only one extremity at a time.

If the victim can move all of the body parts without pain or discomfort and there are no other apparent signs of injury, have him or her attempt to rest for a few minutes in a sitting position (Fig. 3-20). Continue to check the vital signs and monitor the ABCs. If no further difficulty develops, help the victim slowly stand when he or she is ready (Fig. 3-21).

If the person is unable to move a body part or is experiencing pain with movement, or dizziness, recheck the ABCs. Help the person rest in the most comfortable position, maintain normal body temperature, and reassure him or her. Determine what additional care is needed and whether or not to call EMS personnel.

As you do this examination, keep watching the victim's level of consciousness, breathing, and skin color. If any problems develop, *stop* whatever you are doing and give first aid *immediately*. The skill sheets at the end of this chapter give detailed steps for the secondary survey.

Provide care

Once you complete the secondary survey, provide care for any specific injuries you find.

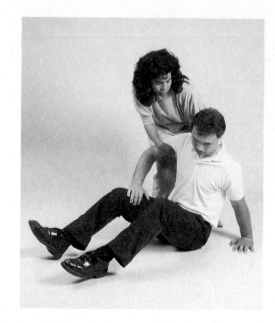

Figure 3-21 Help the victim slowly stand if no difficulties are found.

To provide care for the victim until EMS personnel arrive, follow these general steps:

1. Do no further harm.
2. Monitor the ABCs.
3. Help the victim rest in the most comfortable position.
4. Maintain normal body temperature.
5. Reassure the victim.
6. Provide any specific care needed.

5. If you find in the primary survey that the victim is conscious, has no difficulty breathing, and has no severe bleeding, what should you do next? Why?

6. If you find during the primary survey that the victim is unconscious, what should you do next? Why?

◆ Deciding to Transport the Victim

After completing your check of the victim, you might consider transporting the victim to the hospital yourself if the victim's condition is not severe. This is an important decision. Do not transport a victim with a life-threatening condition or one in whom there is any chance that a life-threatening condition may develop. In these instances, call EMS personnel and wait for help. A car trip can be painful for the victim and may aggravate the injury or cause additional injury.

If you do decide to transport the victim yourself, ask someone else to come with you. One person should drive while the other helps keep the victim comfortable. Be sure you know the quickest route to the nearest medical facility with emergency care capabilities. Pay close attention to the victim, and watch for any changes in his or her condition.

Discourage a victim from driving to the hospital. An injury may restrict movement, or the victim may become groggy or faint. A sudden onset of pain may be distracting. Also, an injured or ill person may drive faster than he or she would normally. Any of these conditions can make driving dangerous for the victim, passengers, pedestrians, and other drivers.

◆ Summary

When you respond to an emergency, remember to follow the four emergency action principles (EAPs). These principles guide your actions in any emergency. They ensure your safety and the safety of others. They also ensure that urgent care is provided for life-threatening emergencies. By following the EAPs, you will give the victim of a serious illness or injury the best chance of survival.

- Survey the scene. Make sure there are no dangers to you, the victim, and bystanders.
- Do a primary survey of the victim. Find out if the victim is conscious. Call EMS if the victim is unconscious. Determine if there are any problems with the airway, breathing, or circulation, and care for them right away. Immediate care is essential for the victim's survival.
- Try to send a bystander to make the call to EMS. Then you can continue to check breathing and circulation and provide care. Give the bystander the necessary information about the victim's condition.
- If you find no life-threatening conditions, do a secondary survey to find and care for any other injuries. Problems that are not an immediate threat to life could become serious if you do not give first aid.

Although the EAPs help you decide what care to give in any emergency, providing care is not an exact science. Because each emergency and each victim is unique, an emergency may not occur exactly as it did in a classroom setting. Even within a single emergency, care needed may change from one moment to the next. For example, the primary survey may indicate the victim is conscious, breathing, has a pulse, and has no severe bleeding. In this instance, there is no need to call EMS personnel immediately. However, during your secondary survey, you may notice that the victim begins to experience breathing difficulty. At this point, there is a need to call EMS personnel.

Many variables exist when dealing with emergencies. You do not need to know exactly what is wrong with the victim to provide appropriate care. Use the EAPs as a tool to help you make decisions. Even though there may not always be a right or wrong answer, following the EAPs ensures that you take care of life-threatening emergencies first.

As you read the following chapters, remember and apply the EAPs to each injury or illness. The EAPs form the basis for providing care in any emergency (Fig. 3-22).

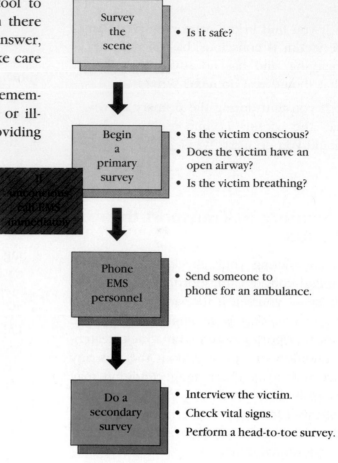

Figure 3-22   Use the EAPs to make care decisions in an emergency.

Answers to Application Questions

1. The check for breathing is a crucial step in your evaluation of the victim's condition. It can mean the difference between life or death. Absence of breathing is a life-threatening emergency that requires immediate care. By using your senses to check for breathing, you can correctly determine the presence or absence of breathing and thus the care that is needed.

2. Checking for a pulse is another crucial step in your evaluation of the victim's condition. Absence of a carotid pulse is the most severe life-threatening emergency that exists. You must start CPR promptly and make sure the EMS system has been called.

3. Severe bleeding is defined as blood that spurts from the wound or cannot be controlled. Normally, oxygen taken into the body through breathing goes to the lungs, is distributed to the heart, and then circulated throughout the body. During severe bleeding, this is not the case. The injury that causes severe bleeding damages the circulatory system—particularly the blood vessels. This damage to the circulatory system impairs the delivery of oxygen-rich blood to all body tissues. Tissues that do not receive oxygen lose their ability to function and will soon die. If severe bleeding is not controlled, the vital organs will not receive the oxygen they need to function and will die. When vital organs fail to function, the victim will die.

4. If the person was conscious and could talk to you, you are assured that he or she is breathing and the heart is beating. The primary survey is complete. If after checking further, you determine there are signals of a life-threatening emergency, call the emergency number immediately.

5. Since no apparent life-threatening emergencies exist, you should do a secondary survey to determine if there are other conditions present that require medical attention and/or EMS personnel.

6. If you find during the primary survey that the victim is unconscious, you should have someone call EMS personnel immediately while you check breathing and circulation. Unconsciousness can be a life-threatening emergency.

Study Questions

1. Match each emergency action principle with the actions it includes.

  a. Survey the scene.
  b. Do a primary survey and care for life-threatening emergencies.
  c. Call EMS personnel.
  d. Do a secondary survey when appropriate.

_____ Open the airway.
_____ Look for bystanders who can help.
_____ Interview the victim and bystanders.
_____ Check for breathing.
_____ Check vital signs.
_____ Do a head-to-toe examination.

_____ Dial 9-1-1 or the local emergency number.
_____ Look for victims.
_____ Check for severe bleeding.
_____ Look for dangers.
_____ Check for a pulse.
_____ Look for clues to determine what happened.

2. List the four emergency action principles (EAPs).

3. List four questions to be answered when surveying the scene.

4. List three things you must tell the victim to get consent.

5. List four important facts you should give EMS personnel when you call.

6. List six conditions that require you to call EMS personnel immediately.

7. List two things you should do if you decide to transport the victim yourself.

8. List the conditions you check for in a primary survey.

9. Describe when and why you would do a secondary survey.

10. You walk into your boss's office for a meeting. You see a cup of coffee spilled on the desk. You find him lying on the floor, motionless. What should you do? Number the following actions in order:

a. _____ Have someone call EMS for help.

b. _____ Check for breathing.

c. _____ Survey the scene.

d. _____ Check for pulse and severe bleeding.

e. _____ Check for consciousness.

f. _____ Shout for help.

In questions 11 through 17, circle the letter of the correct answer.

11. Following the emergency action principles in any emergency situation enables you to—

a. Have a plan of action for the emergency.

b. Assess the situation and provide appropriate care.

c. Enhance the victim's chance of survival or recovery.

d. All of the above.

12. What should you do if you determine that the scene is unsafe?

a. Help anyway, this is an emergency—but, be careful.

b. Get as close as you think is safe, try to see what happened, and then call EMS personnel for help.

c. Do not approach; call EMS personnel for help immediately.

d. Do not approach; wait for someone else to take action.

13. Why is it necessary to complete a primary survey in every emergency situation?

a. To check for minor injuries

b. To determine if there are any life-threatening conditions that need immediate care

c. To get consent from the victim before providing care

d. To ask for information about the cause of the illness or injury

14. Once you determine the victim's life is in no immediate danger, you should—

    a. Call EMS professionals for help.
    b. Transport the victim to the nearest hospital.
    c. Check for other injuries or conditions that could become life-threatening if not cared for.
    d. Check for consciousness and then get consent from the victim to give care.

15. Before beginning a primary survey, you should first—

    a. Position the victim so that you can open the airway.
    b. Survey the scene.
    c. Check for consciousness.
    d. Call EMS professionals for help.

16. After checking for consciousness, you determine that the victim is unconscious. What should you do next?

    a. Call EMS professionals for help.
    b. Give 2 slow breaths.
    c. Check for a pulse and severe bleeding.
    d. Begin a secondary survey.

17. Which of the following actions are performed during the secondary survey?

    a. Gathering additional information about the victim's condition
    b. Asking the victim to move body parts that are not painful
    c. Checking vital signs
    d. All of the above

18. As you walk to lunch, you notice a group of people gathered at the side of the street. As you come to the edge of the street, you see a car stopped in the street and a person lying immediately in front of it. It appears that the person has been struck by the car. Many people have gathered around, but no one seems to be doing anything. What should you do? Should EMS personnel be called? What dangers may be present? How can bystanders help?

Answers are in Appendix A.

PRACTICE SESSION: *Primary Survey*

You find a person lying on the ground, motionless. You should survey the scene to see if it is safe and to get some idea of what happened. If the scene is safe, do a primary survey by checking the ABCs.

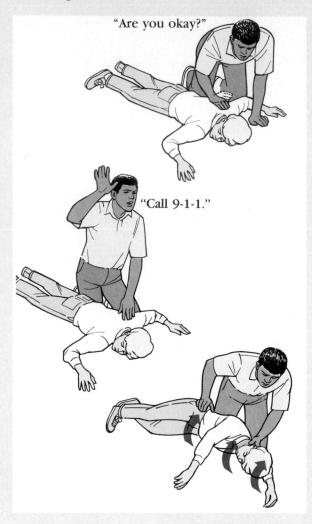

"Are you okay?"

"Call 9-1-1."

☐ **Check for consciousness**
* Tap or gently shake person.
* Shout, "Are you OK?"

If person responds. . .
* Begin a secondary survey.

If person does not respond. . .

☐ **Phone EMS personnel for help**
* Send someone else to call, if possible.

☐ **Roll person onto back** (if necessary)
* Kneel facing person.
* Place one hand on person's shoulder and other hand on person's hip.
* Roll person toward you as a single unit. Move your hand from person's shoulder to support back of head and neck.

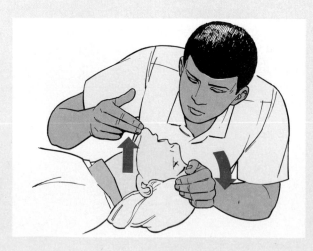

☐ **Open airway** (use head-tilt/chin-lift)
* Tilt head back and lift chin.

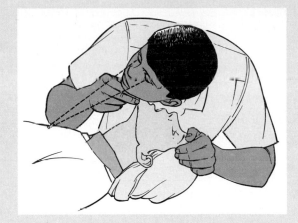

☐ Check for breathing

- ♦ Look, listen, and feel for breathing for about 5 seconds.

If person is breathing. . .
- ♦ Keep airway open.
- ♦ Monitor breathing.
- ♦ Check for and control severe bleeding.
- ♦ Await arrival of EMS personnel.

If person is not breathing. . .

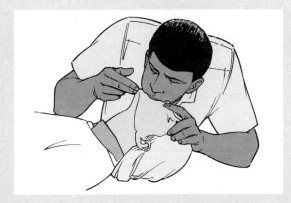

☐ Give 2 slow breaths

- ♦ Keep head tilted back.
- ♦ Pinch nose shut.
- ♦ Seal your lips tightly around person's mouth.
- ♦ Give 2 slow breaths, each lasting about 1½ seconds.
- ♦ Watch chest to see that your breath goes in.

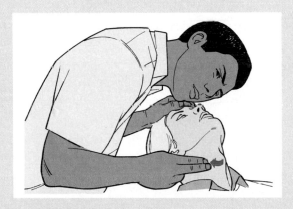

☐ Check for pulse

- ♦ Locate Adam's apple.
- ♦ Slide fingers down into groove of neck on side closer to you.
- ♦ Feel for pulse for about 5 to 10 seconds.

If person has a pulse. . .
- ♦ Check for and control severe bleeding.
- ♦ Recheck breathing.
- ♦ If not breathing, do rescue breathing.

If person does not have a pulse. . .
- ♦ Check for and control severe bleeding.
- ♦ Begin CPR.

PRACTICE SESSION: *Secondary Survey*

You have already surveyed the scene, done a primary survey, and phoned the local emergency number. You are ready to begin a secondary survey of a conscious person.

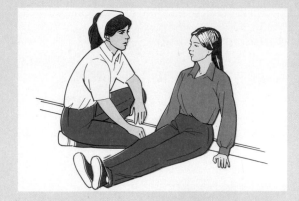

☐ Interview person

- ◆ Ask person. . .
  - ◆ His or her name.
  - ◆ What happened.
  - ◆ If he or she feels pain anywhere.
  - ◆ If he or she has any allergies.
  - ◆ If he or she has any medical conditions or is taking any medications.

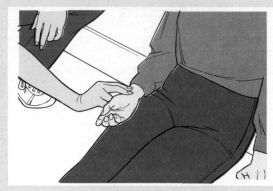

☐ Check vital signs

Determine if pulse is abnormal
- ◆ Tell person you are going to take his or her pulse.
- ◆ Locate pulse on thumb side of wrist.
- ◆ Ask yourself if it is. . .
  - ◆ Regular or irregular.
  - ◆ Hard to find.
  - ◆ Excessively fast or slow.
- ◆ Note any abnormalities.

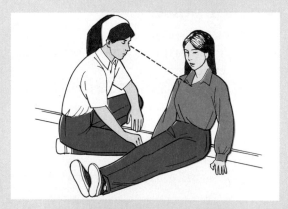

Determine if breathing is abnormal
- ◆ Ask yourself if person is. . .
  - ◆ Gasping for air.
  - ◆ Making unusual noises as he or she breathes.
  - ◆ Breathing excessively fast or slowly.
  - ◆ Experiencing pain when breathing.
- ◆ Note any abnormalities.

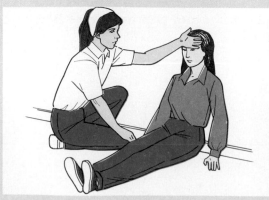

Determine skin appearance and temperature
- ◆ Feel person's forehead with back of your hand.
- ◆ Look at person's face and lips.
- ◆ Ask yourself if skin is. . .
  - ◆ Cold or hot.
  - ◆ Unusually wet or dry.
  - ◆ Pale, bluish, or flushed.
- ◆ Note any abnormalities.

☐ Perform Head-to-Toe Examination

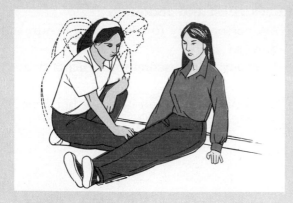

NOTE: DO NOT ASK VICTIM TO MOVE ANY AREA IN WHICH HE OR SHE HAS DISCOMFORT OR PAIN OR IF YOU SUSPECT INJURY TO HEAD OR SPINE.

Visually inspect body
* Look carefully for bleeding, cuts, bruises, and obvious deformities.

Check ears, nose, and mouth
* Look for fluid or blood.

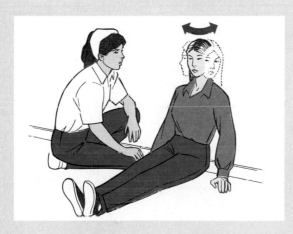

Check neck
* Ask person to try to gently move head from side to side.
* Note pain, discomfort, or inability to move.

Check shoulders
* Ask person to try to shrug shoulders.
* Note pain, discomfort, or inability to move.

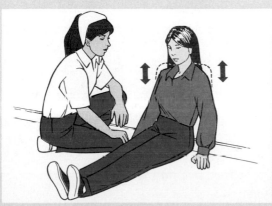

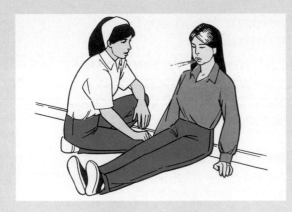

Check chest and abdomen
- Ask person to try to take a deep breath and blow air out.
- Note any pain, discomfort, or inability to move.
- Ask if person has pain in his or her abdomen.

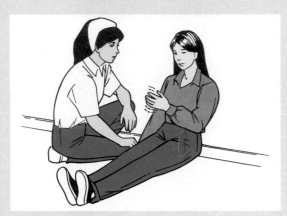

Check arms
- Check one arm at a time.
- Ask person to try to. . .
  - Move hands and fingers.
  - Bend arm.
- Note any pain, discomfort, or inability to move.

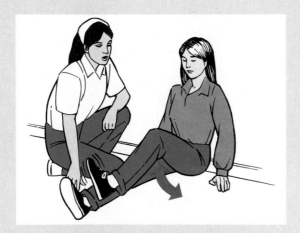

Check hips and legs
- Check one leg at a time.
- Ask person to try to. . .
  - Move foot, toes, ankle.
  - Bend leg.
- Note any pain, discomfort, or inability to move.

If person can move body parts without pain or discomfort and is not dizzy. . .
* Have person sit up and rest for a few minutes.
* If no further difficulty, have person stand slowly.
* Determine if further care is needed.

If person is unable to move a body part or is experiencing pain on movement, and/or dizziness. . .
* Recheck ABCs.
* Have person stay still.
* Maintain normal body temperature.
* Reassure person.
* Call EMS personnel for help if not already done.

NOTE:

WHAT HAPPENED: _____

_____

_____

PAIN: _____

_____

ALLERGIES: _____

_____

MEDICAL CONDITIONS/
MEDICATIONS: _____

_____

_____

BREATHING: _____

PULSE: _____

SKIN TEMPERATURE: _____

MOISTURE: _____

COLOR: _____

FINDINGS: _____

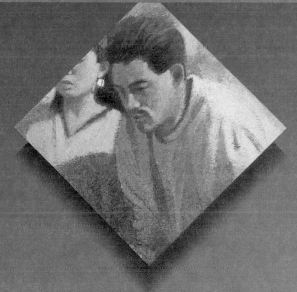

Life-Threatening Emergencies

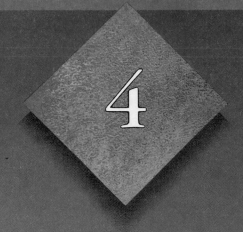

Breathing Emergencies

Objectives

After reading this chapter, you should be able to—

1. List at least four signals of respiratory distress.

2. Describe first aid care for a victim of respiratory distress.

3. Describe the purpose of rescue breathing.

4. Describe when to provide rescue breathing.

5. Describe how to provide rescue breathing.

6. List at least three causes of choking.

7. Describe first aid care for a conscious and an unconscious victim with an obstructed airway.

8. Define the key terms for this chapter.

After reading this chapter and completing the class activities, you should be able to—

1. Demonstrate rescue breathing for an adult.

2. Demonstrate first aid for a conscious victim with an obstructed airway.

3. Demonstrate first aid for an unconscious victim with an obstructed airway.

4. Make appropriate decisions regarding care when given an example of an emergency situation in which a person is having difficulty breathing or is not breathing.

Key Terms

Airway obstruction: Blockage of the airway that prevents air from reaching a person's lungs.

Aspiration (as pĭ RA shun): Taking blood, vomit, saliva, or other foreign material into the lungs.

Breathing emergency: Emergency in which breathing is so impaired that life is threatened.

Finger sweep: Technique used to remove foreign material from a victim's upper airway.

Head-tilt/chin-lift: Technique for opening the airway.

Rescue breathing: The technique of breathing for a nonbreathing victim.

Respiratory (re SPI rah to re *or* RES pah rah tor e) arrest: Condition in which breathing has stopped.

Respiratory distress: Condition in which breathing is difficult.

For Review

Before reading this chapter, you should have a basic understanding of the anatomy of the airway and how the respiratory and circulatory systems function (Chapter 2). You should also know the steps of the primary survey (Chapter 3).

◆ Introduction

In previous chapters, you learned what you can do to help in an emergency. You learned four emergency action principles (EAPs) that guide your actions in any emergency. Remember, the EAPs are—

- Survey the scene.
- Do a primary survey and care for life-threatening problems.
- Call EMS personnel for help.
- Do a secondary survey, when appropriate, and care for additional problems.

In this chapter, you will learn how to care for someone who is in **respiratory distress** or who has stopped breathing.

As you read in Chapter 3, once you are sure the scene is safe, begin a primary survey of the victim. The primary survey detects any life-threatening conditions. First check to see if the victim is conscious. Call EMS if the victim is unconscious. Then complete the primary survey by checking the ABCs:

- *Airway*
- *Breathing*
- *Circulation*

Because oxygen is vital to life, you must always ensure that the victim has an open airway and is breathing. A **breathing emergency** should be detected during the primary survey. It occurs when someone's breathing is so impaired that life is threatened. A breathing emergency can occur in two ways: breathing can become difficult, or breathing can stop. A person who is having difficulty breathing is in respiratory distress. A person who is not breathing is in **respiratory arrest**.

◆ The Breathing Process

Breathing requires the respiratory, circulatory, nervous, and musculoskeletal systems to work together. As you read in Chapter 2, injuries or illnesses that affect any of these systems may impair breathing. For example, if the heart stops beating, the victim will stop breathing. Injury or disease in areas of the brain that control breathing may impair or stop breathing. Damage to muscles or bones of the chest and back can make breathing difficult or painful. All of these situations are, or could result in, breathing emergencies.

The body requires constant oxygen for survival. When you breathe air into your lungs, the oxygen in the air is transferred to the blood. The blood transports the oxygen to the

Secord

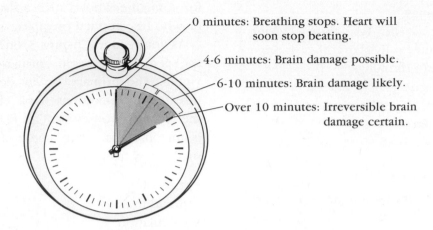

0 minutes: Breathing stops. Heart will
soon stop beating.

4-6 minutes: Brain damage possible.

6-10 minutes: Brain damage likely.

Over 10 minutes: Irreversible brain
damage certain.

Figure 4-1   Time is critical in starting lifesaving measures. Six minutes without
oxygen will generally cause brain damage.

brain, organs, muscles, and other parts of the body where it is used to provide energy. This energy allows the body to perform its many functions such as breathing, walking, talking, digesting food, and maintaining body temperature. Different functions require different levels of energy and, therefore, different amounts of oxygen. For example, sitting in a chair requires less energy than jogging around the block. A body battling disease, even the common cold, uses more energy than a body in its normal healthy state because it must carry out all normal functions of life and simultaneously fight the disease. Does this explain why you are usually tired when you are sick?

Without oxygen, cells begin to die in four to six minutes (Fig. 4-1). Some tissues, such as the brain, are very sensitive to oxygen starvation. Unless the brain receives oxygen within minutes, brain damage or death will result.

Breathing emergencies can be caused by the following:

* An obstructed airway (choking)

* Illness (such as pneumonia)
* Respiratory conditions (such as emphysema, asthma)
* Electrocution
* Shock
* Drowning
* Heart attack or heart disease
* Injury to the chest or lungs
* Allergic reactions to foods, insect stings, and so on
* Drugs
* Poisoning, such as inhaling or ingesting toxic substances

◆ Respiratory Distress

Respiratory distress is the most common type of breathing emergency. Respiratory distress is not always caused by injuries or illnesses, such as those listed in the preceding paragraph. It may also result from excitement or anxiety. Learn to recognize the signals of respiratory distress.

Signals of Respiratory Distress

There are many signals of respiratory distress. Victims may look as if they cannot catch their breath, or they may gasp for air. They may appear to breathe faster or slower than normal. Their breaths may be unusually deep or shallow. They may make unusual noises, such as wheezing or gurgling, or high-pitched sounds like crowing.

The victim's skin appearance may also signal respiratory distress. At first, the victim's skin may be unusually moist and appear flushed. Later, it may appear pale or bluish as the oxygen level in the blood falls.

Victims may say they feel dizzy or lightheaded. They may feel pain in the chest or tingling in the hands and feet. Understandably, the victim may be apprehensive or fearful. Any of these signals is a clue that the victim may be in respiratory distress. Table 4-1 lists the signals of respiratory distress.

Specific Causes of Respiratory Distress

Although respiratory distress is often caused by injury, several other conditions also can cause respiratory distress. These include asthma, hyperventilation, and anaphylactic shock.

Asthma

Asthma is a condition that narrows the air passages and makes breathing difficult. During an asthma attack, the air passages become constricted, or narrowed, due to a spasm of the muscles lining the bronchi or swelling of the bronchi themselves.

Asthma is more common in children and young adults. It may be triggered by an allergic reaction to food, pollen, a drug, or an insect sting. Emotional stress may also trigger it. For some people, physical activity may induce asthma. Normally, someone with asthma easily controls attacks with medication. When taken, these medications stop the muscle spasm, opening the airway and making breathing easier.

Table 4-1	Signals of Respiratory Distress
Condition	**Signals**
Abnormal breathing	Breathing is slow or rapid. Breaths are unusually deep or shallow. Victim is gasping for breath. Victim is wheezing, gurgling, or making high-pitched noises such as crowing.
Abnormal skin appearance	Victim's skin is unusually moist. Victim's skin has a flushed, pale, or bluish appearance.
How the victim feels	Victim feels short of breath. Victim feels dizzy or lightheaded. Victim feels pain in the chest or tingling in hands and feet.

Signals of asthma. A characteristic signal of asthma is wheezing when exhaling. Wheezing occurs because air becomes trapped in the lungs. This trapped air may also make the victim's chest appear larger than normal, particularly a small child's.

1. How can air become trapped in the lungs?

Hyperventilation

Hyperventilation occurs when someone breathes faster than normal. This rapid breathing upsets the body's balance of oxygen and car-

An Altitude Adjustment

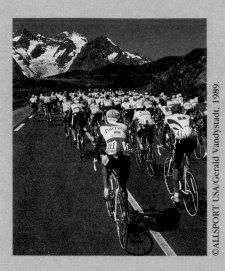

©ALLSPORT USA/Gerald Vandystadt, 1989.

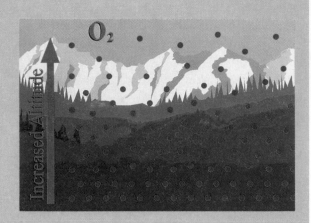

The portion of the Tour de France bicycle race that winds its way through the Alps is a legendary challenge. Each year, some 250,000 fans gather along the road of L'Alpe de Huez to watch professional cyclists attack the most difficult climb of the tour. The tortuous path twists 21 times and reaches a snowy summit of 5,728 feet. Even athletes in superb condition find themselves struggling—legs wobble, shoulders begin to bob, and elbows stick out awkwardly. Many riders drop out.

A secret enemy of the riders is altitude. At higher elevations, the air pressure is lower, allowing oxygen molecules to spread farther apart in the atmosphere. Consequently, the cyclist gets less oxygen with each gulp of air and transports less oxygen to straining muscles. Oxygen is necessary to exercise because it helps release energy the muscles can use.

Endurance sports like bicycle racing are especially difficult at high altitudes. To equal his oxygen intake at sea level, the cyclist must breathe faster, and his heart must pump harder. He risks hyperventilating and fainting. Studies show that the athlete's aerobic capacity, which includes the heart's ability to pump oxygen to the muscles and the muscle's ability to use oxygen efficiently, can drop 5 to 10 percent when a person moves from sea level to 6,500 feet.

To compensate for the change in altitude, the body makes adjustments within a few days. As the athlete becomes accustomed to the new climate, he begins to breathe in a greater volume of air with each breath. The body produces more red blood cells to carry oxygen more efficiently. These adjustments actually improve the aerobic capacity of athletes who train in the mountains or in low-pressure chambers.

Many U.S. Olympic team members live at high altitudes like Colorado Springs to train. U.S. Junior National Team cyclist Eric Harris, who is training for the Olympics, says he can feel a difference in his riding at high altitudes. He rides up to 110 miles a day during endurance training in January through April.

"Each of us has our own aerobic training level—your head pounds, your chest feels like knives are going into it with each breath. If you miss a breath by drinking or talking, it takes 10 to 20 more to make it up. Mountains are where cycling turns into an individual sport.

"You have to train in the mountains to be good in them. That's why I left Texas and moved to Utah and Colorado. No one from the low flatlands will be a great climber in the big mountains, maybe good, but never great."

Eric has accepted the challenge of the mountains—hoping to set cycling records to be listed among those of the Olympic greats.

bon dioxide. Hyperventilation is often the result of fear or anxiety and is likely in people who are tense and nervous. But, it is also caused by injuries such as head injuries, by severe bleeding, or by illnesses such as high fever, heart failure, lung disease, or diabetic emergencies. It can also be triggered by asthma or exercise.

Signals of hyperventilation. A characteristic signal of hyperventilation is shallow, rapid breathing. Despite their efforts to breathe, the victims state that they cannot get enough air or that they are suffocating. Therefore, they are often fearful and apprehensive, or they may appear confused. They may say that they feel dizzy or their fingers and toes feel numb or tingly.

Anaphylactic shock

While working in a wooded area behind your house, you are stung by a hornet. You provide care for the sting and continue to work. A few minutes later, you develop a rash and begin to feel tightness in your chest and throat. You are having difficulty breathing. You feel your neck, face, and tongue begin to swell. You are a victim of a life-threatening condition known as anaphylactic shock.

Anaphylactic shock, also known as anaphylaxis, is a severe allergic reaction. Air passages may swell and restrict the victim's breathing. Anaphylaxis may be caused by insect stings, food, or medications such as penicillin. Some people know that they will have a severe allergic reaction to certain substances. Therefore, they may have learned to avoid these substances and may carry medication to reverse this reaction.

Signals of anaphylactic shock. Signals of anaphylaxis include a rash, a feeling of tightness in the chest and throat, and swelling of the face, neck, and tongue. The person may also feel dizzy or confused. If not cared for quickly, anaphylactic shock can become a life-threatening emergency.

Q
2. Why is anaphylactic shock a life-threatening emergency?

First Aid for Respiratory Distress

Recognizing the signals of respiratory distress and giving first aid are often keys to preventing other emergencies. Respiratory distress may signal the beginning of a life-threatening condition. For example, it can be the first signal of a more serious breathing emergency or even a heart attack. Respiratory distress can lead to respiratory arrest, which, if not immediately cared for, will result in death.

Many of the signals of different kinds of respiratory distress are similar. You do not need to know the specific cause to provide care effectively.

Remember to survey the scene to ensure your own safety before you approach the victim. Respiratory distress can be caused by toxic fumes.

If the victim is breathing, you know the heart is beating. Make sure the person is not bleeding severely. Help him or her rest in a comfortable position. Usually <u>sitting</u> is more comfortable because breathing is easier (see Figure 4-2 on the next page). Provide enough air by opening a window. Have bystanders move back. Make sure someone has called the local emergency number for help, if you have not already done so.

If the victim is conscious, do a secondary survey. As you do this, remember that a person experiencing breathing difficulty may have trouble talking. Therefore, talk to any bystanders who may know about the victim's problem. The victim can confirm answers or answer yes-or-no questions by nodding. If possible, try to help reduce any anxiety that may contribute to the victim's breathing difficulty. If it is available, assist the victim in taking his or her prescribed medication for the condition. This may be oxygen, an inhalant (bron-

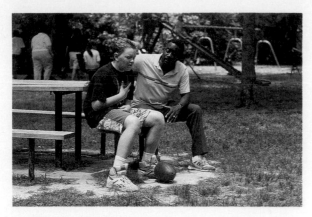

Figure 4-2 Sitting can make breathing easier for victims in respiratory distress.

Table 4-2 First Aid for Respiratory Distress
Complete a primary survey.
Activate the EMS system.
Help the victim rest comfortably.
Do a secondary survey.
Reassure the victim.
Assist with medication.
Maintain normal body temperature.
Monitor vital signs.

chial dilator), or medication in an anaphylaxis kit. Continue to look and listen for any changes in the victim's vital signs. Watch for additional signs of respiratory distress. Calm and reassure the victim. Help maintain normal body temperature by preventing chilling on a cool day or by providing shade on a hot day.

If the victim's breathing is rapid and there are signals of an injury or an underlying illness or condition, call EMS personnel immediately. This person needs advanced care right away. If, however, the victim's breathing is rapid and you are certain that it is caused by emotion, such as excitement, tell him or her to relax and breathe slowly. Reassurance is often enough to correct hyperventilation. If the victim's breathing still does not slow down, have the victim cup both hands around the mouth and nose and breathe into them. When the victim rebreathes exhaled air, the condition will usually correct itself. If the condition does not correct itself or if the victim becomes unconscious from hyperventilating, call EMS personnel immediately. Although breathing usually returns to normal when a person hyperventilating as a result of emotional trauma becomes unconscious, you should not wait to

find out. Call EMS personnel for any person who loses consciousness.

◆ Respiratory Arrest

Respiratory arrest is the condition in which breathing stops. It may be caused by illness, injury, or an obstructed airway. The causes of respiratory distress can also lead to respiratory arrest. In respiratory arrest, the person gets no oxygen to continue body functions. The body can function only for a few minutes without oxygen before body systems begin to fail. Without oxygen, the heart muscle stops functioning, causing the circulatory system to fail. When the heart stops, other body systems will start to fail. However, you can keep the person's respiratory system functioning artificially by **rescue breathing**.

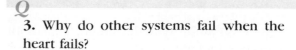

Q
3. Why do other systems fail when the heart fails?

Rescue Breathing

Rescue breathing is a way of breathing air into someone to supply that person with the oxy-

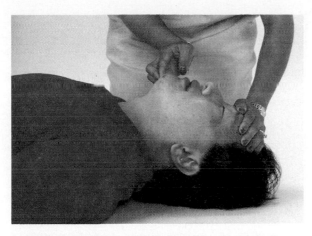

Figure 4-3 The head-tilt/chin-lift opens the victim's airway.

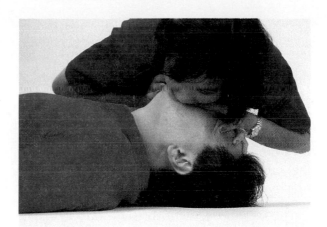

Figure 4-4 To breathe for a nonbreathing victim, pinch the nose shut, seal your mouth around the victim's mouth, and breathe slowly into the victim.

gen he or she needs to survive. Rescue breathing is given to victims who are not breathing but still have a pulse.

Rescue breathing works because the air you breathe into the victim contains more than enough oxygen to keep that person alive. The air you take in with every breath contains about 21 percent oxygen, but your body uses only a small part of that. The air you breathe out of your lungs and into the lungs of the victim contains about 16 percent oxygen. That is enough oxygen to keep someone alive.

You will discover whether you need to give rescue breathing during the first two steps of the ABCs in the primary survey, when you open the airway and check for breathing. If you cannot see, hear, or feel any signs of breathing, give 2 slow breaths immediately to get air into the victim's lungs. Then check circulation by feeling for the pulse and looking for severe bleeding. If you find a life-threatening emergency, call EMS personnel.

If the victim is not breathing but has a pulse, begin rescue breathing. To give breaths, keep the airway open with the **head-tilt/chin-lift** (Fig. 4-3). The head-tilt/chin-lift not only opens the airway by moving the tongue away from the back of the throat, but also

moves the soft tissue flap called the epiglottis from the opening of the trachea. Gently pinch the victim's nose shut with the thumb and index finger of your hand that is on the victim's forehead. Next, make a tight seal around the victim's mouth with your mouth. Breathe slowly into the victim until you see the victim's chest rise (Fig. 4-4). Each breath should last about 1½ seconds, with a pause in between to let the air flow back out. Watch the victim's chest rise each time you breathe in to ensure that your breaths are actually going in.

If you do not see the victim's chest rise and fall as you give breaths, you may not have the head tilted far enough back to open the airway adequately. Retilt the victim's head and try again to give breaths. If your breaths still do not go in, the victim's airway is obstructed. Therefore, you must give first aid for the obstructed airway (described later in this chapter).

Check for a pulse after giving the 2 slow breaths. If the victim has a pulse but is not breathing, continue rescue breathing by giving 1 breath every 5 seconds. A good way to time the breaths is to count, "one one-thousand, two one-thousand, three one-thousand." Then take a breath yourself, and breathe into the victim. Counting this way ensures that you give 1 breath every 5 seconds. Remember, breathe slowly into the victim. Each breath should last about 1½ seconds. After 1 minute of rescue breathing (about 12 breaths), recheck the pulse to make sure the heart is still beating. If the victim still has a pulse but is not breathing, continue rescue breathing. Check the pulse every minute. Do not stop rescue breathing unless one of the following occurs:

• The victim begins to breathe on his or her own.
• The victim has no pulse. Begin CPR (described in next chapter).
• Another trained rescuer takes over for you.
• EMS personnel arrive on the scene and take over.
• You are too exhausted to continue.

Practicing rescue breathing using the skill sheets at the end of this chapter will help you gain confidence in giving rescue breaths.

Q
4. Would rescue breathing alone sustain the life of someone without a pulse? Why or why not?

Special Considerations for Rescue Breathing

Air in the stomach

When you are giving rescue breathing, air normally enters the victim's lungs. Sometimes, however, air may enter the victim's stomach instead. There are several reasons why this may occur. First, breathing into the victim longer than about 1½ seconds may cause extra air to fill the stomach. Do not overinflate the lungs. Stop the breath when the chest has risen. Second, if the victim's head is not tilted back far enough, the airway will not open completely. As a result, the chest may only rise slightly. This will cause you to breathe more forcefully, causing air to enter the stom-

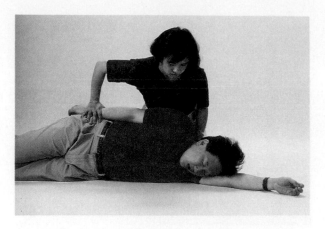

Figure 4-5 If vomiting occurs, turn the victim on his side, and clear the mouth of any matter.

ach. Third, when breaths are given too quickly, increased pressure in the airway is created, causing air to enter the stomach. Long, slow breaths minimize pressure in the air passages.

Air in the stomach can cause gastric distention. Gastric distention can be a serious problem because it can make the victim vomit. When an unconscious victim vomits, stomach contents may get into the lungs, obstructing breathing. This is called **aspiration**. Aspiration can hamper rescue breathing and eventually be fatal.

To avoid forcing air into the stomach, be sure to keep the victim's head tilted far enough back. Breathe slowly into the victim, only enough to make the chest rise. Breaths should not be given too quickly or too hard. Each breath should last about 1½ seconds. Pause between breaths long enough for the victim's lungs to empty and for you to take another breath.

Vomiting

When you give rescue breathing, the victim may vomit, whether or not there is gastric distention. If this happens, turn the victim's head and body together as a unit onto one side (Fig. 4-5). This helps to prevent vomit from enter-

My Baby's Drowning

Connie Danson nearly collapsed when she saw her 18-month-old son in the pool. She pulled his limp, pale body from the water. There were bubbles of water coming out of his nose and mouth and his eyes were open wide.

He had been in the living room when Connie left to put the laundry in the dryer. How had he gotten outside? One of the other children must have left the door open. Hysterical, Connie ran to call 9-1-1. "My baby's drowned," she sobbed into the phone. "I think he's dead."

Connie had already been through a lot with her premature child, Andy. He weighed less than 3 pounds at birth and had stayed in the hospital for three months. Nurses at the hospital taught Connie how to do rescue breathing and CPR in case Andy stopped breathing or his heart stopped. When Andy survived his first year, Connie felt grateful.

Now the sight of her child under the water kept replaying in her mind. She could barely explain the problem to the dispatcher.

"He can't breathe," Connie sobbed.

Dispatcher Anthony Carravaggio notified police and EMS personnel and then, speaking in a slow voice, he tried to calm Connie.

"Ma'am, there's an ambulance on the way," said the dispatcher. "Where is the child now?"

"He's right here on the floor," Connie said.

"Now tilt his head back gently and listen closely for any sounds," the dispatcher said.

"He's not making any sounds and he's not moving at all," Connie cried.

"Connie, you're going to have to breathe for him; do you know how?"

"I learned it in a CPR course, but I'm not sure I remember," Connie said.

"Listen to me. Pinch his nose shut. Put your mouth over his and give two slow breaths," the dispatcher said.

"OK."

Returning to the phone, Connie said, "OK, I did it."

"Now you have to see if he has a pulse. Do you remember how to do that?" the dispatcher asked.

"Yes," Connie said, leaning over to recheck her son. "He has a pulse, but he's still not breathing."

"Connie, you need to keep breathing for him. Give him one breath, count to three and breathe again. Do this for about a minute. I'll stay on the phone. I can hear you."

Connie listened as he explained the rescue breathing procedure. Over and over, she gave a rescue breath to her baby and watched for his chest to rise and fall.

Connie thought she heard the baby wheezing, but she wasn't sure. She leaned closer to his face and saw Andy's face redden and his body twitch. He began to cry.

Connie picked up the phone.

"Is that him?" the dispatcher asked.

"Yes," Connie said tearfully.

"He sounds good," the dispatcher said. "Are the paramedics there yet?"

"I hear the sirens outside," said Connie.

"OK. They will take care of him now."

It is difficult to stay calm in an emergency, even when you have learned first aid. With the help of a dispatcher, Connie overcame her panic and provided lifesaving care for her baby. If you feel yourself panicking in an emergency, remember 9-1-1 or your local emergency number; dispatchers can help you remember your first aid skills.

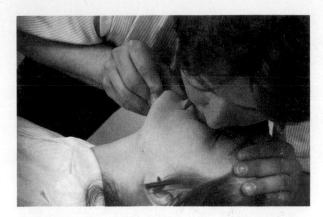

Figure 4-6 For mouth-to-nose breathing, close the victim's mouth, and seal your mouth around the victim's nose. Breathe slow breaths, watching the chest to see that the air goes in.

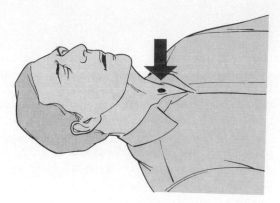

Figure 4-7 You may need to perform rescue breathing on a victim with a stoma.

ing the lungs. Quickly wipe the victim's mouth clean, reposition the victim on his or her back, and continue with rescue breathing.

Mouth-to-nose breathing

Sometimes you may not be able to make an adequate seal over a victim's mouth to perform rescue breathing. For example, the person's jaw or mouth may be injured or shut too tightly to open, or your mouth may be too small to cover the victim's. If so, provide mouth-to-nose rescue breathing as follows:

* Maintain the backward head-tilt position with one hand on the forehead. Use your other hand to close the victim's mouth, making sure to push on the chin and not on the throat.
* Open your mouth wide, take a deep breath, seal your mouth tightly around the victim's nose, and breathe into the victim's nose (Fig. 4-6). Open the victim's mouth between breaths, if possible, to let air come out.

Mouth-to-stoma breathing

Some people have had an operation that removed all or part of the upper end of their windpipe. They breathe through an opening called a stoma in the front of the neck (Fig. 4-7). Air passes directly into the windpipe through the stoma instead of through the mouth and nose.

Most people with a stoma wear a medical alert bracelet or necklace or carry a card identifying this condition. You may not see the stoma immediately. You will probably notice the opening in the neck as you tilt the head back to check for breathing.

To give rescue breathing to someone with a stoma, you must give breaths through the stoma instead of the mouth or nose. Follow the same basic steps as in mouth-to-mouth breathing, except—

1. Look, listen, and feel for breathing with your ear over the stoma (Fig. 4-8, *A*).
2. Give breaths into the stoma, breathing at the same rate as for mouth-to-mouth breathing (Fig. 4-8, *B*).

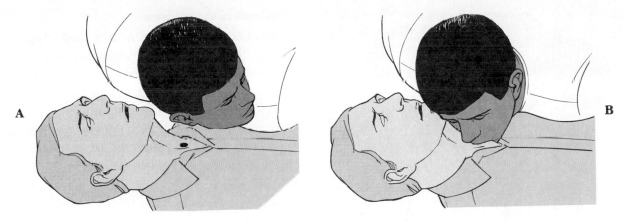

Figure 4-8 A, Look, listen, and feel for breathing with your ear over the stoma. **B,** Seal your mouth around the stoma and breathe at the same rate as for mouth-to-mouth breathing.

Victims with dentures

If you know or see that the victim is wearing dentures, do not automatically remove them. Dentures help rescue breathing by supporting the victim's mouth and cheeks during mouth-to-mouth breathing. If the dentures are loose, the head-tilt/chin-lift may help keep them in place. Remove the dentures *only* if they become so loose that they block the airway or make it difficult for you to give breaths.

Suspected head, neck, or back injuries

Head, neck, or back injuries should be suspected in victims who have sustained a violent force, such as that which results from a motor vehicle crash, a fall, or a diving or other sports-related incident. If you suspect the victim may have an injury to the head, neck, or back, you should try to minimize movement of the head and neck when opening the airway. This requires you to modify your normal technique of head-tilt/chin-lift.

You should first try to open the victim's airway by lifting the chin without tilting the head back (Fig. 4-9). This may be enough to allow

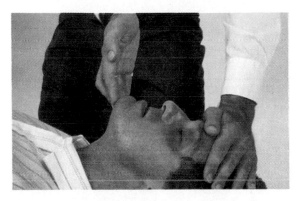

Figure 4-9 If you suspect head, neck, or back injuries, try to open the airway by lifting the chin without tilting the head.

air to pass into the lungs. If you attempt rescue breathing and your breaths are not going in, you should tilt the head back very slightly. In most cases, this will be enough to allow air to pass into the lungs. If air still does not go in, tilt the head farther back. It is unlikely that this action will cause any additional injury to the victim. A person who is not breathing needs oxygen. Therefore, opening the airway is the primary concern.

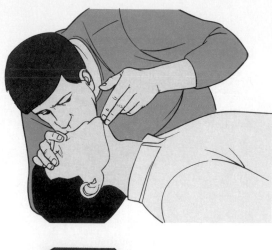

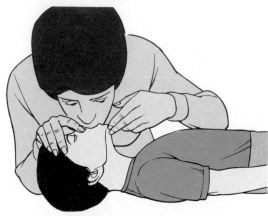

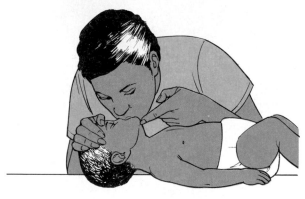

Figure 4-10 Rescue breathing for adults, children, and infants is basically the same.

Infants and children

Rescue breathing for infants and children follows the same general procedure as that for adults. The minor differences in procedure take into account the infant's or child's undeveloped physique and moderately faster heartbeat and breathing rate (Fig. 4-10). Rescue breathing for infants and children uses less air in each breath, and breaths are delivered at a slightly faster rate. You do not need to tilt a child's or infant's head as far back as an adult's. To learn rescue breathing for infants and children, take the American Red Cross Infant and Child CPR course.

◆ Airway Obstruction

Airway obstruction is the most common cause of respiratory emergencies. There are two types of airway obstruction—anatomical and mechanical.

An obstruction is called anatomical if the airway is blocked by an anatomic structure, such as the tongue or swollen tissues of the mouth and throat. This type of obstruction may result from injury to the neck or a medical emergency such as anaphylactic shock. The most common cause of obstruction in an unconscious person is the tongue, which drops to the back of the throat and blocks the airway. This occurs because muscles, including the tongue, relax when deprived of oxygen. The head-tilt/chin-lift not only opens the airway by moving the tongue away from the back of the throat, but also moves the epiglottis from the opening of the trachea.

The epiglottis is a special tissue that covers the opening of the trachea when you swallow to prevent food and liquid from entering the lungs.

An obstruction is called mechanical if the airway is blocked by a foreign object, such as a piece of food, a small toy, or fluids like vomit, blood, mucus, or saliva. Someone with a mechanical obstruction is choking.

Common causes of choking include—

* Trying to swallow large pieces of poorly chewed food.
* Drinking alcohol before or during meals. Alcohol dulls the nerves that aid swallowing, making choking on food more likely.
* Wearing dentures. Dentures make it difficult to sense whether food is fully chewed before swallowing.
* Eating while talking excitedly or laughing, or eating too fast.
* Walking, playing, or running with food or objects in the mouth.

A person whose airway is blocked by a piece of food or other object can quickly stop breathing, lose consciousness, and die. You must be able to recognize that the airway is obstructed and give care immediately. This is why checking the airway comes first in the ABCs of the primary survey. If you mistake an obstructed airway for a heart attack or some other serious condition, you might be slow to give the right kind of care, or you might give the wrong kind of care.

A person who is choking may have either a complete or a partial airway obstruction. A victim with a complete airway obstruction is not able to breathe at all. With a partial airway obstruction, the victim's ability to breathe depends on how much air can get past the obstruction into the lungs.

Q

5. How do food and objects get stuck in your trachea when they should be in the esophagus?

Partial Airway Obstruction

A person with a partial airway obstruction can still move air to and from the lungs. This air

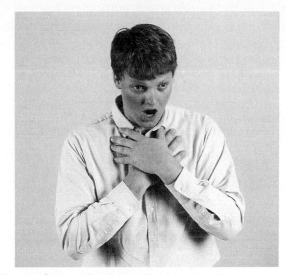

Figure 4-11 Clutching the throat with one or both hands is universally recognized as a distress signal for choking.

allows the person to cough in an attempt to dislodge the object. The person may also be able to move air past the vocal cords to speak. The narrowed airway causes a wheezing sound as air moves in and out of the lungs. The victim may clutch at his or her throat with one or both hands as a natural reaction to choking. This is universally recognized as a distress signal for choking (Fig. 4-11). If the victim is coughing forcefully or wheezing, do not interfere with attempts to cough up the object. A person who is getting enough air to cough or speak also has enough air entering the lungs to breathe. Stay with the victim and encourage him or her to continue coughing to clear the obstruction. If coughing persists, call EMS personnel for help.

Complete Airway Obstruction

A partial airway obstruction can quickly become a complete airway obstruction. A person with a completely blocked airway is unable to speak, breathe, or cough. Sometimes the victim may cough weakly and ineffectively or make high-pitched noises. All of these signals tell you the victim is not getting enough air to sustain life. Act immediately! Have a bystander call EMS personnel while you begin to provide care.

Q
6. How does choking lead to death?

First Aid for Choking

When someone is choking, your goal is to re-establish an open airway as quickly as possible. Give abdominal thrusts, also called the Heimlich maneuver. Abdominal thrusts compress the abdomen, increasing pressure within the lungs and airway. This simulates a cough, forcing air trapped in the lungs to push the object out of the airway, like a cork from a bottle of champagne (Fig. 4-12).

Care for a conscious choking victim

To give abdominal thrusts to a conscious choking victim, stand behind the victim and wrap your arms around his or her waist. (The victim may be seated or standing.) Make a fist with one hand and place the thumb side against the middle of the victim's abdomen just above the navel and well below the lower tip of the breastbone (Fig. 4-13, *A* and *B*). Grab your fist with your other hand and give quick, upward thrusts into the abdomen (Fig. 4-13, *C*). Repeat these thrusts until the object is dislodged or the victim becomes unconscious. The skill sheets at the end of this chapter detail the steps of this technique.

If you are alone and choking

If you are choking and no one is around who can help, you can give yourself abdominal thrusts in one of two ways. (1) Make a fist with one hand and place the thumb side on the middle of your abdomen slightly above your navel and well below the tip of your

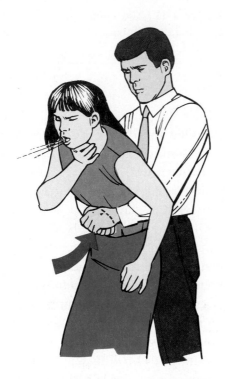

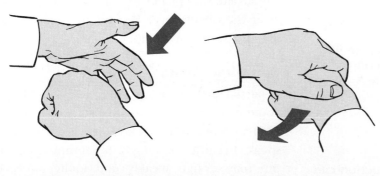

Figure 4-12 Abdominal thrusts simulate a cough, forcing air trapped in the lungs to push the object out of the airway.

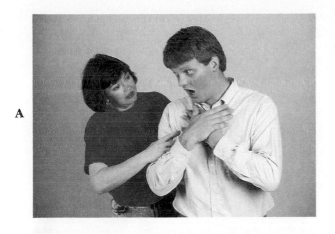

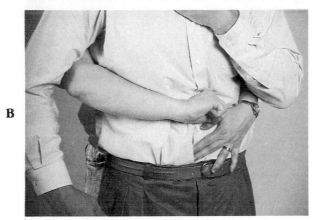

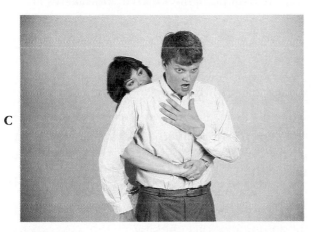

breastbone. Grasp your fist with your other hand and give a quick upward thrust. (2) You can also lean forward and press your abdomen over any firm object such as the back of a chair, a railing, or a sink (Fig. 4-14). Be careful not to lean over anything with a sharp edge or a corner that might injure you.

Care for a conscious choking victim who becomes unconscious

While giving abdominal thrusts to a conscious choking victim, you should anticipate that the victim will become unconscious if the obstruction is not removed. If this occurs, lower the victim to the floor on his or her back. Call EMS personnel. Open the airway by grasping the lower jaw and tongue and lifting the jaw. Attempt to dislodge and remove the object by sweeping it out with your finger. This action is called a **finger sweep** (see Figure 4-15, *A* and *B,* on the next page). When doing a finger sweep, use a hooking action to remove the object. Be careful not to push the

Figure 4-13 A, Stand behind the victim to give abdominal thrusts. **B,** Place the thumb side of your fist against the middle of the victim's abdomen. **C,** Grab your fist with your other hand and give quick, upward thrusts into the abdomen.

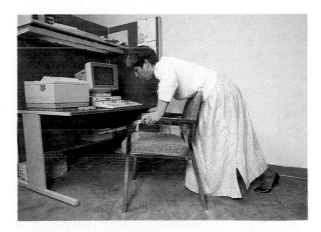

Figure 4-14 To give yourself abdominal thrusts, you can press your abdomen onto a firm object such as the back of a chair.

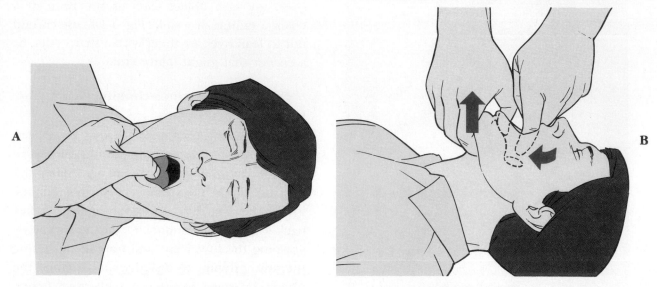

Figure 4-15 A, To do a finger sweep, first lift the lower jaw, and **B,** then use a hooking action to sweep the object out of the airway.

object deeper into the airway. Next, try to open the victim's airway using the head-tilt/chin-lift method and give 2 slow breaths. Often the throat muscles relax enough after the person becomes unconscious to allow air past the obstruction and into the lungs. If air does not go into the lungs, assume that the airway is still obstructed. Give up to 5 abdominal thrusts.

To give abdominal thrusts to an unconscious victim, straddle one or both of the victim's thighs. Place the heel of one hand on the victim's abdomen just above the navel and well below the lower tip of the breastbone. Place the other hand on top of the first. The fingers of both hands should point directly toward the victim's head (Fig. 4-16, *A* and *B).* Give quick, upward thrusts into the abdomen.

After giving abdominal thrusts, do another finger sweep, followed by 2 slow breaths. If you still cannot get breaths into the victim, repeat the sequence: give up to 5 abdominal thrusts, do a finger sweep, and give 2 slow breaths. Continue this sequence until the ob-

ject is expelled, you can breathe into the victim, or EMS personnel arrive and take over.

Care for an unconscious choking victim

During the primary survey, you may discover that an unconscious victim is not breathing and that the 2 slow breaths you give will not go in. If this happens, retilt the head and give 2 slow breaths again. You may not have tilted the victim's head far enough back the first time. If the breaths still will not go in, assume that the victim's airway is obstructed. Make sure EMS has been called. Begin first aid for an unconscious choking victim. Give up to 5 abdominal thrusts as described previously, do a finger sweep, and give 2 slow breaths. Repeat this sequence until the object is dislodged, you can breathe into the victim, or EMS personnel arrive and take over. The skills sheets at the end of this chapter detail the steps of this technique.

If your first attempts to clear the airway do not succeed, *do not stop.* The longer the vic-

A 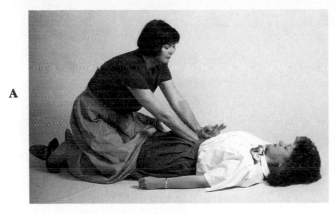 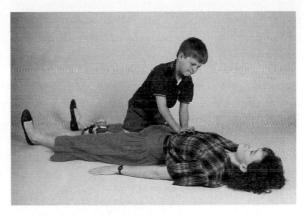 B

Figure 4-16 To give abdominal thrusts to an unconscious victim, **A,** straddle the victim's thighs. Position your hands with your fingers pointing toward the victim's head. Give quick, upward thrusts. **B,** A small rescuer may straddle only one of the victim's thighs.

tim goes without oxygen, the more the muscles will relax, making it more likely that you will still be able to clear the airway.

Once you are able to breathe air into the victim's lungs, give 2 slow breaths. Then complete the primary survey by checking the victim's pulse and checking and caring for severe bleeding. If there is no pulse, begin CPR. (Chapter 5 describes CPR for an adult.) If there is a pulse but the victim is not breathing on his or her own, continue rescue breathing.

If the victim starts breathing on his or her own, monitor both breathing and pulse until EMS personnel arrive and take over. This means you should maintain an open airway; look, listen, and feel for breathing; and keep checking the pulse.

When to stop thrusts

Stop giving thrusts immediately if the object is dislodged or if the person begins to breathe or cough. Make sure the object is cleared from the airway, and watch that the person is breathing freely again. Even after the object is coughed up, the person may still have breathing problems that you do not immediately see. You should also realize that both abdominal thrusts and chest thrusts may cause internal injuries. *Therefore, whenever*

thrusts are used to dislodge an object, the person should be taken to the nearest hospital emergency department for follow-up care, even if he or she seems to be breathing without difficulty.

Special Considerations for Choking Victims

In some circumstances, you should give chest thrusts to choking victims instead of abdominal thrusts, for example, if you cannot reach far enough around the victim to give effective abdominal thrusts or for noticeably pregnant choking victims.

Chest thrusts for a conscious victim

To give chest thrusts to a conscious victim, stand behind the victim, and place your arms under the victim's armpits and around the chest. As in abdominal thrusts, make a fist with one hand, and place the thumb side against the center of the victim's breastbone. Be sure that your fist is centered on the breastbone, not on the ribs. Also make sure that your fist is not near the lower tip of the breastbone. Grab your fist with your other hand and thrust inward (see Figure 4-17 on the next page). Repeat these thrusts until the object is dislodged or the victim becomes unconscious.

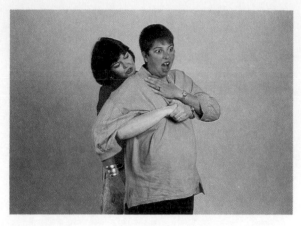

Figure 4-17 Give chest thrusts if you cannot reach around the victim to give abdominal thrusts or if the victim is noticeably pregnant.

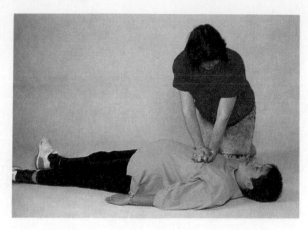

Figure 4-18 If the victim is unconscious, position her on her back.

Chest thrusts for an unconscious victim

With a noticeably pregnant unconscious victim or any victim to whom you cannot effectively deliver abdominal thrusts, give chest thrusts. Kneel facing the victim. Place the heel of one hand on the center of the victim's breastbone and your other hand on top of it (Fig. 4-18). Give up to 5 quick thrusts. Each thrust should compress the chest 1½ to 2 inches and then release. After giving chest thrusts, do a finger sweep, open the airway, and give 2 slow breaths as you normally would for an unconscious choking victim. Repeat the sequence until the obstruction is dislodged, you can breathe into the victim, or EMS personnel arrive and take over.

Table 4-3   How to Differentiate Among Breathing Emergencies

Problem	Signals	Care
Respiratory distress	Gasping, wheezing Fast or slow breathing Deep or shallow breathing	Call emergency number. Help victim rest comfortably.
Respiratory arrest	No apparent breathing	Call emergency number. Begin rescue breathing.
Choking—conscious victim, partial obstruction	Coughing forcefully Can speak and breathe Wheezing	Encourage victim to continue coughing. Call emergency number if coughing persists.
Choking—conscious victim, complete obstruction	Coughing weakly Cannot speak or breathe	Call emergency number. Begin abdominal thrusts.
Choking—unconscious victim	No breathing Breaths won't go in	Call emergency number. Begin cycles of abdominal thrusts, finger sweep, and rescue breaths.

When an Infant Is Choking
(Birth to One Year)

For a Conscious Infant

1 **Is Infant Choking?**

2 **Shout, "Help!"**

Call for help if infant:
- Cannot cough, cry, or breathe.
- Is coughing weakly.
- Is making high-pitched noises.

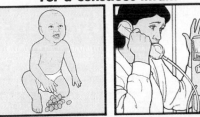

3 **Phone EMS for Help**
- Send someone to call an ambulance.

4 **Turn Infant Facedown**
- Support infant's head and neck.
- Turn infant facedown on your forearm.

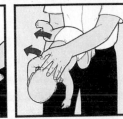
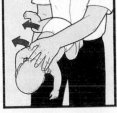

5 **Give 5 Backblows**
- Lower your forearm onto thigh.
- Give 5 backblows forcefully between infant's shoulder blades with heel of hand.

6 **Turn Infant Onto Back**
- Support back of infant's head and neck.
- Turn infant onto back.

7 **Give 5 Chest Thrusts**
- Place middle and index fingers on breastbone.
- Quickly compress breastbone ½ to 1 inch with each thrust.

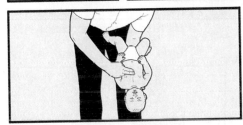

Repeat steps 5, 6, and 7 until object is coughed up or infant starts to cough, cry, or breathe.

If infant becomes unconscious, send someone to call 9-1-1. Place infant on a firm, flat surface.

8 **Look for Object in Infant's Throat**
- Grasp tongue and lower jaw and lift jaw.
- If you can see object in throat, try to remove it with a finger sweep.

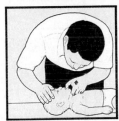
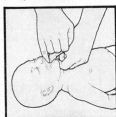

To Do a Finger Sweep
- Slide finger down inside of cheek to base of tongue.
- Sweep object out.

9 **Open Airway**
- Tilt head gently back and lift chin.

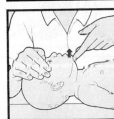
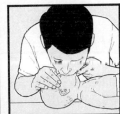

10 **Give 2 Slow Breaths**
- Keep head tilted.
- Seal your lips tight around infant's nose and mouth.
- Give 2 slow breaths for about 1½ seconds each.
- If air won't go in—

11 **Give 5 Back Blows**

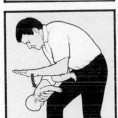
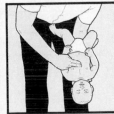

12 **Give 5 Chest Thrusts**

Repeat steps 8, 9, 10, 11, and 12 until airway is cleared or ambulance arrives.

Figure 4-19

When a Child Is Choking

(Ages 1 Through 8)

For a Conscious Child

1 Ask, "Are You Choking?"

2 Shout, "Help!"

Call for help if child—
- Cannot cough, speak, or breathe.
- Is coughing weakly.
- Is making high-pitched noises.

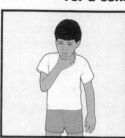

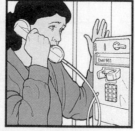

3 Phone EMS for Help
- Send someone to call an ambulance.

4 Do Abdominal Thrusts
- Wrap your arms around child's waist.
- Make a fist.
- Place thumbside of fist on middle of child's abdomen just above navel and well below lower tip of breastbone.
- Grasp fist with your other hand.
- Press fist into child's abdomen with a quick upward thrust.

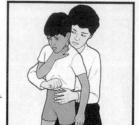
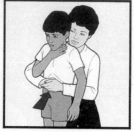

Repeat abdominal thrusts until object is coughed up, or child starts to breathe or cough.

If child becomes unconscious, lower child to floor. Send someone to call 9-1-1.

5 Look for Object in Throat
- Grasp tongue and lower jaw and lift jaw.
- If you can see object in throat, try to remove it with a finger sweep.

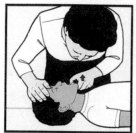
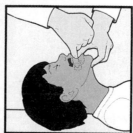

To Do a Finger Sweep—
- Slide finger down inside of cheek to base of tongue.
- Sweep object out.

6 Open Airway
- Tilt head gently back and lift chin.

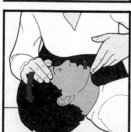
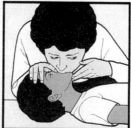

7 Give 2 Slow Breaths
- Keep head tilted back.
- Pinch nose shut.
- Seal your lips tight around child's mouth.
- Give 2-slow breaths for about 1½ seconds each.

8 Give Up to 5 Abdominal Thrusts

If air won't go in—
- Place heel of one hand against middle of child's abdomen.
- Place other hand on top of first hand.
- Press into abdomen with quick upward thrusts.

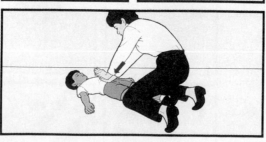

Repeat steps 5, 6, 7, and 8, until airway is cleared, or ambulance arrives.

Figure 4-20

Care for choking infants and children

First aid for a child who is choking is similar to that for an adult (Fig. 4-19). The only significant differences involve considering the child's size when you provide care. Obviously, you cannot use the same force when giving abdominal thrusts to expel the object. First aid for an infant who is choking includes a combination of chest thrusts given with two fingers, and back blows (Fig. 4-20).

You can learn more about first aid for choking infants and children by taking the American Red Cross Infant and Child CPR course.

◆ Summary

In this chapter, you have learned how to recognize and provide first aid for breathing emergencies. You now know to look for a breathing emergency in the primary survey because it can be life-threatening. You have learned the signals of respiratory distress and respiratory arrest and the appropriate care for each condition. You have also learned the basic techniques for rescue breathing, and for special situations. Finally, you have learned how to give first aid for choking victims, both conscious and unconscious. By knowing how to care for breathing emergencies, you are now better prepared to care for cardiac and other emergencies. You will learn about cardiac emergencies in Chapter 5.

Answers to Application Questions

1. During an asthma attack, air can become trapped in the lungs because the swollen bronchial passages will not allow a sufficient amount of air to pass through and be exhaled.

2. Swollen tissues of the mouth and throat that result from anaphylaxis impair breathing. Impaired breathing is a life-threatening emergency. Any time breathing is impaired, the body tissues may be deprived of oxygen, causing body systems to fail.

3. When the heart fails, blood is not circulated to body tissues. Without the oxygen carried in the blood, tissues die and systems malfunction.

4. Rescue breathing provides a victim with oxygen. However, once oxygen is in the body, it is the heart's job to deliver oxygen picked up by the blood to body tissues. Without a working heart, blood does not circulate, and, although the oxygen is present in the lungs, it remains there and never reaches the body tissues.

5. During breathing, the epiglottis opens, allowing air to enter the trachea and move on to the lungs. When you eat, the epiglottis functions to cover the opening of the trachea so that food and liquids cannot enter the lungs. Choking can occur when a person tries to breathe and swallow at the same time. When this happens, the epiglottis receives mixed signals. It receives messages to protect the trachea from food and objects, but also to allow air to enter. The epiglottis cannot do both. In these situations, the epiglottis opens, resulting in air, food, and liquids entering the trachea.

6. Choking can result in respiratory arrest, cutting off the oxygen supply to the body. If care does not begin immediately, body tissues will begin to die, and body systems will fail. If the condition is not corrected, body systems failure will result in death.

Study Questions

1. Match each term with the correct definition.

    a. Airway obstruction
    b. Aspiration
    c. Breathing emergency
    d. Finger sweep
    e. Head-tilt/chin-lift
    f. Rescue breathing
    g. Respiratory arrest
    h. Respiratory distress

    _____ Taking blood, vomit, saliva, or other foreign material into the lungs; a danger when an unconscious victim vomits.

    _____ Process of breathing for a nonbreathing victim.

    _____ Blockage of the airway that prevents air from reaching the victim's lungs.

    _____ Condition in which breathing stops.

    _____ Condition in which breathing becomes difficult.

    _____ Technique for opening the airway.

    _____ Technique used to remove foreign material from a victim's airway.

    _____ Emergency in which breathing is so impaired that life is threatened.

2. List four signals of respiratory distress.

3. List three causes of choking.

4. Match each type of care with its purpose.

    a. Abdominal thrusts
    b. Recognizing and caring for respiratory distress
    c. Rescue breathing

    _____ Supply(ies) oxygen to the lungs when someone has stopped breathing.

    _____ Force(s) a foreign object out of the airway.

    _____ May prevent respiratory arrest from occurring.

In questions 5 through 16, circle the letter of the correct answer.

5. Which of the following are signals of respiratory distress?

    a. Gasping for air
    b. Breathing that is slower than normal
    c. Wheezing
    d. a and c
    e. a, b, and c

6. Asthma, hyperventilation, and anaphylactic shock—

    a. Are causes of respiratory distress.
    b. Require rescue breathing.
    c. Are always life-threatening.
    d. a and c
    e. a, b, and c

7. First aid care for victims of respiratory distress always includes the following:

    a. Helping the victim rest in a comfortable position
    b. Calling EMS personnel for help
    c. Giving rescue breathing
    d. a and b
    e. a, b, and c

8. Which of the following statements about rescue breathing is/are true?

    a. Rescue breathing supplies the body with oxygen necessary for survival.
    b. Rescue breathing always requires the use of a finger sweep to clear the airway.
    c. Rescue breathing is given to victims who are not breathing but still have a pulse.
    d. a and c
    e. a, b, and c

9. You discover the need for rescue breathing during the primary survey when you determine the victim is—

    a. Unconscious.
    b. Unconscious and having difficulty breathing.
    c. Unconscious, not breathing, but has a pulse.
    d. Unconscious, not breathing, and has no pulse.

10. When you give rescue breaths, how much air should you breathe into the victim?

a. Enough to make the stomach rise
b. Enough to make the chest rise
c. Enough to feel resistance
d. Enough to fill the victim's cheeks

11. Which actions are part of the care for an unconscious victim with an obstructed airway?

a. Retilting the head and repeating 2 slow breaths
b. Giving up to 5 abdominal thrusts
c. Calling EMS personnel
d. b and c
e. a, b, and c

12. What should you do for a conscious victim who is choking and cannot speak, cough, or breathe?

a. Give abdominal thrusts.
b. Give 2 slow breaths.
c. Do a finger sweep.
d. Lower the victim to the floor and open the airway.
e. a, b, and c

13. After giving your first series of abdominal thrusts to an unconscious victim with an obstructed airway, you should—

a. Do a finger sweep and then give 2 slow breaths.
b. Give 2 slow breaths and then do a finger sweep.
c. Check for pulse, give 2 slow breaths, and do a finger sweep.
d. Do a finger sweep and check for pulse.

14. After 1 minute of rescue breathing, you check the victim's pulse. The victim still has a pulse but still is not breathing. You should—

a. Continue rescue breathing by giving 2 slow breaths.
b. Continue rescue breathing by giving 1 breath every 5 seconds.
c. Stop rescue breathing for 1 minute.
d. Check vital signs.

15. While eating dinner, a friend suddenly starts to cough weakly and make high-pitched noises. You should—

   a. Lower him to the floor, do a finger sweep, give 2 slow breaths and up to 5 abdominal thrusts.
   b. Give abdominal thrusts until the object is dislodged or he becomes unconscious.
   c. Encourage him to continue coughing to try to dislodge the object.
   d. Open the airway using the head-tilt/chin-lift.

16. A woman is choking on a piece of candy, but is conscious and coughing forcefully. What should you do?

   a. Slap her on the back until she coughs up the object.
   b. Give abdominal thrusts.
   Ⓒ Encourage her to continue coughing.
   d. Do a finger sweep.

---

17. Sequence the following actions for performing rescue breathing from the time you discover that the victim is not breathing.

   2 Check for pulse and severe bleeding.
   3 Give 1 breath every 5 seconds.
   1 Give 2 slow breaths.
   4 Recheck pulse after 1 minute.

18. Sequence the following actions for providing care to an unconscious choking victim from the time you realize your breaths will not go in.

   4 Do a finger sweep.
   1 Repeat 2 slow breaths.
   3 Give up to 5 abdominal thrusts.
   2 Reposition the victim's head.
   5 Repeat the sequence of care if air still will not go in.

Answers are in Appendix A.

PRACTICE SESSION: *Rescue Breathing for an Adult*

You find a person lying motionless on the ground. You should survey the scene to see if it is safe and to get some idea of what happened. If the scene is safe, do a primary survey by checking the ABCs.

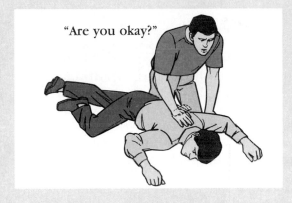

"Are you okay?"

☐ Check for consciousness
- Tap or gently shake person.
- Shout, "Are you OK?"

If person responds. . .
- Begin a secondary survey.

If person does not respond. . .

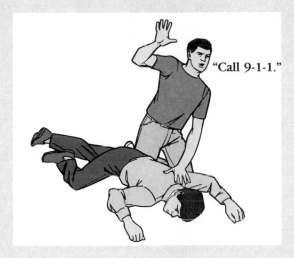

"Call 9-1-1."

☐ Phone EMS personnel for help
- Call for an ambulance or send someone else to call.

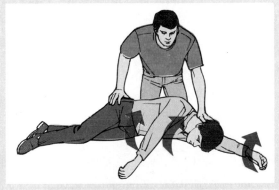

☐ Roll person onto back (if necessary)
- Roll person toward you by pulling slowly.

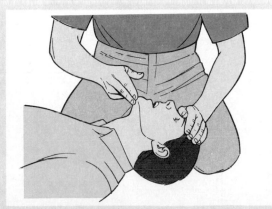

☐ Open airway (use head-tilt/chin-lift)
- Tilt head back and lift chin.

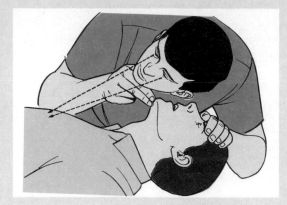

☐ Check for breathing
- Look, listen, and feel for breathing for about 5 seconds.

If person is breathing. . .
- Keep airway open.
- Monitor breathing.
- Check and control severe bleeding.
- Await arrival of EMS personnel.

If person is not breathing. . .

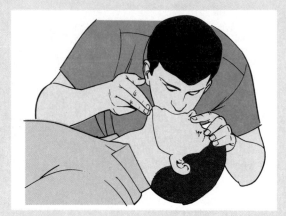

☐ Give 2 slow breaths
- Keep head tilted back.
- Pinch nose shut.
- Seal your lips tightly around person's mouth.
- Give 2 slow breaths, each lasting about 1½ seconds.
- Watch chest to see that your breaths go in.

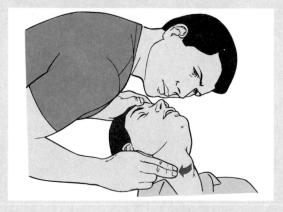

☐ Check for pulse
- Locate Adam's apple.
- Slide fingers down into groove of neck on side closer to you.
- Feel for pulse for about 5 to 10 seconds.

If person has a pulse. . .
- Check for and control severe bleeding.
- Recheck breathing.
- If not breathing, do rescue breathing.

If person does not have a pulse. . .
- Check for and control severe bleeding.
- Begin CPR.

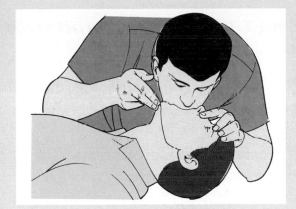

☐ Begin rescue breathing

- Maintain open airway with head-tilt/chin-lift.
- Pinch nose shut.
- Give 1 slow breath about every 5 seconds.
- Watch chest to see that your breaths go in.
- Continue for 1 minute—about 12 breaths.

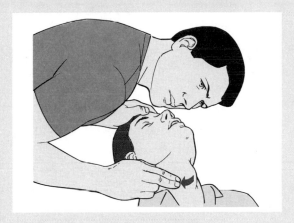

☐ Recheck pulse and breathing every minute

- Feel for pulse for about 5 to 10 seconds.

If person has a pulse and is breathing. . .
- Keep airway open.
- Monitor breathing.
- Await arrival of EMS personnel.

If person has a pulse but is still not breathing. . .
- Continue rescue breathing until EMS personnel arrive.

If person does not have a pulse and is not breathing. . .
- Begin CPR.
- Await arrival of EMS personnel.

101

PRACTICE SESSION: *First Aid for an Unconscious Adult with a Complete Airway Obstruction*

You find a person lying motionless on the ground. You should survey the scene to see if it is safe and to get some idea of what happened. If it is safe, do a primary survey by checking the ABCs.

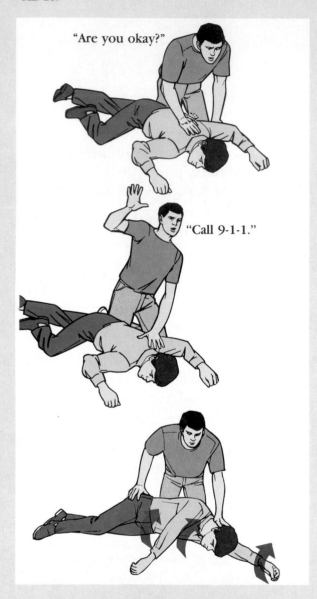

☐ **Check for consciousness**
- Tap or gently shake person.
- Shout, "Are you OK?"

If person responds. . .
- Begin a secondary survey.

If person does not respond. . .

☐ **Phone EMS personnel for help**
- Call for an ambulance or send someone else to call.

☐ **Roll person onto back** (if necessary)
- Roll person toward you by pulling slowly.

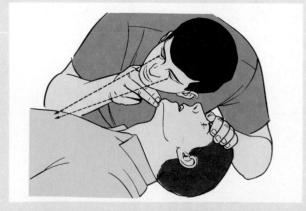

☐ **Open airway and check for breathing**
- Tilt head back and lift chin.
- Look, listen, and feel for breathing for about 5 seconds.

If person is breathing. . .
+ Keep airway open.
• Monitor breathing.
• Check for and control severe bleeding.
• Await arrival of EMS personnel.

If person is not breathing. . .

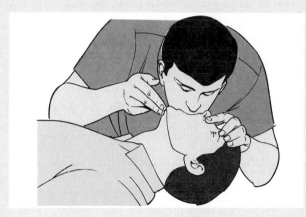

☐ Give 2 slow breaths
• Pinch nose shut and seal lips tightly around person's mouth.
• Give 2 slow breaths, each lasting about 1½ seconds.
• Watch chest to see that your breaths go in.

If breaths go in. . .
• Check pulse and breathing.
• If person has a pulse but is not breathing, do rescue breathing.
• If person has no pulse and is not breathing, do CPR.

If breaths do not go in. . .

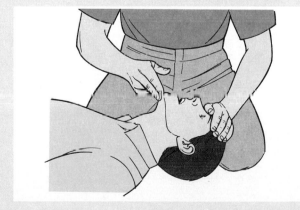

☐ Retilt person's head and repeat breaths
• Tilt person's head farther back.
• Pinch nose shut and seal your lips tightly around person's mouth.
• Give 2 slow breaths, each lasting about 1½ seconds.

If breaths still do not go in. . .

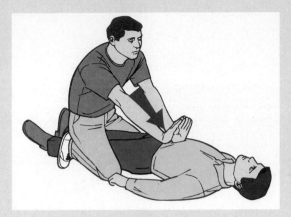

☐ Give up to 5 abdominal thrusts

- ◆ Place heel of one hand against middle of person's abdomen.
- ◆ Place other hand directly on top of first hand.
- ◆ Press into person's abdomen with upward thrusts.

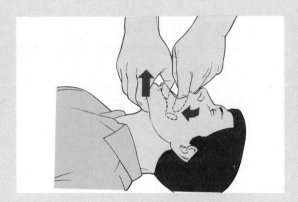

☐ Do finger sweep (simulate)

- ◆ Grasp both tongue and lower jaw between your thumb and fingers and lift jaw.
- ◆ Slide finger down inside of cheek to base of tongue.
- ◆ Attempt to sweep object out.

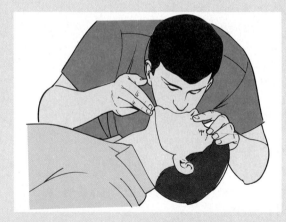

☐ Open airway and give 2 slow breaths

- ◆ Tilt head back.
- ◆ Pinch nose shut.
- ◆ Seal your lips tightly around person's mouth.
- ◆ Give 2 slow breaths, each lasting about 1½ seconds.
- ◆ Watch chest to see if your breaths go in.

If breaths go in. . .

* Check pulse and breathing.
* If person has a pulse but is not breathing, do rescue breathing.
* If person has no pulse and is not breathing, do CPR.
* Check for and control severe bleeding.
* Await arrival of EMS personnel.

If breaths do not go in. . .

* Repeat thrusts, finger sweep, and breathing steps until. . .
* Obstruction is removed.
* Person starts to breathe or cough.
* EMS personnel take over.

PRACTICE SESSION: *First Aid for a Conscious Adult with a Complete Airway Obstruction*

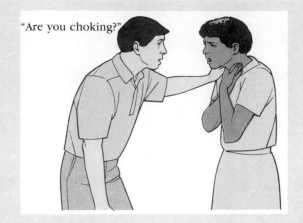

☐ Determine if person is choking
  ◆ Ask, "Are you choking?"

If person is not choking . . .
  ◆ Encourage person to continue coughing.
  ◆ Continue to monitor situation.

If person is choking . . .

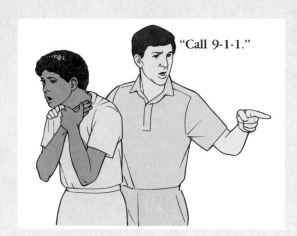

☐ Phone EMS personnel for help
  ◆ Send someone to call for ambulance.
  ◆ Tell them to give dispatcher person's condition.

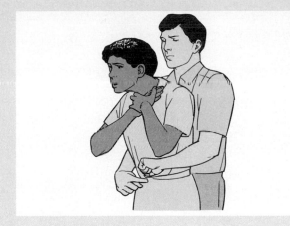

☐ Give abdominal thrusts

- ◆ Wrap your arms around person's waist.
- ◆ Make a fist.
- ◆ Place thumb side of fist against middle of person's abdomen just above navel and well below lower tip of breastbone.
- ◆ Grasp fist with your other hand.
- ◆ Press fist into person's abdomen with a quick upward thrust.
- ◆ Each thrust should be a separate and distinct attempt to dislodge object.

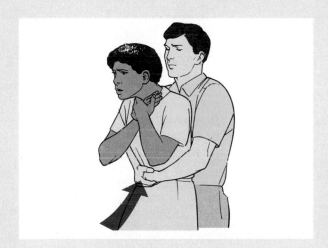

Repeat abdominal thrusts until. . .
- ◆ Object is coughed up.
- ◆ Person starts to breathe or cough forcefully.
- ◆ Person becomes unconscious.
- ◆ EMS or other trained person takes over.

Cardiac Emergencies

Key Terms

Cardiac (KAR de ak) arrest: Condition in which the heart has stopped or beats too irregularly or too weakly to pump blood effectively.

Cardiopulmonary (kar de o PUL mo ner e) resuscitation (re sus i TA shun): The technique combining rescue breathing and chest compressions for a victim whose breathing and heart have stopped.

Cardiovascular (kar de o VAS ku lar) disease: Disease of the heart and blood vessels; commonly known as heart disease.

Cholesterol (ko LES ter ol): A fatty substance made by the body and found in certain foods. Too much cholesterol in the blood can cause fatty deposits on artery walls that may restrict or block blood flow.

Coronary (KOR ŏ ner e) arteries: Blood vessels that supply the heart muscle with oxygen-rich blood.

Heart: The muscular organ that pumps blood throughout the body.

Heart attack: A sudden illness involving the death of heart muscle tissue when it does not receive enough oxygen-rich blood.

Risk factors: Conditions or behaviors that increase the chance that a person will develop a disease.

For Review

Before reading this chapter, you should have a basic understanding of how the respiratory and circulatory systems function (Chapter 2) and of how rescue breathing works (Chapter 4). You should also know the steps of the primary survey discussed in Chapter 3.

♦ Introduction

In the primary survey, you identify and care for immediate threats to a victim's life. Your first aid priorities are the victim's airway, breathing, and circulation (the ABCs). In Chapter 4, you learned how to open a victim's airway and how to provide rescue breathing for a victim who has a pulse but is not breathing.

In this chapter, you will learn how to recognize and provide care for sudden illnesses involving the **heart**. You will learn first aid for a victim having a **heart attack** and for a victim whose heart stops beating. The condition in which the heart stops, known as **cardiac arrest**, sometimes results from a heart attack. To provide first aid for a cardiac arrest victim, you need to learn how to perform **cardiopulmonary resuscitation** (CPR). Properly performed CPR can keep a victim's vital organs supplied with oxygen-rich blood until EMS personnel arrive to provide advanced care.

This chapter also identifies the important **risk factors** for **cardiovascular disease**, because you can do more to promote good cardiovascular health than learning CPR. People too often focus only on what to do after a cardiac arrest occurs. Learn to modify your behavior in order to prevent cardiovascular disease.

♦ Heart Attack

The heart is a muscular organ about the size of your fist that functions like a pump. It lies between the lungs, in the middle of the chest, behind the lower half of the sternum (breastbone). The heart is protected by the ribs and sternum in front and by the spine in back (see Figure 5-1 on the next page). It is separated into right and left halves. Oxygen-poor blood enters the right side of the heart and is pumped to the lungs, where it picks up oxygen. The now oxygen-rich blood returns to the left side of the heart, from which it is pumped to all parts of the body.

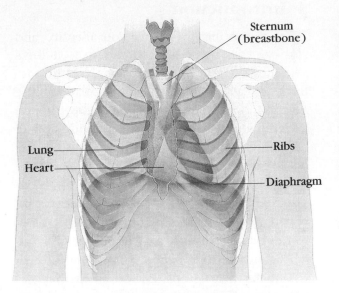

Figure 5-1 The heart is located in the middle of the chest, behind the lower half of the sternum.

One-way valves direct the flow of blood as it moves through the heart (Fig. 5-2). For the circulatory system to be effective, the respiratory system must also be working so that the blood can pick up oxygen in the lungs.

Like all living tissue, the cells of the heart need a continuous supply of oxygen. The **coronary arteries** supply the heart muscle with oxygen-rich blood (Fig. 5-3, *A*). If heart muscle tissue is deprived of this blood, it dies. If enough tissue dies, the heart cannot pump effectively. When heart tissue dies, it is called a heart attack.

A heart attack interrupts the heart's electrical system. This may result in an irregular heartbeat and may therefore prevent blood from circulating effectively.

Common Causes of Heart Attack

Heart attack is usually the result of cardiovascular disease. Cardiovascular disease—disease of the heart and blood vessels—is the leading cause of death for adults in the United States. It is estimated that approximately 66 million Americans suffer some form of cardiovascular disease. In 1987, cardiovascular disease caused 974,045 deaths. Of these, more than 500,000 were due to heart attack, most of which were sudden deaths.

Cardiovascular disease develops slowly. Fatty deposits of **cholesterol** and other material may gradually build up on the inner walls of the arteries. This condition, called atherosclerosis, causes progressive narrowing of these vessels. Narrowing of the coronary arteries is called coronary artery disease. When coronary arteries narrow, a heart attack may occur (Fig. 5-3, *B*). Atherosclerosis can also involve arteries in other parts of the body such as the brain. Diseased arteries of the brain can lead to stroke.

Because atherosclerosis develops gradually, it can go undetected for many years. Even with significantly reduced blood flow to the heart muscle, there may be no signals of heart trouble. Most people with atherosclerosis are unaware of it. As the narrowing progresses, some people experience early warning signals when the heart does not receive enough blood. Others may suffer a heart attack or even cardiac arrest without any previous warning. Fortunately, this process can be slowed or stopped by lifestyle changes, such as forming healthy eating habits. Later in this chapter and in Chapter 18, you will learn what you can do to keep your heart healthy.

The Heart as a Pump

Too often we take our hearts for granted. As a mechanical pump, the heart is extremely reliable. The heart beats about 70 times each minute, or more than 100,000 times a day. During the average lifetime, the heart will beat nearly three billion times. The heart pumps about a gallon of blood per minute, or about 40 million gallons in an average lifetime. The heart pumps blood through about 60,000 miles of blood vessels.

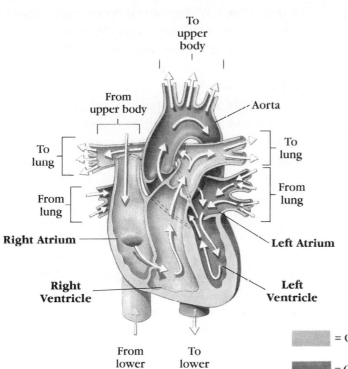

From upper body

To upper body

Aorta

To lung

To lung

From lung

From lung

Right Atrium

Left Atrium

Right Ventricle

Left Ventricle

From lower body

To lower body

Figure 5-2 The heart is separated into right and left halves. The right side receives blood from the body and sends it to the lungs. The left side receives blood from the lungs and pumps it out through the body. One-way valves direct the flow of blood through the heart.

= Oxygen-poor blood pumped from the body to the lungs

= Oxygen-rich blood pumped from the lungs to the body

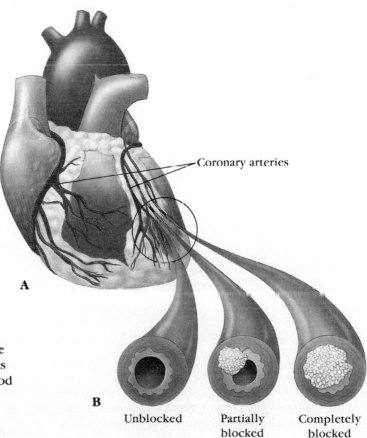

Coronary arteries

A

B

Unblocked

Partially blocked

Completely blocked

Figure 5-3 **A,** The coronary arteries supply the heart muscle with blood. **B,** Buildup of materials on the inner walls of these arteries reduces blood flow to the heart muscle and may cause a heart attack.

Q

1. How does atherosclerosis result in a heart attack?

Signals of a Heart Attack

The most prominent signal of a heart attack is persistent chest pain or discomfort. However, it is not always easy for you to distinguish between the pain of a heart attack and chest pain caused by indigestion, muscle spasms, or other conditions. Brief, stabbing chest pains or pain that feels more intense when the victim bends or breathes deeply is usually not caused by a heart attack.

The pain of a heart attack can range from discomfort to an unbearable crushing sensation in the chest. The victim may describe it as an uncomfortable pressure, squeezing, tightness, aching, constricting, or heavy sensation in the chest. Often, the pain is felt in the center of the chest behind the sternum. It may spread to the shoulder, arm, neck, or jaw (Fig. 5-4). The pain is constant and usually not re-

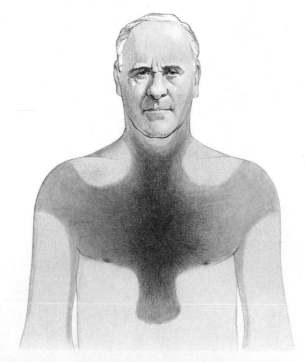

Figure 5-4 Heart attack pain is most often felt in the center of the chest, behind the sternum. It may spread to the shoulder, arm, neck, or jaw.

lieved by resting, changing position, or taking oral medication. Any severe chest pain, chest pain that lasts longer than 10 minutes, or chest pain that is accompanied by other heart attack signals should receive emergency medical care immediately.

Although a heart attack is often dramatic, heart attack victims can have relatively mild symptoms. The victim often mistakes the signals for indigestion or gas. Some heart attack victims feel no chest pain or discomfort.

Some people with coronary artery disease may experience chest pain or pressure that comes and goes at different times. This type of pain is called angina pectoris, a medical term for pain in the chest. Angina pectoris develops when the heart needs more oxygen than it gets. When the coronary arteries are narrow and the heart needs more oxygen, such as during physical activity or emotional stress, heart muscle tissues may not get enough oxygen. This lack of oxygen can cause a constricting chest pain that may spread to the neck, jaw, and arms. Pain associated with angina usually lasts less than 10 minutes. A victim who knows that he or she has angina will tell you he or she has prescribed medication that will help relieve the pain. Reducing the heart's demand for oxygen, such as by stopping physical activity and taking prescribed medication, often relieves angina symptoms.

Another signal of a heart attack is difficulty breathing. The victim may be breathing faster than normal because the body tries to get much-needed oxygen to the heart. The victim's pulse may be faster or slower than normal, or irregular. The victim's skin may be pale or bluish, particularly around the face. The face may also be moist from perspiration. Some heart attack victims sweat profusely. These signals result from the stress the body experiences when the heart does not work effectively.

Since any heart attack may lead to cardiac arrest, it is important to recognize and act on these signals. Prompt action may prevent cardiac arrest. A heart attack victim whose heart is still beating has a far better chance of living than a victim whose heart has stopped. Most people who die from a heart attack die within one to two hours after the first signals. Many could have been saved if bystanders or the victim had been aware of the signals of a heart attack and acted promptly. Since most heart attacks result from clotting within arteries, early treatment with medication that dissolves clots has proven to be helpful in minimizing the damage to the heart.

Many heart attack victims delay seeking care. Nearly half of all heart attack victims wait two or more hours before going to the hospital. Victims often do not realize they are having a heart attack. They may dismiss the signals as indigestion or muscle soreness.

Remember, the key signal of a heart attack is persistent chest pain. If the chest pain is severe or chest discomfort does not go away within 10 minutes, call EMS personnel immediately and begin care for a heart attack.

Q
2. Why do some heart attack victims end up in cardiac arrest?

Caring for a Heart Attack

The most important first aid measure is to recognize that any of the signals listed in Table 5-1 may be those of a heart attack. Therefore, you must take immediate action if any of these signals appear. A heart attack victim will probably deny the seriousness of the signals he or she is experiencing. Do not let this influence you. If you think that he or she might be having a heart attack, you must act. First, have the victim stop what he or she is doing and rest comfortably. Many heart attack victims find it easier to breathe while sitting (Fig. 5-5).

Continue with your secondary survey. Talk to bystanders and the victim, if possible, to get more information. If the victim is experiencing persistent chest pain, ask him or her the following:

Table 5-1 Signals of a Heart Attack	
Condition	**Signals**
Persistent chest pain or discomfort	Persistent pain or pressure in the chest that is not relieved by resting, changing position, or oral medication. Pain may range from discomfort to an unbearable crushing sensation.
Breathing difficulty	Victim's breathing is noisy. Victim feels short of breath. Victim breathes faster than normal.
Changes in pulse rate	Pulse may be faster or slower than normal, or may be irregular.
Skin appearance	Victim's skin may be pale or bluish in color. Victim's face may be moist, or victim may sweat profusely.

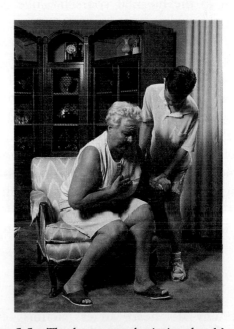

Figure 5-5 The heart attack victim should rest in a position that helps breathing.

- When did the pain start?
- What brought it on?
- Does anything lessen it?
- What does it feel like?
- Where does it hurt?

Then call EMS personnel for help.

Ask the victim if he or she has a history of heart disease. Some victims who have heart disease have prescribed medications for chest pain. You can help by getting the medication for the victim. A medication often prescribed for angina is nitroglycerin. Nitroglycerin is a small tablet that is dissolved under the tongue. Sometimes nitroglycerin patches are placed on the chest. Once absorbed into the body, nitroglycerin enlarges the blood vessels to make it easier for blood to reach heart muscle tissue. The pain is relieved because the heart does not have to work so hard and oxygen delivery to the heart is increased.

If you still think that the victim may be having a heart attack, or if you are unsure about the victim's condition, ask a bystander to call EMS personnel for help. If you are alone, make the call yourself. Surviving a heart attack often depends on how soon the victim receives advanced medical care. Do not try to drive the victim to the hospital yourself, since cardiac arrest can occur at any time. Call the emergency number right away, before the condition worsens and the heart stops beating.

Keep a calm and reassuring manner when caring for a heart attack victim. Comforting the victim helps reduce anxiety and eases some of the discomfort. Watch the victim closely until EMS personnel arrive. Continue to monitor the vital signs. Watch for any changes in appearance or behavior. Since the heart attack victim's condition may deteriorate into cardiac arrest, be prepared to give CPR.

Q

3. Why do heart attack victims often deny that they are having a heart attack?

Table 5-2   Care for a Heart Attack

Recognize the signals of a heart attack.

Convince the victim to stop activity and rest.

Help the victim to rest comfortably.

Try to obtain information about the victim's condition.

Comfort the victim.

Call the local emergency number for help.

Assist with medication, if prescribed.

Monitor vital signs.

Be prepared to give CPR if victim's heart stops beating.

◆ Cardiac Arrest

Cardiac arrest occurs when the heart stops beating or beats too irregularly or too weakly to circulate blood effectively. Breathing soon ceases. Cardiac arrest is a life-threatening emergency because the vital organs of the body are no longer receiving oxygen-rich blood. Every year, more than 300,000 heart attack victims die of cardiac arrest before reaching a hospital.

Common Causes of Cardiac Arrest

Cardiovascular disease is the most common cause of cardiac arrest. Drowning, suffocation, and certain drugs can cause breathing to stop, which will soon lead to cardiac arrest. Severe injuries to the chest or severe loss of blood can also cause the heart to stop. Electrocution disrupts the heart's own electrical activity and causes the heart to stop. Stroke or other types of brain damage can also stop the heart.

Signals of Cardiac Arrest

A victim in cardiac arrest is not breathing and has no pulse. The victim's heart has either stopped beating or is beating so weakly or irregularly that it cannot generate a pulse. The absence of a pulse is the primary signal of cardiac arrest. No matter how hard you try, you

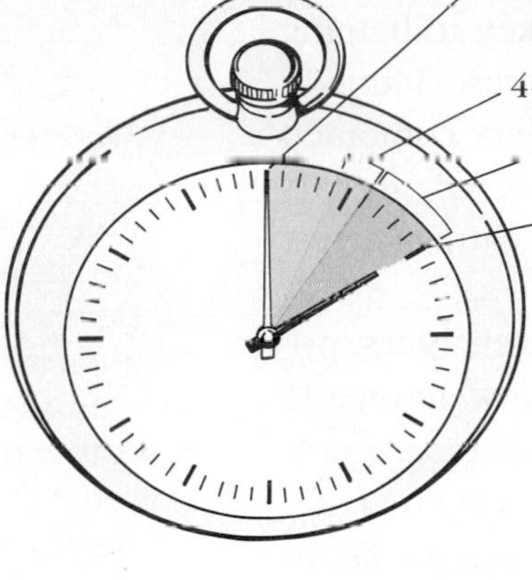

0 minutes: Breathing stops. Heart will
soon stop beating.

4-6 minutes: Brain damage possible.

6-10 minutes: Brain damage likely.

Over 10 minutes: Irreversible brain
damage certain.

Figure 5-6 Clinical death is a condition in which the heart and breathing stop. Clinical death can result in biological death. Biological death is the irreversible death of brain cells.

will not be able to feel a pulse. If you cannot feel a carotid pulse, no blood is reaching the brain. The victim will be unconscious and breathing will stop.

Although cardiac arrest can result from a heart attack, cardiac arrests can occur suddenly, independent of a heart attack. Therefore, the victim may not have shown the signals of a heart attack before the cardiac arrest. This is called sudden death.

Care For Cardiac Arrest

A victim who is not breathing and has no pulse is considered clinically dead. However, the cells of the brain and other vital organs will continue to live for a short period of time until oxygen in the bloodstream is depleted. This victim needs cardiopulmonary resuscitation (CPR). The term "cardio-" refers to the heart, and "pulmonary" refers to the lungs. CPR is a combination of rescue breathing and chest compressions. Chest compressions are a method of making the blood flow when the heart is not beating. Given together, rescue breathing and chest compressions artificially take over the functions of the lungs and heart. CPR increases a cardiac arrest victim's chances of survival by keeping the brain supplied with oxygen until advanced medical care can be given. Without CPR, the brain will begin to die within four to six minutes. The irreversible damage caused by brain cell death is known as biological death (Fig. 5-6). Be aware, however, that even under the best of

conditions, CPR only generates about one third of the normal blood flow to the brain.

Despite the best efforts of the rescuer, CPR alone is not enough to help someone survive cardiac arrest. Advanced medical care is also needed. This is why it is so important to call EMS personnel immediately if you determine that an adult is unconscious. Trained emergency personnel can provide advanced cardiac life support (ACLS) wherever they are called. EMTs and paramedics act as an extension of hospital emergency departments. For example, they can administer medications or use a defibrillator (Fig. 5-7). A defibrillator is a device that sends an electric shock through the chest to the heart to enable the heart to

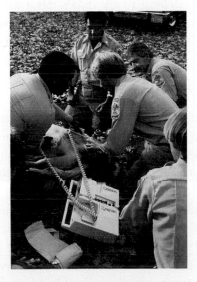

Figure 5-7 Use of a defibrillator and other advanced measures may restore a heartbeat in a victim of cardiac arrest.

resume a functional heartbeat. Defibrillation given as soon as possible is the key to helping some victims survive cardiac arrest. Immediate initiation of CPR by bystanders combined with early defibrillation administered by EMS professionals gives the victim of cardiac arrest the best chance for survival.

Some professionals, such as firefighters, police officers, and lifeguards, use new automatic defibrillators that require little training. Automatic defibrillators, for use by trained responders, are now being placed in some factories, stadiums, and other places where large numbers of people gather. In the near future, automatic defibrillators may be used even more commonly.

It is important to start CPR promptly and continue to provide CPR until EMS personnel arrive. Effective rescue breathing and chest compressions can help keep the brain, heart, and other vital organs supplied with oxygen-rich blood until the heart can be restarted. Any delay in starting CPR or advanced medical care reduces the victim's chance for survival. As someone trained in first aid, you are the first link in the victim's chain of survival.

Review of first aid care for cardiac arrest

As in any emergency, you care for cardiac arrest according to the EAPs. First aid for cardiac arrest always begins with a primary survey of the victim. Take about 5 to 10 seconds to check the pulse to be *sure* the heart is not beating. Unneeded chest compressions may cause harm. If there is no pulse, begin CPR immediately. Identify yourself to bystanders as someone trained in CPR, and make sure someone calls EMS for an ambulance immediately. If you are alone, find the nearest phone, call EMS for help, then begin CPR.

It might help you to know that, even in the best of situations, when CPR is started promptly and EMS personnel arrive quickly, victims of cardiac arrest rarely survive. Controlling your emotions and accepting death are not easy. Remember that any attempt to help is worthwhile. Since performing CPR and

A Shocking Discovery

Every year, 300,000 to 400,000 Americans collapse in cardiac arrest in their homes and on the streets. Ninety-five percent will not survive, but the development of a simple, computerized electric-shocking device offers an opportunity to increase survival.

In two thirds of all cardiac arrests, the heartbeat flutters chaotically before it stops, a condition called ventricular fibrillation. The electrical impulses that cause the heart muscle to pump are no longer synchronized and fail to create the strong pumping action needed to circulate the blood.

Electric-shocking devices, or defibrillators, were introduced onto mobile coronary units in 1966.[1] The machines allowed emergency personnel to monitor the heart's electrical rhythm. A doctor attached electrodes to the victim and reviewed the heart's rhythm. If necessary, an electric shock was delivered to the heart to try to restore its proper rhythm. Paramedics eventually took the place of doctors in evaluating rhythms and administering shocks. Because there were too few trained personnel across the United States, cardiac arrest victims were not always able to get the lifesaving help they needed.

Fortunately, a new, easy-to-use Automatic External Defibrillator (AED) allows emergency medical technicians, First Responders, and even citizen responders to provide the lifesaving shocks. With the new defibrillators, a computer chip, rather than an advanced medical professional, analyzes the heart's rhythm. Typically the First Responder places the two electrodes on the victim's chest and then presses two buttons—first "ANALYZE," then "SHOCK." The machine does the rest.

AEDs monitor the heart's electrical activity through two electrodes placed on the chest. On a heart monitor, ventricular fibrillation looks like a chaotic, wavy line, whereas a normal heartbeat shows a pattern of evenly spaced, well-defined spiked points. The computer chip determines the need for a shock by looking at the pattern, size, and frequency of the electrocardiogram waves.

If the rhythm resembles ventricular fibrillation, the machine readies an electrical charge. When the electric charge disrupts the irregular heartbeat, it is called defibrillation. This allows the heart's natural electrical system to begin to fire off electrical impulses correctly so the heart can beat normally.

When First Responders are trained to use AEDs, they can drastically reduce the amount of time it takes to administer a shock in a cardiac emergency, researchers say. By extending training to First Responders, communities increase the numbers of emergency personnel trained to use AEDs. In Eugene, and Springfield, Oregon, AEDs were placed on every firetruck and all firefighters were trained to use them. Researchers saw these communities' survival rates for cardiac arrest increase by 18 percent in the first year.[2]

More than 23 states recognize defibrillator training for EMTs. AEDs also are being introduced in areas that hold large groups of people, such as convention centers, stadiums, large businesses, and industrial complexes. Some health experts hope that someday AEDs will be as commonplace as fire alarms.

REFERENCES

1. Pantridge, J.F., and Geddes, J. S. A mobile intensive care unit in the treatment of myocardial infarction. *Lancet* 2(1967):271-273.

2. Graves, J.R., Austin, D., Jr., and Cummins, R.O. *Rapid Zap: Automated Defibrillation.* Englewood Cliffs, N.J.: Prentice-Hall, Inc., 1989.

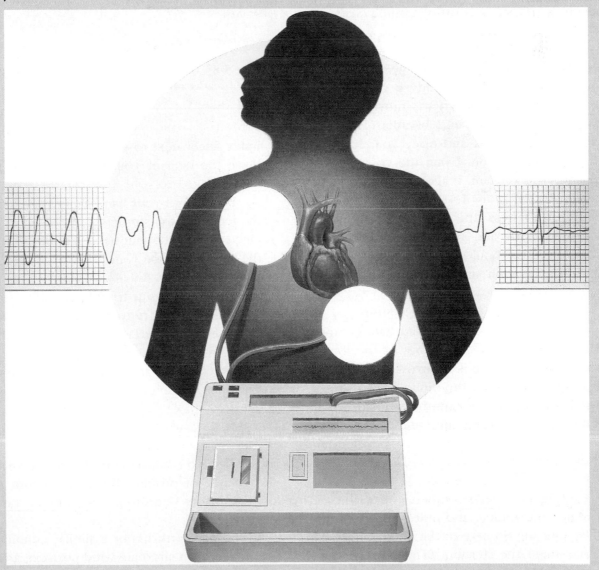

calling for help are only two of the several factors that determine whether a cardiac arrest victim survives, you should feel assured that you did everything you could to help.

◆ CPR for Adults

The theory that is most widely held today is that chest compressions create pressure within the chest cavity that moves blood through the circulatory system.

For CPR to be the most effective, the victim should be flat on his or her back on a firm surface. The victim's head should be on the same level as the heart or lower. CPR is much less effective if the victim is on a soft surface, like a sofa or mattress, or is sitting up in a chair.

Chest Compressions

To give chest compressions, kneel beside the victim. Position yourself midway between the chest and the head in order to move easily between compressions and breaths (Fig. 5-8). Lean over the chest and place your hands in the correct position. Using the correct hand position is important. It allows you to give the most effective compressions without adding injury. Compress the chest by alternately pressing down and releasing. Ideally, chest compressions should be delivered straight down in a smooth, uniform pattern.

Finding the correct hand position

The correct position for your hands is over the lower half of the sternum. At the lowest point of the sternum is an arrow-shaped piece of hard tissue called the xiphoid. You should avoid pressing directly on the xiphoid, which can break and injure underlying tissues.

To locate the correct hand position for chest compressions—

◆ Find the lower edge of the victim's rib cage. Slide your middle and index fingers up the edge of the rib cage to the notch where the ribs meet the sternum (Fig. 5-9, *A).* Place your middle finger on this notch. Place your

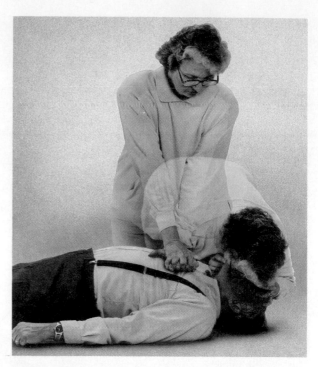

Figure 5-8 Position yourself so that you can give rescue breaths and chest compressions without having to move.

index finger next to your middle finger.
◆ Place the heel of your other hand on the sternum next to your index finger (Fig. 5-9, *B).* The heel of your hand should rest along the length of the sternum.
◆ Once the heel of your hand is in position on the sternum, place your other hand directly on top of it (Fig. 5-9, *C).*
◆ Use the heel of your hand to apply pressure on the sternum. Try to keep your fingers off the chest by interlacing them or holding them upward. Applying pressure with your fingers can lead to inefficient chest compressions or unnecessary damage to the chest.

The correct hand position provides the most effective compressions. It also decreases the chance of pushing the xiphoid into the delicate organs beneath it, although this rarely occurs.

If you have arthritis or a similar condition, you may use an alternate hand position, grasping the wrist of the hand on the chest with the

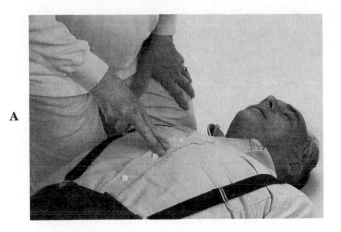

A

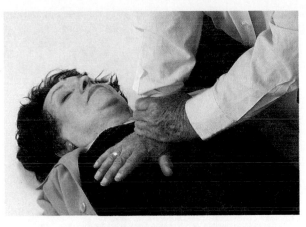

Figure 5-10 Grasping the wrist of the hand positioned on the chest is an alternate hand position for giving chest compressions.

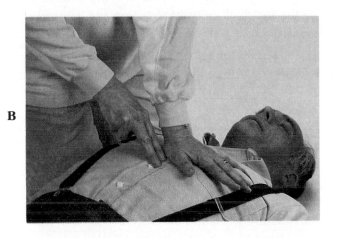

B

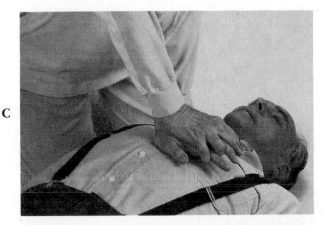

C

Figure 5-9 **A,** Find the notch where the lower ribs meet the sterum. **B,** Place the heel of your hand on the sternum, next to your index finger. **C,** Place your other hand over the heel of the first. Use the heel of your bottom hand to apply pressure on the sternum.

other hand (Fig. 5-10). You find the correct hand position in the same way.

The victim's clothing will not necessarily interfere with your ability to position your hands correctly to give chest compressions. If you can find the correct position without removing thin clothing, such as a T-shirt, do so. Sometimes a layer of thin clothing will help keep your hands from slipping, since the victim's chest may be moist with sweat. If you are not sure that you can find the correct hand position, bare the victim's chest. You should not be overly concerned about being able to find the correct hand position if the victim is obese, since fat does not accumulate as much over the sternum as it does elsewhere.

Position of the rescuer

Your body position is important when giving chest compressions. Compressing the chest straight down provides the best blood flow. The correct body position is also less tiring for you.

Kneel at the victim's chest with your hands in the correct position. Straighten your arms and lock your elbows so that your shoulders are directly over your hands (see Figure 5-11 on the next page). When you press down in this position, you will be pushing straight down onto the sternum. Locking your elbows keeps your arms straight and prevents you from tiring quickly.

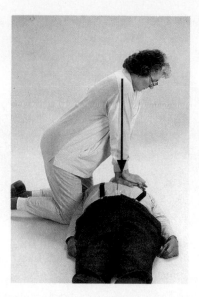

Figure 5-11 With your hands in place, position yourself so that your shoulders are directly over your hands, arms straight and elbows locked.

Compressing the chest requires little effort in this position. When you press down, the weight of your upper body creates the force needed to compress the chest. Push with the weight of your upper body, not with the muscles of your arms. Push straight down. Do not rock back and forth. Rocking results in less effective compressions and unnecessarily uses much needed energy. If your arms and shoulders tire quickly, you are not using the correct body position. After each compression, release the pressure on the chest without losing con-

tact with it and allow the chest to return to its normal position before starting the next compression (Fig. 5-12).

Compression technique

Each compression should push the sternum down from 1½ to 2 inches (3.8 to 5 centimeters). The downward and upward movement should be smooth, not jerky. Maintain a steady down-and-up rhythm, and do not pause between compressions. Spend half of the time pushing down and half of the time coming up. When you press down, the chambers of the heart empty. When you come up, release all pressure on the chest. This lets the chambers of the heart fill with blood between compressions.

Keep your hands in their correct position on the sternum. If your hands slip, find the notch as you did before, and reposition your hands correctly.

Give compressions at the rate of 80 to 100 per minute. As you do compressions, count aloud, "One and two and three and four and five and six and. . ." up to 15. Counting aloud will help you pace yourself. Push down as you say the number and come up as you say "and." You should be able to do the 15 compressions in about 9 to 11 seconds. Even though you are compressing the chest at a rate of 80 to 100 times per minute, you will only actually per-

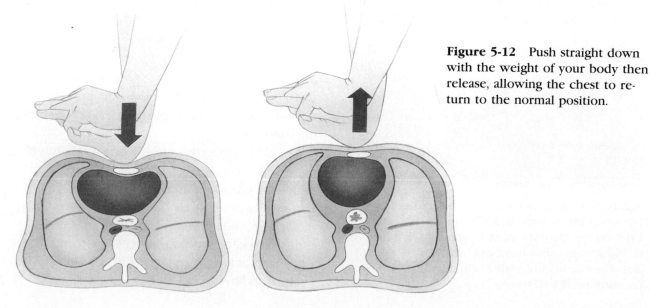

Figure 5-12 Push straight down with the weight of your body then release, allowing the chest to return to the normal position.

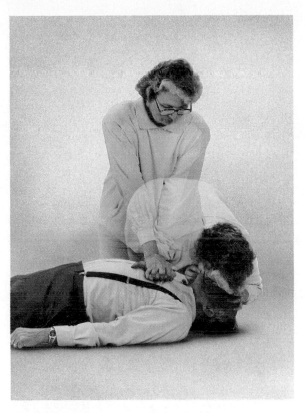

Figure 5-13 Give 15 compressions, then 2 breaths.

form 60 compressions in a minute. This is because you must take the time to do rescue breathing, giving 2 breaths between groups of 15 compressions.

Compression/breathing cycles

When you give CPR, do cycles of 15 compressions and 2 breaths. For each cycle, give 15 chest compressions, then open the airway with a head-tilt/chin-lift and give 2 slow breaths (Fig. 5-13). This cycle should take about 15 seconds. For each new cycle of compressions and breaths, use the correct hand position by first finding the notch at the lower end of the sternum.

After doing 4 cycles of continuous CPR, check to see if the victim has a pulse. These 4 cycles should take about 1 minute. Check the pulse at the end of the fourth cycle of 15 compressions and 2 breaths (Fig. 5-14). Tilt the victim's head to open the airway, and check the carotid pulse. If there is no pulse, continue CPR with 15 compressions. Check the pulse again every few minutes. If you find a pulse, check for breathing. Give rescue breathing if necessary. If the victim is breathing, keep his or her airway open, and monitor breathing and pulse closely until EMS personnel arrive. The skill sheets at the end of this chapter provide for step-by-step practice of CPR.

Q

4. Why are chest compressions and rescue breathing both necessary for CPR to be effective?

5. Why would chest compressions alone not sustain the life of a person without a pulse?

Figure 5-14 Check the pulse at the end of the fourth cycle of 15 compressions and 2 breaths.

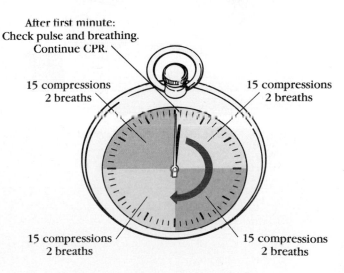

After first minute: Check pulse and breathing. Continue CPR.

15 compressions 2 breaths

15 compressions 2 breaths

15 compressions 2 breaths

15 compressions 2 breaths

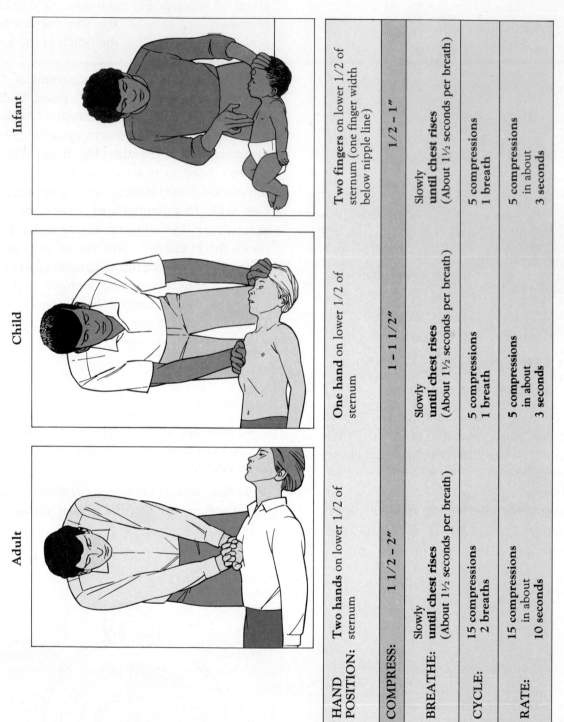

	Adult	**Child**	**Infant**
HAND POSITION:	**Two hands** on lower 1/2 of sternum	**One hand** on lower 1/2 of sternum	**Two fingers** on lower 1/2 of sternum (one finger width below nipple line)
COMPRESS:	1 1/2 – 2"	1 – 1 1/2"	1/2 – 1"
BREATHE:	Slowly **until chest rises** (About 1½ seconds per breath)	Slowly **until chest rises** (About 1½ seconds per breath)	Slowly **until chest rises** (About 1½ seconds per breath)
CYCLE:	15 compressions 2 breaths	5 compressions 1 breath	5 compressions 1 breath
RATE:	15 compressions in about 10 seconds	5 compressions in about 3 seconds	5 compressions in about 3 seconds

Figure 5-15   The technique for chest compressions differs for adults, children, and infants.

CPR for Infants and Children

The technique of CPR for infants and children is similar to the technique for adults. Like CPR for adults, CPR for infants and children consists of a series of alternating compressions and breaths. Because of their smaller bodies, infants and children have faster heart and breathing rates. Therefore, you must adjust your hand position to give compressions, as well as your compressions and breaths. Figure 5-15 compares these techniques for adults, children, and infants. To learn more about CPR for infants and children, take the American Red Cross Infant and Child CPR course.

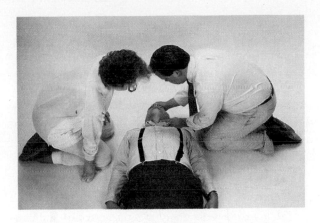

Figure 5-16 The second rescuer should again check the victim's pulse before resuming CPR.

More About CPR

If a second trained rescuer is at the scene

If two rescuers trained in CPR are at the scene, you should both identify yourselves as CPR-trained rescuers. One of you should phone EMS personnel for help, if this has not been done, while the other provides CPR. Then one should take over CPR when the other is tired. If the first rescuer is tired and needs help, follow these steps:

* The first rescuer stops CPR at the end of a cycle of 15 compressions and 2 breaths.
* The second rescuer kneels next to the victim on the other side. The second rescuer tilts the head and feels for the carotid pulse (Fig. 5-16). If there is no pulse, the second rescuer continues CPR with 15 compressions.
* The first rescuer then checks that the victim's chest is rising and falling during rescue breathing and feels the carotid pulse for an artificial pulse during chest compressions. This artificial pulse tells you that blood is being moved through the victim's body with each compression.

When to stop CPR

Once you begin CPR, you should try not to interrupt the blood flow being created artificially. However, there are several conditions under which you can stop CPR:

* If another trained person takes over CPR for you (Continue to assist by calling EMS personnel for help if this has not already been done.)
* If EMS personnel arrive and take over care of the victim
* If you are exhausted and unable to continue
* If the scene suddenly becomes unsafe

If the victim's heartbeat returns but he or she is still not breathing, continue giving rescue breathing. If the victim is breathing and has a heartbeat, keep the airway open and watch the vital signs closely until EMS personnel arrive.

◆ Preventing Cardiovascular Disease

Although a heart attack may seem to strike suddenly, many Americans' lifestyles may

ET Says, "Phone First if. . . ."

Scene:

"Grandpa, are you okay?" Liz Davis, a college freshman visiting her 65-year-old grandfather yells these words as her grandfather collapses to the floor. Liz is stunned. Receiving no answer, she quickly runs to her grandfather. She checks to see if he is conscious. He is not. Liz knows she must quickly decide what to do. She remembers that time is critical. What should she do next?

Dilemma:

Liz is faced with many options. Should she run across the street to a local physician's office? Should she try to get help from her grandfather's visiting nurse who lives about two blocks away? Should she call her grandmother who is visiting some friends? Maybe she should call her mom or dad. Should she call for an ambulance? Should she try to do CPR even though she is not sure she remembers how?

Liz's dilemma is natural. She is faced with an extremely stressful situation, and thoughts are racing through her mind. She wants to help but is not sure how. What should Liz do first? Which is the correct choice? Is there one right answer?

Response:

Since her grandfather's survival depends largely on the speed with which advanced medical care arrives, Liz needs to get an ambulance rolling. She should waste no time in picking up the phone and calling for help. Calling the local emergency number will get medical personnel en route to her grandfather immediately. The dispatcher will give Liz instructions over the phone on how to care for her grandfather until help arrives.

Rationale:

A small number of cardiac arrests occur in public places. In this situation, there are usually witnesses who can be sent immediately to call for help while a rescuer begins CPR. Therefore, CPR followed by advanced cardiac care by trained professionals can occur rapidly. With most cardiac arrests, however, this is not the case. Most arrests occur in the home, and witnesses, like Liz, are rarely trained in CPR.

Data gathered in the last few years have shown that most people faced with situations like Liz's are slow to call EMS personnel for help. Most people tend to confer with friends, neighbors, or family before deciding to call. Any delay has been shown to decrease the victim's chances of survival. Because of the realization that most victims collapse in their homes and in the presence of individuals with little or no CPR training, a new educational concept called "Phone First" has emerged. The primary objective of "Phone First" is to eliminate any delay in phoning for help—to make target groups that are likely to have no CPR training, such as children or the elderly, aware that they need to call EMS personnel immediately.

A by-product of the "Phone First" concept is the controversy this creates for an individual like *you*, trained in CPR, who may be the sole witness of a cardiac arrest. The question arises. . . do you perform CPR first and then call, or vice versa?

If the victim is unconscious, go to the nearest phone and call your local emergency number, which in many areas of the country is 9-1-1. After making the call, go back to the victim, check breathing and pulse, and begin CPR, if necessary.

What You Can Do:

You can do more than just remember the "Phone First" concept. You can help spread the message. Encourage people to take at least one CPR course. Educate those who have not taken a CPR course about when and how to activate the EMS system in their area. Since very few of the elderly take CPR, you can help educate them through your personal contacts. If you talk with your grandparents or have an opportunity to work or socialize with elderly people, explain the importance of calling EMS personnel for help right away. This message is also appropriate for others, like children, who do not know CPR and are unlikely to take a course and keep their skills current.

You can do even more. Encourage others to find out their local EMS number, place it by the phone, and develop a plan of action for an emergency. Tell them that the dispatcher will instruct them on how to provide care until help arrives. But above all, help spread the word. Deliver the message that can help save more lives: *Don't Delay, Phone First.*

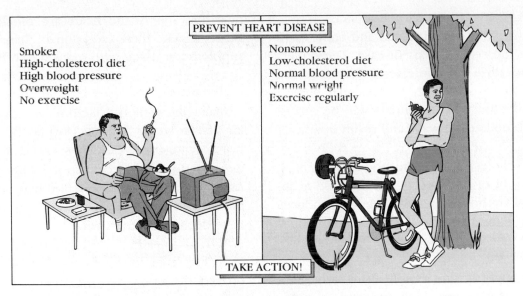

Figure 5-17 Control risk factors; do not let them control you.

gradually be endangering their hearts. This can eventually result in cardiovascular disease. Potentially harmful behaviors frequently begin early in life. For example, many children develop tastes for "junk" foods high in cholesterol with little or no nutritional value. Sometimes, children are not encouraged to exercise.

Several studies have shown that coronary artery disease actually begins in the teenage years, when most smoking begins. Teenagers are more likely to begin smoking if their parents smoke. Smoking contributes to cardiovascular disease, as well as to other diseases.

Risk Factors for Heart Disease

Scientists have identified numerous factors that increase the chances of a person developing heart disease. These are known as risk factors. Some risk factors for heart disease cannot be changed. For instance, men have a higher risk for heart disease than women. Having a history of heart disease in your family also increases your risk.

But many risk factors for heart disease can be controlled. Smoking, diets high in fats, high blood pressure, obesity, and lack of routine exercise are all linked to increased risk of heart disease. When one risk factor, such as high blood pressure, is combined with other risk factors, such as obesity or cigarette smoking, the risk of heart attack or stroke is greatly increased.

Controlling risk factors

Controlling your risk factors involves adjusting your lifestyle to minimize the chance of future cardiovascular disease (Fig. 5-17). The three major risk factors you can control are cigarette smoking, high blood pressure, and high blood cholesterol levels.

Cigarette smokers have more than twice the chance of having a heart attack than nonsmokers and two to four times the chance of cardiac arrest. The earlier a person starts using tobacco, the greater the risk to his or her future health. Giving up smoking will rapidly reduce the risk of heart disease. After a number of years, the risk becomes the same as if the person never smoked. If you do not smoke, do not start. If you do smoke, quit.

Uncontrolled high blood pressure can damage blood vessels in the heart and other organs. You can often control high blood pressure by losing excess weight and changing your diet. When these are not enough, medications can be prescribed. It is important to have regular checkups to guard against high blood pressure and its harmful effects.

Diets high in saturated fats and cholesterol increase the risk of heart disease. These diets raise the level of cholesterol found in the blood and increase the chances that cholesterol and other fatty materials will be deposited on blood vessel walls and result in atherosclerosis.

Some cholesterol in the body is essential. The amount of cholesterol in the blood is determined by how much your body produces and by the food you eat. Foods high in cholesterol include egg yolks, organ meats, shrimp, and lobster.

More important to an unhealthy blood cholesterol level is saturated fat. Saturated fats raise the blood cholesterol level by interfering with the body's ability to remove cholesterol from the blood. Saturated fats are found in beef, lamb, veal, pork, ham, whole milk, and whole milk products.

Rather than eliminating saturated fats and cholesterol from your diet, limit your intake. This is easier than you think. Moderation is the key. Make changes whenever you can by substituting low fat milk or skim milk for whole milk, margarine for butter, trimming visible fat from meats, and broiling or baking rather than frying. Read labels carefully. A "cholesterol free" product may be high in unwanted saturated fat. For further information on a healthy diet, see Chapter 18.

Two additional ways to help prevent heart disease are to control your weight and exercise regularly. Excess calories in the diet are stored as fat. In general, overweight people have a shorter life expectancy. Obese middle-aged men have nearly three times the risk of a fatal heart attack than normal-weight middle-aged men.

Routine exercise has many benefits, including increased muscle tone and weight control. Exercise may also help you survive a heart attack because the increased circulation of blood through the heart develops additional channels for blood flow. If the primary channels that supply the heart are blocked in a heart attack, these additional channels can supply heart tissue with oxygen-rich blood.

Results of managing risk factors

Managing your risk factors for cardiovascular disease really works. During the past 20 years, deaths from cardiovascular disease have decreased by 33 percent in the United States. As a result, as many as 250,000 lives may have been saved each year. Also, deaths from stroke have declined 50 percent.

Why did deaths from these causes decline? Probably, they declined as a result of improved detection and treatment, as well as lifestyle changes. People are becoming more aware of their risk factors for heart disease and taking action to control them. If you do this, you can improve your chances of living a long and healthy life.

If you suffer a cardiac arrest, your chances of survival are poor. Waiting to suffer a cardiac arrest is like placing an ambulance at the bottom of a 100-foot cliff. Once you fall off the cliff, there is little likelihood that even the best of care can save your life. Conversely, preventing cardiovascular disease is like placing a blockade at the top of the cliff to keep you from tumbling to your death. Begin today to reduce your risk of cardiovascular disease.

♦ Summary

It is important to recognize signals that may indicate a heart attack. If you think someone is suffering from a heart attack or if you are unsure, call EMS personnel without delay. Then provide care by helping the victim rest in the most comfortable position until help arrives.

When heartbeat and breathing stop, it is called cardiac arrest. A person who suffers cardiac arrest is dying, since no oxygen is reaching body cells. Irreversible brain damage will occur from lack of oxygen. When the brain dies, it is called biological death.

Prompt action can help prevent biological

death. By starting CPR immediately, you can help keep the brain supplied with oxygen. By calling EMS quickly, you can increase the cardiac arrest victim's chances for survival until EMS personnel arrive to give advanced cardiac life support (ACLS).

If the victim does not have a pulse, start CPR. Always remember these simple guidelines for CPR:

* Use the correct hand position.
* Compress down and up smoothly.
* Give 15 compressions in approximately 10 seconds.
* Give 2 breaths.
* Repeat this cycle of compressions and breaths 3 more times.
* Check for the return of a pulse.

* If there is no pulse, continue CPR, starting with 15 compressions.
* Check the pulse every few minutes.
* If the victim's pulse returns, stop CPR and check to see if the person has started to breathe.
* If the victim is still not breathing, begin rescue breathing.

Once you start CPR, do not stop unnecessarily. Continue CPR until the victim's heart starts beating, you are relieved by another trained person, you are exhausted, or EMS personnel arrive and take over.

In the next two chapters, you will learn how to care for bleeding and shock, two other life-threatening conditions you may find in the primary survey.

Answers to Application Questions

1. The narrowing of coronary arteries from atherosclerosis severely restricts or completely cuts off the delivery of oxygen-rich blood to the heart. When heart muscle does not receive enough oxygen, it dies. The death of heart muscle limits the heart's ability to pump effectively. This is a heart attack.

2. A heart attack becomes cardiac arrest when so much of the heart muscle is destroyed that the heart is unable to contract regularly and subsequently stops beating. There is no way to predict the extent of the damage sustained by the heart during a heart attack or to predict when a heart attack might become cardiac arrest. Therefore, it is very important to recognize and acknowledge signals of a heart attack and to seek professional help quickly.

3. Victims deny they are having a heart attack for a variety of reasons. No one wants to have a heart attack. In fact, most people are so afraid of having a heart attack that they deny symptoms. Still others do not want their families and loved ones to worry about them. They may be embarrassed about being ill or by the commotion a hospital visit causes.

4. CPR is only effective if it replaces the circulatory and respiratory functions of the heart and lungs, respectively. Chest compressions function in place of the heart to circulate oxygen-rich blood to the body. Rescue breathing functions in place of the lungs, breathing air into the body.

5. A person without a pulse is not breathing. Although chest compressions deliver blood throughout the body, they cannot sustain life if oxygen is unavailable. CPR—the combination of rescue breathing and chest compressions—not only provides the body with oxygen, but also delivers it to the body tissues.

Study Questions

1. Match each term with the correct definition.

a. Cardiac arrest   f. Heart attack
b. Cardiopulmonary resuscitation (CPR)   g. Cardiovascular disease
c. Cholesterol   h. Risk factors
d. Coronary arteries   i. Angina
e. Heart

_____ A muscular organ that pumps blood throughout the body.
_____ A fatty substance that builds up on the inner walls of arteries.
_____ The leading cause of death for adults in the United States.
_____ Temporary chest pain caused by a lack of oxygen to the heart.
_____ Blood vessels that supply the heart with oxygen-rich blood.
_____ A combination of chest compressions and rescue breaths.
_____ Conditions or behaviors that increase the chance of developing disease.
_____ Condition that results when the heart stops beating.
_____ A sudden illness involving the death of heart muscle tissue caused by insufficient oxygen-rich blood reaching the cells.

2. Name the primary signal of cardiac arrest.

3. List the conditions in which a rescuer may stop CPR.

4. List four risk factors for heart disease that are controllable.

In questions 5 through 12, circle the letter of the correct answer.

5. The most prominent signal of a heart attack is—

a. Profuse sweating.
b. Pale skin.
c. Persistent chest pain.
d. Difficulty breathing.

6. Chest pain associated with heart attack is—

a. An uncomfortable pressure.
b. Persistent pain that may spread to the shoulder, arm, neck, or jaw.
c. Usually relieved by changing positions.
d. a and b
e. a, b, and c

7. During a heart attack—

a. The heart may function inadequately.
b. Some heart muscle dies from lack of oxygen.
c. The heart stops.
d. a and b
e. b and c

8. To care effectively for a person having a heart attack, you should—

a. Position the victim for CPR.
b. Call EMS personnel immediately.
c. Begin rescue breathing.
d. All of the above

9. You know a person's heart is beating if he or she—

a. Has a pulse.
b. Is breathing.
c. Is conscious.
d. Is speaking.
e. All of the above

10. CPR is needed—

a. When the victim is not breathing.
b. When the victim's heart stops beating.
c. For every heart attack victim.
d. When the heart attack victim loses consciousness.

11. The purpose of CPR is to—

a. Keep a victim's airway open.
b. Identify any immediate threats to life.
c. Supply the vital organs with oxygen-rich blood.
d. All of the above

12. CPR artificially takes over the functions of two body systems. They are the—

    a. Nervous and respiratory systems.
    (b.) Respiratory and circulatory systems.
    c. Circulatory and nervous systems.
    d. Circulatory and musculoskeletal systems.

Use the following scenario to answer question 13:

It is Saturday afternoon; you are at home with your parents. You and your father start to watch a tennis match on television. At the commercial break, your father mumbles something about indigestion and heads to the medicine cabinet to get an antacid. Twenty minutes later, you notice that your dad does not respond to a great play made by his favorite player. You ask what is wrong, and he complains that the antacid has not worked. He states that his chest and shoulder hurt. He is perspiring heavily. You notice that he is breathing fast and he looks ill.

13. List the signals of a heart attack you find in the scenario.

14. To continue the scenario—while waiting for EMS personnel to arrive, your father loses consciousness. You discover that he is not breathing. You give 2 breaths. He also has no pulse. Sequence the following actions you would now take to care for your father.

    _2_ Give 15 compressions.
    _3_ Give 2 slow breaths.
    _1_ Locate the compression position.
    _4_ Repeat cycle of 15 compressions and 2 breaths.
    _5_ Recheck the pulse after 1 minute.

15. After 1 minute of CPR, you recheck to see if your father has a pulse. He does not. What should you do next?

    a. Give abdominal thrusts.
    b. Keep the airway open until EMS personnel arrive.
    c. Check for breathing, and begin rescue breathing if needed.
    (d.) Continue CPR.
    e. None of the above

Answers are in Appendix A.

PRACTICE SESSION: *CPR for an Adult*

You find a person lying motionless on the ground. You should survey the scene to see if it is safe and to get some idea of what happened. If the scene is safe, do a primary survey by checking the ABCs.

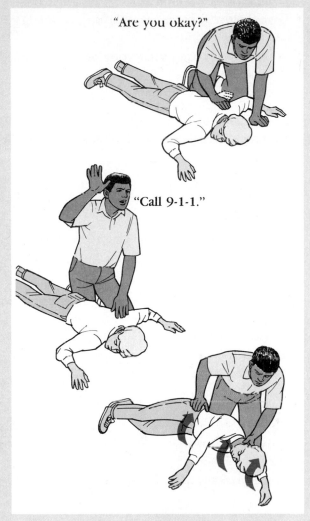

"Are you okay?"

"Call 9-1-1."

☐ Check for consciousness
- ◆ Tap or gently shake person.
- ◆ Shout, "Are you OK?"

If person responds. . .
- ◆ Begin a secondary survey.

If person does not respond. . .

☐ Phone EMS personnel for help
- ◆ Call for an ambulance or send someone else to call.

☐ Roll person onto back (if necessary)
- ◆ Roll person toward you by pulling slowly.

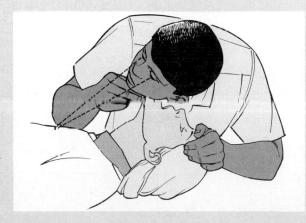

☐ Open airway and check for breathing
- ◆ Tilt head back and lift chin.
- ◆ Look, listen, and feel for breathing for about 5 seconds.

If person is breathing. . .
- ◆ Keep airway open.
- ◆ Monitor breathing.
- ◆ Check for and control severe bleeding.
- ◆ Await arrival of EMS personnel.

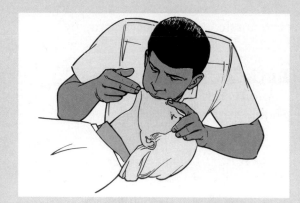

If person is not breathing. . .

☐ Give 2 slow breaths

- ◆ Pinch nose shut and seal your lips tightly around person's mouth.
- ◆ Give 2 slow breaths, each lasting about 1½ seconds.
- ◆ Watch chest to see that your breaths go in.

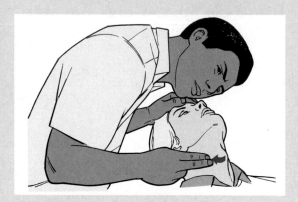

☐ Check for pulse

- ◆ Feel for pulse for about 5 to 10 seconds.

If person has a pulse. . .
- ◆ Check for and control severe bleeding.
- ◆ Recheck breathing.
- ◆ If not breathing, do rescue breathing.
- ◆ Await arrival of EMS personnel.

If person does not have a pulse. . .
- ◆ Check for and control severe bleeding.
- ◆ Begin CPR.
- ◆ Await arrival of EMS personnel.

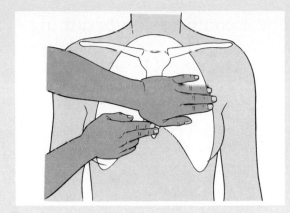

☐ Find hand position

- ◆ Locate notch at lower end of sternum.
- ◆ Place heel of other hand on sternum next to fingers.
- ◆ Remove hand from notch and put it on top of other hand.
- ◆ Keep fingers off chest.

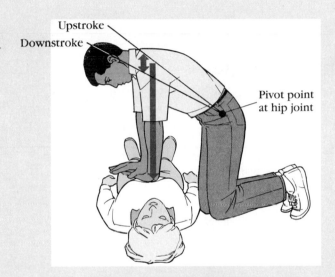

Upstroke
Downstroke
Pivot point at hip joint

☐ Give 15 compressions

- ◆ Position shoulders over hands.
- ◆ Compress sternum 1½ to 2 inches.
- ◆ Do 15 compressions in approximately 10 seconds.
- ◆ Compress down and up smoothly, keeping hand contact with the chest at all times.

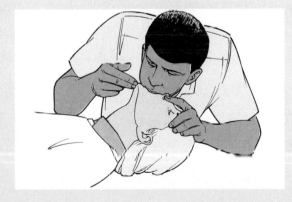

☐ Give 2 slow breaths

- ◆ Open airway with head-tilt/chin-lift.
- ◆ Pinch nose shut and seal your lips tightly around person's mouth.
- ◆ Give 2 slow breaths, each lasting about 1½ seconds.
- ◆ Watch chest to see that your breaths go in.

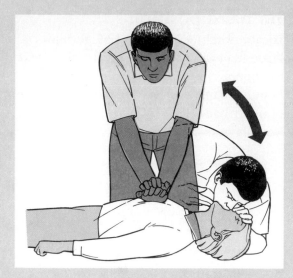

☐ Repeat compression/breathing cycles

◆ Do 3 more cycles of 15 compressions and 2 breaths.

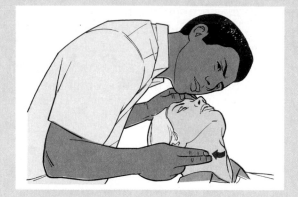

☐ Recheck pulse

◆ Feel for pulse for about 5 seconds.

If person has a pulse and is breathing. . .
◆ Keep airway open.
◆ Monitor breathing.
◆ Await arrival of EMS personnel.

If person has a pulse but is still not breathing. . .
◆ Do rescue breathing until EMS personnel arrive.

If person does not have a pulse and is not breathing. . .
◆ Continue CPR until EMS personnel arrive.

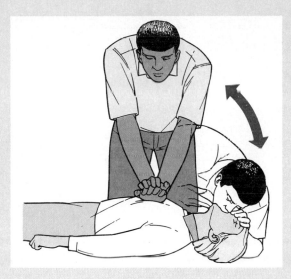

☐ Continue compression/ breathing cycles

- Locate correct hand position.
- Continue cycles of 15 compressions and 2 breaths.
- Recheck pulse every few minutes.

Bleeding

Objectives

After reading this chapter, you should be able to—

1. Explain why severe bleeding must be controlled.

2. List the three major functions of blood.

3. Describe two signals of life-threatening external bleeding.

4. Describe how to control external bleeding.

5. Describe how to minimize the risk of disease transmission when controlling external bleeding.

6. Describe at least five signals of internal bleeding.

7. Describe how to control internal bleeding.

8. Define the key terms for this chapter.

After reading this chapter and completing the class activities, you should be able to—

1. Make appropriate decisions regarding care when given an example of an emergency situation in which a person is bleeding.

Key Terms

Arteries: Large blood vessels that carry oxygen-rich blood from the heart to all parts of the body.

Blood volume: The total amount of blood circulating within the body.

Capillaries (KAP ĭ ler ēz): Tiny blood vessels linking arteries and veins that transfer oxygen and other nutrients from the blood to all body cells and remove waste products.

Clotting: The process by which blood thickens at a wound site to seal an opening in a blood vessel and stop bleeding.

Direct pressure: The pressure applied by one's hand on a wound to control bleeding.

External bleeding: Visible bleeding.

Hemorrhage (HEM or ij): A loss of a large amount of blood in a short period of time.

Internal bleeding: Bleeding inside the body.

Pressure bandage: A bandage applied snugly to create pressure on a wound to aid in controlling bleeding.

Pressure points: Sites on the body where pressure can be applied to major arteries to slow the flow of blood to a body part.

Veins: Blood vessels that carry oxygen-poor blood from all parts of the body to the heart.

For Review

Before reading this chapter, you should have a basic understanding of how the circulatory system functions and how it interacts with other body systems (Chapter 2). You will also need to recall the emergency action principles (Chapter 3).

◆ Introduction

Bleeding is the escape of blood from **arteries, veins**, or **capillaries**. A large amount of bleeding occurring in a short amount of time is called a **hemorrhage**. Bleeding is either internal or external. **Internal bleeding** is often difficult to recognize. **External bleeding** is usually obvious because it is visible (see Figure 6-1 on the next page). Uncontrolled bleeding, whether internal or external, is a life-threatening emergency. As you learned in the previous chapters, severe bleeding can result in death. You check for severe bleeding during the primary survey. You may not identify internal bleeding, however, until you perform the secondary survey. In this chapter, you will learn how to recognize and care for both internal and external bleeding.

◆ Blood and Blood Vessels

Blood Components

Blood consists of liquid and solid components and comprises approximately 8 percent of the body's total weight. The liquid part of the blood is called plasma. The solid components are the red and white blood cells and cell fragments called platelets.

Plasma is a fluid that makes up about half of the total **blood volume**. Composed mostly of water, plasma maintains the blood volume needed for normal function of the circulatory system. Plasma also contains nutrients essential for energy production, growth, and cell maintenance, and carries waste products for elimination.

White blood cells are a key disease-fighting part of the immune system. They defend the body against invading microorganisms. They also aid in producing antibodies that help the body resist infection.

Red blood cells account for most of the solid components of the blood. They are produced in the marrow in the hollow center of large bones such as the large bones of the arm

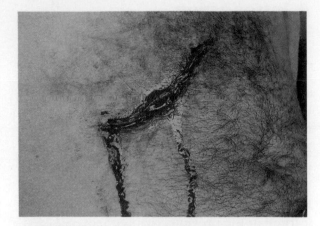

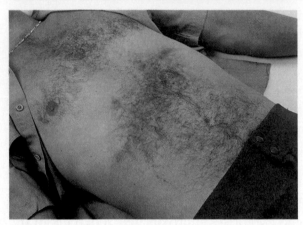

Figure 6-1 External bleeding is more easily recognized than internal bleeding.

(humerus) and thigh (femur). Red blood cells number nearly 260 million in each drop of blood. The red blood cells transport oxygen from the lungs to the body cells and carbon dioxide from the cells to the lungs. Red blood cells outnumber white blood cells about 1,000 to 1.

Platelets are disk-shaped structures in the blood that are made up of cell fragments. Platelets are an essential part of the blood's **clotting** mechanism because of their tendency to bind together. They help stop bleeding by forming blood clots at wound sites. Blood clots form the framework for healing. Until blood clots form, bleeding must be controlled artificially.

Blood Functions

The blood has three major functions:

1. Transporting oxygen, nutrients, and wastes
2. Protecting against disease by producing antibodies and defending against germs
3. Maintaining constant body temperature by circulating throughout the body

Blood Vessels

Blood is channeled through blood vessels. There are three major types of blood vessels: arteries, capillaries, and veins (Fig. 6-2). Arteries carry oxygen-rich blood away from the heart. Arteries become smaller throughout the body until they connect to the capillaries. Capillaries are microscopic blood vessels linking arteries and veins. They transfer oxygen and other nutrients from the blood into the cells. Capillaries pick up waste products, such as carbon dioxide, from the cells and move them into the veins. The veins carry waste products from the cells to the kidneys, intestines, and lungs, where waste products are eliminated.

Because the blood in the arteries is closer to the pumping action of the heart, blood in the arteries travels faster and under greater

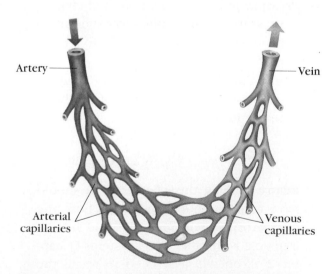

Figure 6-2 Blood flows through the three major types of blood vessels: arteries, capillaries, and veins.

pressure than blood in the capillaries or veins. Blood flow in the arteries pulses with the heartbeat; blood in the veins flows more slowly and evenly.

◆ When Bleeding Occurs

When bleeding occurs, the body begins a complex chain of events. The brain, heart, and lungs immediately attempt to compensate for blood loss in order to maintain the flow of oxygen-rich blood to the body, particularly to the vital organs.

Other important reactions also occur on a microscopic level. Platelets collect at the wound site in an effort to stop blood loss through clotting. White blood cells prevent infection by attacking microorganisms that commonly enter through breaks in the skin. The body manufactures extra red blood cells to help transport more oxygen to the cells.

Blood volume is also affected by bleeding. Normally, excess fluid is absorbed from the bloodstream by the kidneys, lungs, intestinal tract, and skin. However, when bleeding occurs, this excess fluid is reabsorbed into the bloodstream as plasma. This helps to maintain the critical balance of fluids needed by the body to keep blood volume constant.

Bleeding severe enough to critically reduce the blood volume is life-threatening. Life-threatening bleeding can be either internal or external.

Q

1. How do the brain, heart, and lungs attempt to compensate for blood loss?

2. Why will severe bleeding result in death if not controlled?

External Bleeding

External bleeding occurs when a blood vessel is opened externally, such as through a tear in the skin. You can usually see this type of

bleeding. Most external bleeding you will encounter will be minor. Minor bleeding, such as a scraped knee, usually stops by itself within 10 minutes when the blood clots. Sometimes, however, the damaged blood vessel is too large, or the blood is under too much pressure for effective clotting to occur. In these cases, bleeding can be life-threatening, and you will need to recognize and control it promptly. You look for severe bleeding during the check for circulation that is part of the primary survey.

Signals of external bleeding

The signals of life-threatening external bleeding include—

- Blood spurting from a wound.
- Blood that fails to clot after all measures have been taken to control bleeding.

Each type of blood vessel bleeds differently. Arterial bleeding is often rapid and profuse. It is life-threatening. Because arterial blood is under more pressure, it usually spurts from the wound, making it difficult for clots to form. Because clots do not form as rapidly, arterial bleeding is harder to control. Its high concentration of oxygen gives arterial blood a bright red color.

Venous bleeding (bleeding from the veins) is easier to control than arterial bleeding. Veins are damaged more often because they are closer to the skin's surface. Venous blood is under less pressure than arterial blood and flows from the wound at a steady rate without spurting. Only damage to veins deep in the body, such as those in the trunk or thigh, produces profuse bleeding that is hard to control. Because it is oxygen-poor, venous blood is dark red or maroon.

Capillary bleeding, the most common type of bleeding, is usually slow because the vessels are small and the blood is under low pressure. It is often described as "oozing" from the wound. Clotting occurs easily with capillary bleeding. The blood is usually less red than arterial blood.

Blood: The Beat Goes On

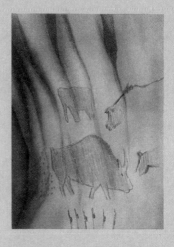

The Ice Age—Prehistoric Man

Primitive man draws a giant mammoth on a cave, with a red ochre marking resembling a heart in its chest.

500 B.C.—Greek Civilization

Ancient Greek physicians propound the theory of the humours, associating man's personality and health with four substances in the body—blood, black bile, yellow bile, and phlegm. An imbalance can cause diseases or emotional problems. A curious practice called bloodletting develops in which physicians open a patient's vein and let him or her bleed to fix an imbalance in the humours.

900 to 1400—The Middle Ages

Bloodletting flourishes during the Middle Ages. Astrology's influence grows, leading doctors to use astrological charts to determine when and where to open a vein. Medical schools sprout up in England, France, Belgium, and Italy.

3000 B.C.—The Fifth Dynasty

Egyptians believe that blood is created in the stomach and that vessels running from the heart are filled with blood, air, feces, and tears.

Circa 200 A.D.—Late Roman Civilization

Galen, doctor of Roman Emperor Marcus Aurelius, theorizes that blood is continuously formed in the liver and then moves in two systems—one that combines with the air and a second that forms from food to nourish the body.

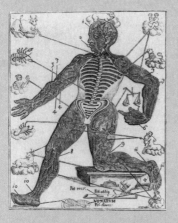

1628—The Renaissance Period

Dr. William Harvey cuts into live frogs and snakes to observe the heart. Through his studies, Harvey determines that blood circulates through the heart, the lungs, and rest of the body.

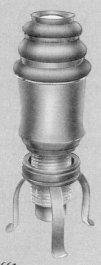

Early 1900s   The Twentieth Century

Dr. Karl Landsteiner discovers that all human blood is not compatible and names the blood types. His work helps make blood transfusions commonplace.

1982

Dr. William DeVries implants the first artificial heart in Barney Clark. The Seattle dentist survives 112 days, and the Jarvik-7 beats 12,912,499 times before Clark dies. In the 1980s, five artificial hearts are implanted. The longest survival period lasts 620 days. The body continues to treat the artificial heart as a "foreign body" and rejects it.

1953

Dr. John H. Gibbon invents a heart-lung machine to recirculate blood and provide oxygen during open-heart surgery, enabling more complex surgical techniques to develop.

1661

The invention of the microscope allows Italian-born physician Malpighi to see the tiny capillaries that link veins and arteries.

1665

The first blood transfusion mixes the blood of one dog with another. Transfusions range from successful to disastrous. One scientist proposes a transfusion between unhappily married people to try to reconcile the couple. After a man who receives sheep's blood dies, transfusion is outlawed in France.

1967

The first heart transplant is attempted by Dr. Christiaan Barnard in Cape Town, South Africa. Louis Washansky, a 54-year-old grocer, receives the heart of a woman hit by a speeding car. Washansky survives 18 days.

The Future

Through the ages, medical science has made extensive progress in saving lives. Two to three million Americans receive blood transfusions each year. More than 5,000 Americans are living with another person's heart inside their chest. About 160,000 Americans are kept alive with an artificial kidney or a kidney transplant. The early medical experiments of yesterday have become commonplace life-saving procedures today.

1944

When kidneys fail, poisons are released into the bloodstream that can cause vomiting, coma, and eventually death. Dr. Willem Kolff, a Dutch physician, develops one of the first artificial kidneys by sending the blood through a cellophane tubing that filters out the poisons.

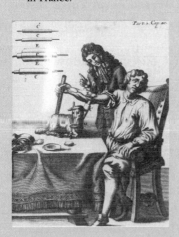

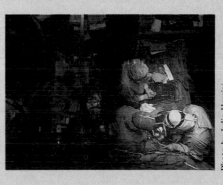

Photo by Julie Harris/
THE GEORGE WASHINGTON UNIVERSITY.

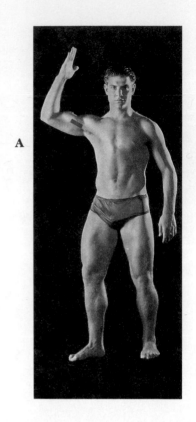

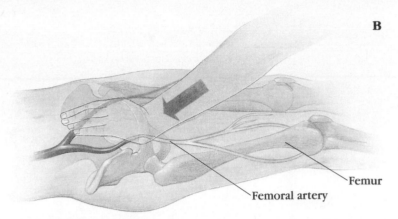

Femur

Femoral artery

Figure 6-3 **A,** Pressure points are specific sites on the body where arteries lie close to the bone. **B,** Blood flow to an area can be controlled by applying pressure at one of these sites, compressing the artery against the bone.

Q

3. Why is arterial bleeding extremely dangerous?

Controlling external bleeding

External bleeding is usually easy to control. Generally, the pressure created by placing a hand on the wound can control bleeding. This is called applying **direct pressure**. Pressure placed on the wound restricts the blood flow through the wound and allows normal clotting to occur. Elevating the injured area also slows the flow of blood and encourages clotting. Pressure on a wound can be maintained by snugly applying a bandage to the injured area. A bandage applied to control bleeding is called a **pressure bandage**.

Although rare, in some cases of severe bleeding, direct pressure on the wound and elevation of the wounded area may not control bleeding. In these cases, you will have to resort to other measures. In an effort to further slow bleeding, you can compress the ar-

tery supplying the area against an underlying bone at specific sites on the body. These sites are called **pressure points** (Fig. 6-3, *A*). The main pressure points used to control bleeding in the arms and legs are found at specific areas of the brachial and femoral arteries (Fig. 6-3, *B*). Pressure points in other areas of the body also control blood flow, but you are unlikely to need to use them. A tourniquet, a tight band placed around an arm or leg to help constrict blood flow to a wound, is no longer used because it too often does more harm than good.

To control external bleeding, follow these general steps:

1. Place direct pressure on the wound with a sterile gauze pad or any clean cloth, such as a washcloth, towel, or handkerchief. Using a pad or cloth will help keep the wound free from germs. Place a hand over the pad and apply firm pressure (Fig. 6-4, *A*). If you do not have a pad or cloth available, have the injured person apply pressure with his

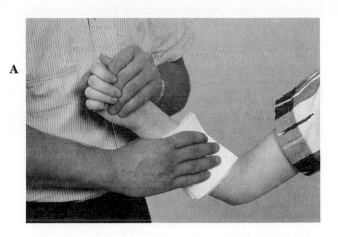
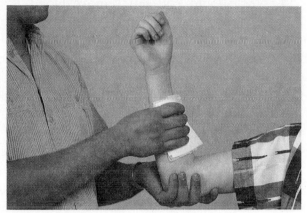
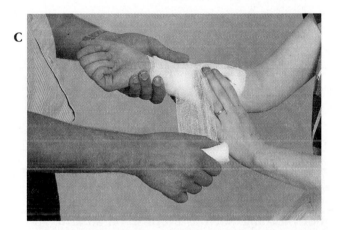
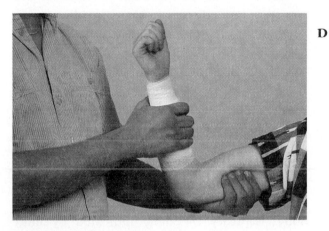

Figure 6-4 **A,** Apply direct pressure to the wound using a sterile gauze pad or clean cloth. **B,** Elevate the injured area above the level of the heart if there is no fracture. **C,** Apply a pressure bandage. The victim may be able to help you. **D,** If necessary, slow the flow of blood by applying pressure to the artery with your hand at the appropriate pressure point.

or her hand. As a last resort, use your own bare hand.

2. Elevate the injured area above the level of the heart if you do not suspect a broken bone (Fig. 6-4, *B*).

3. Apply a pressure bandage to hold the gauze pads or cloth in place (Fig. 6-4, *C*).

4. If blood soaks through the bandage, add more pads to help absorb the blood. Do not remove any blood-soaked pads.

5. If bleeding continues, apply pressure at a pressure point to slow the flow of blood (Fig. 6-4, *D*). Make sure that EMS personnel are called.

6. Continue to monitor airway and breathing. Observe the victim closely for signals that may indicate that the victim's condition is worsening. If bleeding is not severe, provide additional care as needed.

Q

4. Why should you not remove blood-soaked pads from a wound when trying to control bleeding?

Preventing disease transmission

To reduce the risk of disease transmission when controlling bleeding, you should—

- Place an effective barrier between you and the victim's blood when you give first aid. Examples of such barriers are the victim's hand, a piece of plastic wrap, rubber or disposable gloves, or even a clean, folded cloth.
- Wash your hands thoroughly with soap and water immediately after providing care, even if you wore gloves or used another barrier. Use a utility or rest room sink, not one in a food preparation area.
- Avoid eating, drinking, and touching your mouth, nose, or eyes while providing care or before washing your hands.

Internal Bleeding

Internal bleeding is the escape of blood from arteries, veins, or capillaries into spaces in the body. Capillary bleeding, indicated by mild bruising, is beneath the skin and is not serious. However, deeper bleeding involves arteries and veins and results in severe blood loss.

Severe internal bleeding usually occurs in injuries caused by a violent blunt force, such as in a car crash when the driver is thrown against the steering wheel, or when someone falls from a height. Internal bleeding may also occur when an object such as a knife penetrates the skin and damages internal structures. In any serious injury, suspect internal bleeding. For example, if you find a motorcycle rider thrown from a bike, you may not see any serious external bleeding, but you should consider that the violent forces involved indicate the likelihood of internal injuries. Internal

bleeding could also occur from a fractured bone that ruptures an organ or blood vessels. The body's inability to adjust to severe internal bleeding will eventually produce signals that indicate shock. Shock is discussed in more detail in the next chapter.

Signals of internal bleeding

Internal bleeding is more difficult to recognize than external bleeding because the signals are less obvious and may take time to appear. These signals include—

- Discoloration of the skin (bruising) in the injured area.
- Soft tissues, such as those in the abdomen, that are tender, swollen, or hard.
- Anxiety or restlessness.
- Rapid, weak pulse.
- Rapid breathing.
- Skin that feels cool or moist or looks pale or bluish.
- Nausea and vomiting.
- Excessive thirst.
- Declining level of consciousness.

Controlling internal bleeding

Controlling internal bleeding depends on the severity and site of the bleeding. For minor bleeding, such as a bruise on an arm, apply ice or a chemical cold pack to the injured area to help reduce pain and swelling. When applying ice, always remember to place something, such as a gauze pad or a towel, between the source of cold and the skin to prevent skin damage.

If you suspect internal bleeding caused by serious injury, call EMS personnel immediately. There is little you can do to control serious internal bleeding effectively. Activating the EMS system is the best help that you can provide. EMS personnel must transport the victim rapidly to the hospital. Usually, the victim needs immediate surgery to correct the problem. While waiting for EMS personnel to arrive, the best you can do is follow the general guidelines for care for any emergency. These are—

1. Do no further harm.
2. Monitor the ABCs
3. Help the victim rest in the most comfortable position.
4. Maintain normal body temperature.
5. Reassure the victim.
6. Provide care for other specific conditions.

Q
5. How does the application of ice reduce pain?

◆ **Summary**

One of the most important things you can do in any emergency is to recognize and control life-threatening bleeding. External bleeding is easily recognized and should be cared for immediately. Check for severe bleeding during the primary survey. Although internal bleeding is less obvious, it can also be life-threatening. Recognize when a serious injury has occurred, and suspect the presence of internal bleeding. You may not identify internal bleeding until you perform the secondary survey. When you identify or suspect life-threatening bleeding, activate the EMS system immediately, and provide care until EMS personnel arrive and take over.

Answers to Application Questions

1. When bleeding occurs, the brain, heart, and lungs strive to supply adequate oxygen to all body tissues. First, body tissues that are not receiving adequate oxygen notify the brain. Then the brain sends instructions to the heart to beat faster so that it can pump more blood and deliver the needed oxygen. Simultaneously, the brain instructs the lungs to breathe faster to bring in the needed oxygen.

2. Severe bleeding results in death because blood loss decreases blood volume and deprives body tissues of the oxygen they need for survival.

3. Arterial bleeding is dangerous because bleeding under pressure potentially causes more blood loss than venous or capillary bleeding. The greater the blood loss, the faster the heart beats to meet the body's demands for oxygen. However, by increasing its rate, the heart also increases the rate of blood loss. Arterial bleeding results in a large amount of blood loss in a short time, rapidly reducing the supply of oxygen body tissues need for survival. It is also dangerous because the pressure in the arteries causes the surging of blood, which impedes clotting.

4. When bleeding occurs, platelets congregate at the wound site, forming a clot and controlling bleeding. Dressings absorb the blood and may stick to the wound. If a blood-soaked dressing is removed, part or all of the clot is torn away with it. If the clot is torn, bleeding will begin again.

5. Think of how your fingers respond to the cold. If exposed for long, they become numb. Why? Cold interferes with nerve impulses. In this instance, cold deadens nerve impulses to your fingers. The result is numbness. The same principle holds true for ice applied to a recent injury. Ice deadens nerve impulses to the injured area and reduces pain.

Study Questions

1. Match each term with the correct definition.

   a. Hemorrhage
   b. Arteries
   c. Capillaries
   d. Veins
   e. Internal bleeding
   f. External bleeding
   g. Direct pressure
   h. Pressure points
   i. Pressure bandage

   _____ Vessels that transport oxygen and other nutrients to cells and remove waste products.

   _____ Using your hand to apply pressure on the wound.

   _____ The loss of a large amount of blood in a short period of time.

   _____ Visible bleeding.

   _____ The escape of blood from an artery, vein, or capillary into spaces in the body.

   _____ Sites on the body where pressure can be applied to major arteries to control bleeding.

   _____ Vessels that transport oxygen-poor blood containing waste products.

   _____ Vessels that transport oxygen-rich blood to the capillaries for distribution to cells.

   _____ Used to maintain pressure on the wound to control bleeding.

2. List two functions of the blood.

3. List two signals of life-threatening external bleeding.

4. Describe how to control external bleeding.

5. List five signals of internal bleeding.

6. Describe how to control minor internal bleeding.

7. Match the step of care for controlling external bleeding with its specific task.

   a. Apply direct pressure
   b. Elevate
   c. Apply pressure bandage
   d. Apply pressure at a pressure point

   _____ Uses principles of gravity to slow blood flow to the injured area to help control bleeding.
   _____ Places pressure on the major artery supplying the injured area, which limits blood flow.
   _____ Maintains pressure on the wound and helps prevent infection.
   _____ Places pressure on the wound to slow blood flow and aid clotting.

Use the following scenario to answer questions 8 and 9:

Your dad returns home from a day of fishing. He caught a half dozen trout and decides to clean the fish for dinner. He takes out his knife and begins to clean the fish. He is in the middle of a story when he accidently cuts his hand severely. Screaming, he grabs his hand. Despite the pressure he places on the wound, bleeding continues. He becomes anxious, starts breathing faster, and looks pale.

8. Sequence the actions you would take to care for your father's wound.

   _____ Apply a pressure bandage to maintain pressure on the wound.
   _____ Find any clean material, place it on the injury, and apply direct pressure.
   _____ Find the pressure point for the brachial artery and apply pressure.
   _____ Hold or have him hold his injured arm above the level of his heart.

9. Describe how someone close by can help in this emergency.

10. What should you do if you suspect serious internal bleeding? (Circle the letter of the correct answer.)

    a. Call EMS personnel immediately.
    b. Apply pressure at the closest pressure point.
    c. Place an ice pack on the affected area.
    d. Wrap a pressure bandage around the affected area.

11. List three things you can do to reduce the risk of disease transmission when controlling bleeding.

Answers are in Appendix A.

7

Shock

Objectives

After reading this chapter, you should be able to—

1. List two conditions that can result in shock.

2. List at least four signals of shock.

3. Describe what care to give to minimize shock.

4. Define the key terms for this chapter.

After reading this chapter and completing the class activities, you should be able to—

1. Make appropriate decisions regarding care when given an example of an emergency situation in which shock is likely to occur.

◆ Introduction

10:55 p.m. On an isolated road, a large deer leaps into the path of an oncoming car traveling 55 mph. The driver, a 21-year-old college student and track star, cannot avoid the collision. In the crash, both of her legs are broken and are pinned in the wreckage.

11:15 p.m. Another car finally approaches. Seeing the crashed car, the driver stops and comes forward to help. He finds the woman conscious but restless and in obvious pain. He says he will go to call an ambulance at the nearest house a mile or two down the road. He assures her he will return.

11:25 p.m. When the driver returns, he sees that the woman's condition has changed. She is now breathing faster, looks pale, and appears drowsy. He takes hold of her hand in an effort to comfort her and feels that her skin is cold and moist. Her pulse is fast but so weak he can hardly feel it.

11:30 p.m. The rescue squad arrives 10 minutes after receiving the phone call. The man explains that the woman became drowsy and is no longer conscious. Her breathing has become very irregular. The EMTs go to work immediately.

11:40 p.m. Finally, the rescuers free her legs and remove her from the car. The man notices that she looks worse. He knows the hospital is still 10 minutes away.

12:00 midnight Despite the best efforts of everyone involved, the woman is pronounced dead slightly more than an hour after the crash. Her heart stopped beating en route to the hospital. Although the EMTs gave CPR and advanced cardiac life support measures, they were unable to save her. She was a victim of a progressively deteriorating condition called **shock.**

Emergencies fall into two general types: injuries and medical emergencies (see Figure 7-1 on the next page). An injury is damage to the body caused by an external force, such as a blow, a fall, or a collision. Most injuries, such as cuts or minor bruises, are not emergencies. More violent forces, such as those that commonly occur in car crashes and other types of collisions, can damage internal organs, tissues, and bones, causing severe blood loss.

A medical emergency, on the other hand, is a sudden illness that results from problems that occur within the body. For instance, a heart attack, which is caused by heart disease, is a medical emergency. Many medical problems can become emergencies. Those involving the circulatory, respiratory, or nervous systems are often life-threatening. Such problems can severely hamper the body's ability to circulate oxygen-rich blood to all parts of the body.

In preceding chapters, you learned that both medical emergencies and injuries can cause life-threatening conditions such as car-

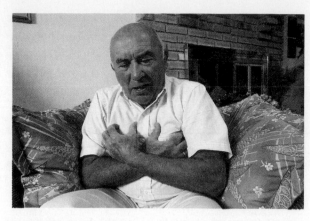 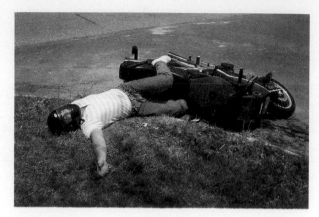

Figure 7-1   Emergencies result from both sudden illness and injury.

diac and respiratory arrest and severe bleeding. Medical emergencies and injuries can also become life-threatening in another way—as a result of shock. When the body experiences injury or sudden illness, it responds in a number of ways. Survival depends on the body's ability to adapt to the physical stresses of illness or injury. When the body's measures to compensate fail, the victim can progress into a life-threatening condition called shock. Shock complicates the effects of injury or sudden illness. In this chapter, you will learn to recognize and give care to minimize shock.

◆ Shock

Shock is a condition in which the circulatory system fails to circulate oxygen-rich blood to all parts of the body. When **vital organs** do not receive oxygen-rich blood, they fail to function properly. This triggers a series of responses that produce specific signals, known as shock. These responses are the body's attempt to maintain adequate blood flow to the vital organs, preventing their failure.

When the body is healthy, three conditions are needed to maintain adequate blood flow:
◆ The heart must be working well.
◆ An adequate amount of oxygen-rich blood must be circulating in the body.
◆ The blood vessels must be intact and able to adjust blood flow.

When someone is injured or becomes suddenly ill, these normal body functions may be interrupted. In cases of minor injury or illness, this interruption is brief because the body is able to compensate quickly. With more severe injuries or illnesses, however, the body may be unable to adjust. When the body is unable to meet its demands for oxygen because blood fails to circulate adequately, shock occurs.

What Causes Shock?

You learned in Chapter 2 that the heart pumps blood by contracting and relaxing in a consistent rhythmic pattern. The heart adjusts its speed and the force of its contractions to meet the body's changing demands for oxygen. For instance, when a person exercises, the heart beats faster and more forcefully because the working muscles demand more oxygen (Fig. 7-2).

Similarly, when someone suffers a severe injury or sudden illness that affects the flow of blood, the heart beats faster and stronger at first to adjust to the increased demand for more oxygen. Because the heart is beating faster, breathing must also speed up to meet the increased demands of the body for oxygen (Fig. 7-3). You can detect these changes by feeling the pulse and listening to breathing when you check vital signs during the secondary survey.

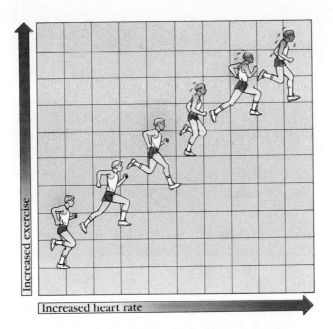

Figure 7-2 The heartbeat changes as necessary to adjust to the body's demands for oxygen.

Regardless of the cause, any significant decrease in body fluids affects the function of the heart. The heart will eventually fail to beat rhythmically. The pulse may become irregular or be absent altogether. With some irregular heart rhythms, blood does not circulate at all.

The blood vessels act as pipelines, transporting oxygen and nutrients to all parts of the body and removing wastes. For the circulatory system to function properly, blood vessels must remain intact, preventing loss of blood volume. Normally, blood vessels decrease or increase the flow of blood to different areas of the body by constricting (decreasing their diameter) or dilating (increasing their diameter). This ability ensures that blood reaches the areas of the body that need it most, such as the vital organs. Injuries or illnesses, especially those that affect the brain and spinal cord, can cause blood vessels to lose this ability to change size. Blood vessels can also be affected if the nervous system is damaged by infections, drugs, or poisons.

Q

1. Why does the body's need for oxygen increase with injury or illness?

For the heart to do its job properly, an adequate amount of blood must circulate within the body. As you learned in Chapter 6, this amount is referred to as **blood volume**. The body can compensate for some decrease in blood volume. Consider what happens when you donate blood. You can lose one pint of blood over a 10- to 15-minute period without any real stress to the body. Fluid is reabsorbed from the kidneys, lungs, and intestines to replace lost blood volume. In addition, the body immediately begins to manufacture the blood's solid components. With severe injuries involving greater or more rapid blood loss, the body may not be able to adjust adequately. Body cells do not receive enough oxygen, and shock occurs. Any significant fluid loss from the body, even with diarrhea or vomiting, can precipitate shock.

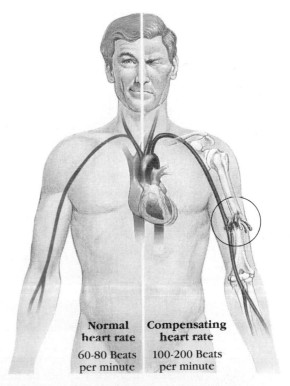

Normal heart rate	Compensating heart rate
60-80 Beats per minute	100-200 Beats per minute

Figure 7-3 The heart beats faster to compensate for significant blood loss.

Q

2. How can damage to the nervous system affect the blood vessels' ability to function?

If the heart is damaged, it cannot pump blood properly. If blood vessels are damaged, the body cannot adjust blood flow. Regardless of the cause, when body cells receive inadequate oxygen, it triggers shock.

When shock occurs, the body attempts to prioritize its needs for blood by ensuring adequate flow to the vital organs, such as the heart, brain, lungs, and kidneys. The body does this by reducing the amount of blood circulating to the less important tissues of the arms, legs, and skin. This is why the skin of a person in shock appears pale and feels cool. In later stages of shock, the skin, especially the lips and around the eyes, may appear blue from a prolonged lack of oxygen. Increased sweating is also a natural reaction to stress

caused by injury or illness. This makes the skin feel moist.

Q

3. Why is sweating a natural reaction to stress from injury or illness?

4. Knowing that shock is a progressive failure of body systems, explain how emotional stress might affect the onset and pace of shock.

Signals of Shock

Although you may not always be able to determine the cause, remember that shock is a life-threatening condition. You should learn to recognize the signals of shock (Fig. 7-4).

Shock victims usually show many of the same signals. A common signal is restlessness

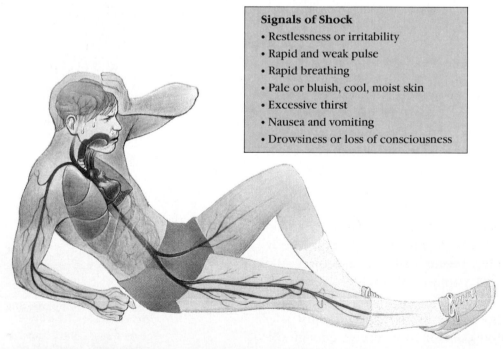

Signals of Shock
- Restlessness or irritability
- Rapid and weak pulse
- Rapid breathing
- Pale or bluish, cool, moist skin
- Excessive thirst
- Nausea and vomiting
- Drowsiness or loss of consciousness

Figure 7-4 The signals of shock may not be immediately obvious. Be alert for these signals in cases of injury or sudden illness. Provide care at once to help reduce the effects of shock.

Shock: The Domino Effect

• An injury causes severe bleeding.

• The heart attempts to compensate for the disruption of blood flow by beating faster. The victim first has a rapid pulse. More blood is lost. As blood volume drops, the pulse becomes weak or hard to find.

• The increased work load on the heart results in an increased oxygen demand. Therefore, breathing becomes faster.

• To maintain circulation of blood to the vital organs, blood vessels in the arms and legs and in the skin constrict. Therefore, the skin appears pale and feels cool. In response to the stress, the body perspires heavily and the skin feels moist.

• Since tissues of the arms and legs are now without oxygen, cells start to die. The brain now sends a signal to return blood to the arms and legs in an attempt to balance blood flow between these body parts and the vital organs.

• Vital organs are now without adequate oxygen. The heart tries to compensate by beating even faster. More blood is lost and the victim's condition worsens.

• Without oxygen, the vital organs fail to function properly. As the brain is affected, the person becomes restless, drowsy, and eventually loses consciousness. As the heart is affected, it beats irregularly, resulting in an irregular pulse. The rhythm then becomes chaotic and the heart fails to pump blood. There is no longer a pulse. When the heart stops, breathing stops.

• The body's continuous attempt to compensate for severe blood loss eventually results in death.

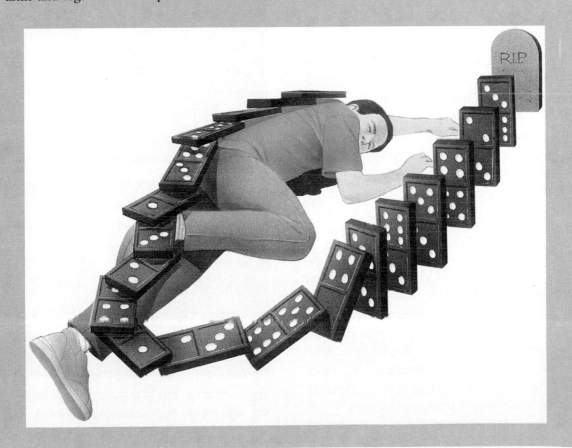

or irritability. This is often the first indicator that the body is experiencing a significant problem. More clearly recognizable signals are pale, cool, moist skin; rapid breathing; and a rapid and weak pulse. If the victim does not show the telltale signals of specific injury or illness, such as the persistent chest pain of heart attack, or obvious external bleeding, it can be difficult to know what is wrong. Remember, *you do not have to identify the specific nature of an illness or injury to provide care that may help save the victim's life.* If the signals of shock are present, assume there is a potentially life-threatening injury or illness.

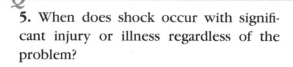

5. When does shock occur with significant injury or illness regardless of the problem?

Care for Shock

Care for shock according to the emergency action principles. First, do a primary survey by checking the ABCs. The care, such as rescue breathing, that you provide for life-threatening conditions will minimize the effects of shock. If you do not find any life-threatening conditions, perform a secondary survey. During the secondary survey, the signals of shock are most likely to become evident. Provide the general care you learned in Chapter 3:

* Do no further harm.
* Monitor the ABCs, and provide care for any airway, breathing, or circulation problem you find (Fig. 7-5, *A*).
* Help the victim rest comfortably. Helping the victim rest comfortably is important because pain can intensify the body's stress and accelerate the progression of shock. Helping the victim rest in a more comfortable position may minimize the pain.
* Help the victim maintain normal body temperature (Fig. 7-5, *B*).

* Reassure the victim.
* Provide care for specific conditions.

The general care you provide in any emergency will always help the body adjust to the stresses imposed by any injury or illness, thus reducing the effects of shock.

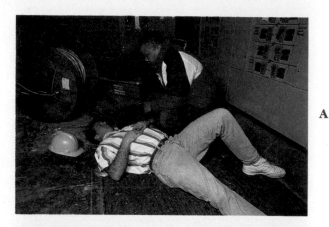

A

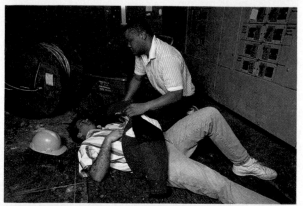

B

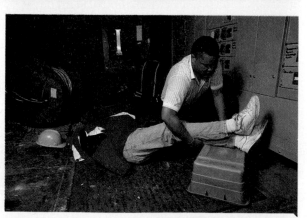

C

Figure 7-5 **A,** Monitor the victim's ABCs if he or she is in shock. **B,** Maintain normal body temperature. **C,** Elevate the victim's legs to keep blood circulating to the vital organs.

You can further help the victim manage the effects of shock if you—

- Control any external bleeding as soon as possible to minimize blood loss.
- Elevate the legs about 12 inches to keep blood circulating to vital organs, unless you suspect head, neck, or back injuries, or possible broken bones involving the hips or legs (Fig. 7-5, *C*). If you are unsure of the victim's condition, leave him or her lying flat.
- Do not give the victim anything to eat or drink, even though he or she is likely to be thirsty. The victim's condition may be severe enough to require surgery, in which case it is better that the stomach be empty.
- Call EMS personnel immediately. Shock cannot be managed effectively by first aid alone. A victim of shock requires advanced life support as soon as possible.

◆ Summary

Do not wait for shock to develop before providing care to a victim of injury or sudden illness. Always follow the emergency action principles to minimize the progressive stages of shock. Care for life-threatening conditions, such as breathing problems or severe external bleeding, before caring for lesser injuries. Remember that the key to managing shock effectively is calling EMS personnel and starting to give care as soon as possible.

Remember that shock is an inevitable factor in serious injuries and illnesses, particularly if there is blood loss or if the normal function of the heart is interrupted. With serious injuries or illnesses, shock is often the final stage before death. You cannot stop shock by administering first aid, but you can slow its progression. Call your emergency number for an ambulance immediately if you notice signs of shock. Shock can be reversed only by advanced medical care, and only if the victim is reached in time.

Answers to Application Questions

1. The body's oxygen needs increase with injury and illness because the body uses more energy in attempting to compensate for the effects of injury or illness while also performing all normal functions.

2. Blood vessel function depends on the vessels receiving accurate instructions from the nervous system. Any time there is damage to the nervous system (brain, spinal cord, or nerves), the transmission of impulses to the blood vessels may be impaired or completely cut off. Without adequate instructions, the blood vessels' ability to function effectively, specifically to change size, is greatly reduced.

3. As activity within the body increases to compensate for injury or illness, body temperature rises. As you read in Chapter 2, the body strives to maintain a constant temperature. Any rise in body temperature results in an attempt to cool the body, as in sweating.

4. Think about the effect of emotional stress on the body under normal circumstances. How does your body respond when you are very angry, worried, or afraid? Your heart rate may increase, you may have trouble breathing, you may sweat profusely. The degree of stress determines how severely the body is affected. Emotional stress can speed the onset of shock by placing additional demands on your body at a time when your body may be struggling to survive.

5. Shock occurs with any significant illness or injury when the body cannot compensate for the injury or illness *and* maintain normal body functions.

Study Questions

1. Match each term with the correct definition.

   a. Blood volume
   b. Injury
   c. Medical emergency

   _____ Condition occurring when the body is subjected to external force.
   _____ Sudden illness resulting from problems occurring within the body.
   _____ Amount of blood circulating within the body.

2. From the scenario at the beginning of the chapter, list four signals of shock.

3. List two conditions that result in shock.

4. List at least five things you can do to care for shock.

In questions 5 through 9, circle the letter of the correct answer.

5. Shock can occur as a result of—

   a. Inadequate blood volume.
   b. Severe diarrhea.
   c. Fatigue.
   d. Overexertion.
   e. a and b

6. When shock occurs, the body prioritizes its needs for blood by sending blood first to—

   a. The arms and legs.
   b. The brain and heart.
   c. The skin.
   d. a and c

7. The skin appears pale during shock as a result of—

    a. Constriction of blood vessels near the skin's surface.

    b. The majority of blood being sent to vital organs.

    c. Profuse sweating.

    d. a and b

    e. a, b, and c

8. Early intervention is the key to managing shock effectively. Which of the following are included in the care for shock?

    a. Maintaining normal body temperature

    b. Monitoring airway, breathing, and circulation

    c. Helping the victim rest comfortably

    d. b and c

    e. a, b, and c

9. Which body systems are affected by shock?

    a. Circulatory and respiratory

    b. All body systems

    c. Circulatory, respiratory, and nervous

    d. Respiratory and nervous

10. Why is shock a life-threatening condition?

11. Why does elevating the victim's legs help manage shock?

Answers are in Appendix A.

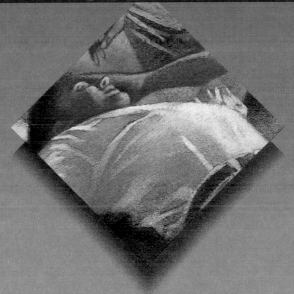

Injuries

◆ Introduction

It is a hot, muggy day in May. The forecast of rain has not seemed to dampen the spirits of the four beach goers headed for the coast. After a week of all-night studying and grueling exams, the soon-to-be graduates are anxious to join their friends.

As they approach the bridge, Joe, the driver, decides he can no longer ignore the car's continually climbing temperature gauge. He pulls over to the side of the road, explaining that, at the end of the term, he had to decide between a new radiator or beach week. After a few minutes, Joe argues that he can safely open the radiator, since the water has had time to cool down.

Despite his friends' objections, Joe takes off his T-shirt and wraps it around the radiator cap. Slowly he releases the cap, a quarter turn at a time. Suddenly, on the last turn, the cap blows off, and scalding water and steam burst out of the radiator, burning his chest and arms. As he turns away from the steam, his back is also burned. His friends use water from the cooler to cool the burned area. However, first aid care is not enough for his blistering skin. They know that Joe needs professional medical care soon.

Predictably, Joe is not the first of the holiday's injuries and will not be the last. As he passes through the hospital's emergency department, his medical records will become part of the statistics that account for one of our nation's most significant health problems—injuries.

* Since the end of World War II, 6 million United States citizens have died of injuries at the rate of approximately 400 a day. Injuries claim thousands of lives each year.
* Approximately 9,100,000 suffered a disabling injury in 1988—an injury that prevented them from immediately returning to their daily routine.
* Injury is a leading cause of death and disability in people age 1 to 44 years.
* Injury is the leading cause of people contacting physicians and the most common cause of hospitalization among people less than 45 years old.
* Injury greatly surpasses all major disease groups (cancer, heart disease, stroke) as a cause of death and disability for people age 1 to 44.

Statistics indicate that most people will have a significant injury at some time in their lives. Researchers predict that few will escape the experience of a fatal or permanently disabling injury to a relative or friend. In the few minutes it will take you to read this introduction, it is estimated that 2 people will be killed and 170 will suffer a disabling injury at the cost of $2,700,000 in lost wages, medical expenses, insurance, property damage, and other indirect costs.

◆ Injuries

How Injuries Occur

The body has a natural resistance to injury. Injuries cause damage when certain external forms of energy produce forces that the body cannot tolerate. These forms of energy are mechanical energy and the energy from heat, electricity, chemicals, and radiation. Damage from these forms of energy injures body tissues and often changes body functions. Injuries can be superficial or deep, penetrating or nonpenetrating, and can affect one or more areas of the body. Some tissues, such as the soft tissues of the skin, have less resistance and are at greater risk if exposed to injury than the deeper, stronger tissues of muscle and bone. Some organs, such as the brain, heart, and lungs, are better protected by bones than other organs such as the digestive or reproductive organs.

Mechanical energy

Mechanical energy produces direct forces, indirect forces, twisting, and contracting forces (see Figure IV-1 on the next page). A direct force is the force of an object striking the body and causing injury at the point of impact. Direct forces can either be blunt or penetrating. For example, a fist striking the chin can break the jaw, or penetrating objects such as bullets and knives can injure structures beneath the skin at the point where they penetrate.

An indirect force is a force that travels through the body when a blunt object strikes the body and causes injury to a body part away from the point of impact. For example, a fall on an outstretched hand may result in an injury to the shoulder or collarbone.

In twisting, one part of the body stays in one position while another part of the body turns. The twisting action can force body parts beyond their normal range of motion, causing injury. For example, if a ski and its binding keep the lower leg in one position while the body falls in another, the knee may be forced beyond its normal range of motion. Twisting injuries are not always this complex. They more often occur as a result of simply stepping off a curb or turning to reach for an out-of-the-way object.

Sudden or powerful muscle contractions can result in musculoskeletal injuries. These commonly occur in sports activities such as throwing a ball long or hard without warming up or sprinting when out of shape. However, our daily routines also require sudden and powerful muscle contractions, for example, when we suddenly turn to catch a heavy object such as a falling child. Although it happens rarely, sudden, powerful muscle contractions can even pull a piece of bone away from the point at which it is normally attached.

These four forces, products of mechanical energy, cause the majority of all injuries. Soft tissue injuries and injuries to muscle and bone (musculoskeletal injuries) are most often the result. Soft tissue injuries outnumber musculoskeletal injuries. Combined they are the major cause of work loss and eligibility for social security and unemployment compensation in the working age group (16 to 65).

Energy from heat, electricity, chemicals, and radiation

Together, the energy from heat, electricity, chemicals, and radiation accounts for only 25 percent of all injuries. Exposure to any of these can result in burns to the skin and other body tissues. Thermal burns, burns caused by heat, are the most common. Sources of electricity, such as common household current or lightning, can penetrate the body, causing external and internal burn damage. Electrical current can also affect the part of the brain that controls breathing and heartbeat. When certain chemicals contact the skin, they cause burns. Solar radiation from the sun's rays causes sunburn. The average citizen is rarely exposed to other forms of radiation.

In 1988, 5,000 people died from fires and burns, making burns the fifth leading cause of unintentional death. Most of those occurred in the home. Over 1 million burn injuries a year require medical attention or result in restricted activity. About one third of those are treated at hospital emergency departments, and over 90,000 people are hospitalized for an average of 12 days. Fires cause 66 percent of all deaths from burns. Hot liquids cause 27 percent, and electricity only 1 percent of burn deaths. The most common causes of nonfatal burns are scalds from hot liquids or foods and contact with hot surfaces.

Factors Affecting Injury

A number of factors affect injuries—age, gender, geographic location, economic status, and alcohol. Technology also affects the type and frequency of injuries. As certain activities, such as skateboarding, gain and lose popularity, the injury statistics reflect the changes.

Injury rates are higher among people under age 45. The elderly and people age 15 to 24

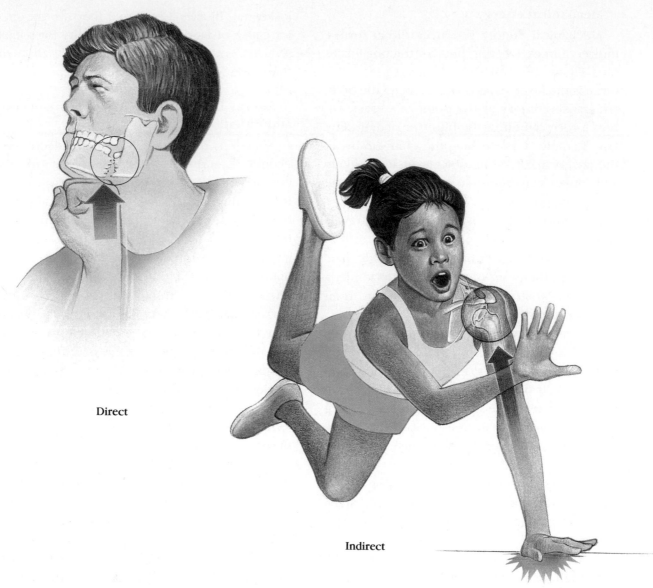

Direct

Indirect

Figure IV-1   The four forces—direct forces, indirect forces, twisting forces, and contracting forces—cause 76 percent of all injuries.

have the highest rate of deaths from injury.

In addition to age, gender is also a significant factor in risk of injury. Males are at greater risk than females for any type of injury. In general, men are 2.5 times more likely to suffer a fatal injury than women.

Many environmental factors influence injury statistics. Whether you live on a farm or in the city, whether your home is built out of wood or brick, the type of heat used in your home, and the climate all affect your degree of risk. For instance, death rates from injury are higher in rural areas. The death rate from injuries is twice as high in low-income areas as in high-income areas.

The use and abuse of alcoholic beverages is a significant factor in many injuries and fatalities, even in young teenagers. The deaths of almost half of all fatally injured drivers involve alcohol, as do those of many adult passengers and pedestrians. Over 40 percent of the deaths of 15- to 19-year-olds are the result of motor vehicle crashes. About half of these fatalities involve alcohol. It is estimated that an

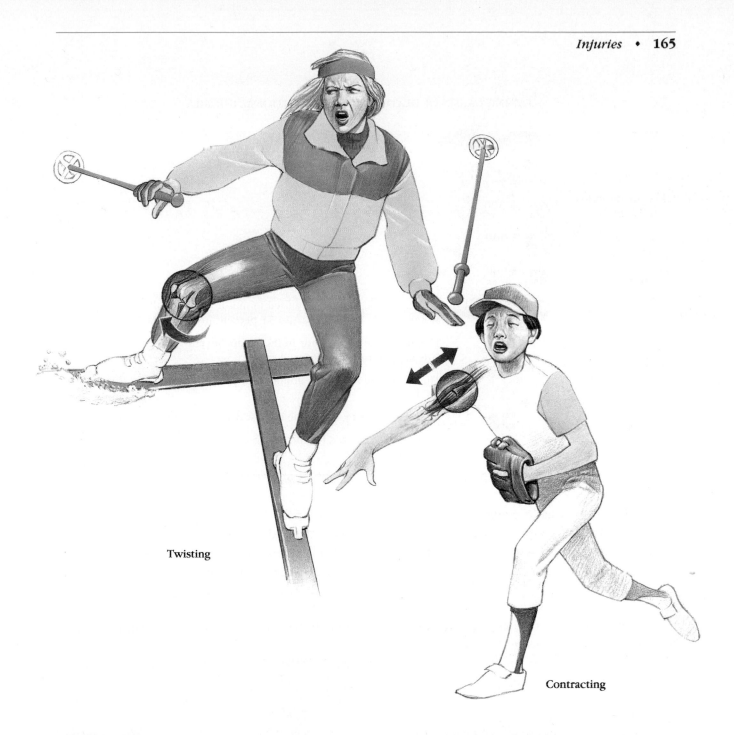

Twisting

Contracting

average of one alcohol-related fatality occurs every 22 minutes.

Alcohol also contributes to other injuries. It is estimated that a significant number of victims who die as a result of falls, drownings, fires, assaults, and suicides have blood alcohol concentrations over the legal limit. In one study of emergency department patients, alcohol was present in the blood of 30 percent of the patients injured while driving or walking on the road, in 22 percent injured at home, in 16 percent injured on the job, and in 56 percent injured in fights and assaults.

Figure IV-2 on the next page shows the leading causes of death from injuries in 1988.

Injury Prevention

Many people believe that injuries just happen—their targets are unfortunate victims of circumstance. However, overwhelming evidence exists that injuries, like disease, do not occur at random. Rather, many injuries are

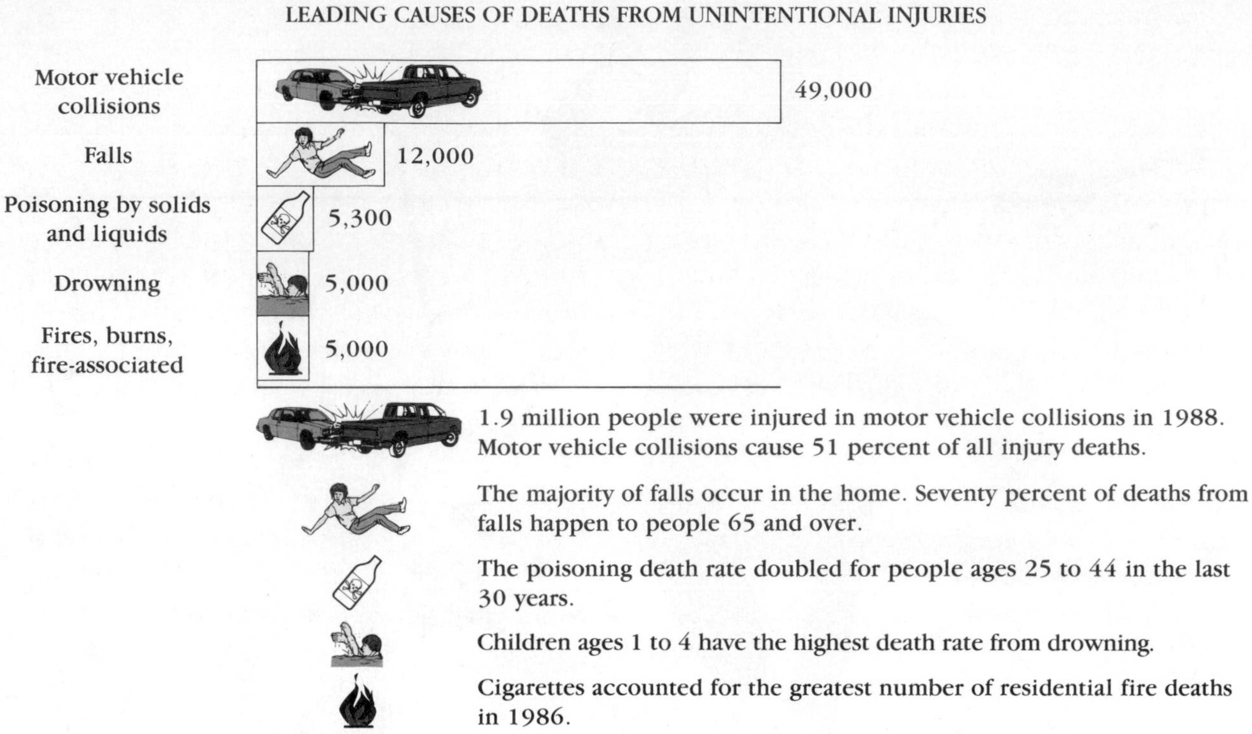

LEADING CAUSES OF DEATHS FROM UNINTENTIONAL INJURIES

Motor vehicle collisions		49,000
Falls		12,000
Poisoning by solids and liquids		5,300
Drowning		5,000
Fires, burns, fire-associated		5,000

1.9 million people were injured in motor vehicle collisions in 1988. Motor vehicle collisions cause 51 percent of all injury deaths.

The majority of falls occur in the home. Seventy percent of deaths from falls happen to people 65 and over.

The poisoning death rate doubled for people ages 25 to 44 in the last 30 years.

Children ages 1 to 4 have the highest death rate from drowning.

Cigarettes accounted for the greatest number of residential fire deaths in 1986.

Figure IV-2 Data from National Safety Council, *Accident Facts,* 1989 edition.

predictable, preventable events resulting from the interaction of people and hazards in the environment.

There are three general strategies for preventing injuries:

- Persuade people at risk to alter behavior
- Require behavior change by law
- Provide automatic protection by product and environmental design

Although laws that require you to conform to safety measures, such as wearing seat belts, are moderately effective, the most successful injury-prevention strategy is the built-in protection of product design. Automatic protection, such as airbags in motor vehicles, does not allow people to make choices (Fig. IV-3).

Typically, behaviors of members of high-risk groups tend to be the hardest to influence, regardless of whether the behavior is voluntary or required. For example, despite the overwhelming number of traffic fatalities in the 15 to 19 age group, teenagers are less likely than adults to wear seat belts.

Many people view laws that require certain behaviors as an infringement of their rights—even though the laws are intended to protect them from injury. Product designs are equally difficult to influence because of manufacturers'

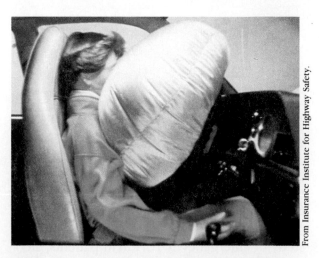

From Insurance Institute for Highway Safety.

Figure IV-3 Airbags provide automatic protection.

reluctance to bear the costs of design changes. For instance, the evidence favoring seat belts was largely irrefutable some time ago. However, it took over 20 years of fighting to get a federal regulation requiring automobile manufacturers to begin to install automatic restraints by 1990.

The American Trauma Society contends that, if existing information about prevention were applied, the injury rate could be reduced by 50 percent. The following steps could significantly reduce your risk of personal injury:

- Know your risk—If you have not already done so, complete the Healthy Lifestyles Awareness Inventory in Appendix D of this text. Note the areas that indicate where you are at risk.

- Take measures that can make a difference—Change behaviors that decrease your risk of injury and the risk of others.

- Think safety—Be alert for and avoid potentially harmful conditions or activities that increase your injury risk. Take precautions such as wearing appropriate protective devices—helmets, padding, and eyewear—and buckle up when driving or riding in motor vehicles. Let your state and congressional representatives know that you support legislation that ensures a safer environment for us all.

- Learn first aid—Despite dramatic improvements in the last decade in emergency medical systems nationwide, the person who can most often make the difference between death and life is you—the citizen responder.

Soft Tissue Injuries

Objectives

After reading this chapter, you should be able to—

1. List two signals of closed wounds.

2. Describe the best defense against infection of an open wound.

3. List at least four signals of an infected wound.

4. Describe how to care for an infected wound.

5. List two purposes of bandaging.

6. Describe how to care for open and closed wounds and wounds with an impaled object.

7. List the four causes of burn injury.

8. Describe the three types of burns.

9. Explain when to call EMS for a burn injury.

10. List the basic steps for burn care.

11. Describe how to care for thermal, chemical, electrical, and radiation burns.

12. Define the key terms for this chapter.

After reading this chapter and completing the class activities, you should be able to—

1. Demonstrate techniques for controlling severe bleeding.

2. Make appropriate decisions for care when given an example of an emergency situation involving soft tissue injuries.

Key Terms

Bandage: Material used to wrap or cover a part of the body; commonly used to hold a dressing or splint in place.

Burn: An injury to the skin or other body tissues caused by heat, chemicals, electricity, or radiation.

Closed wound: A wound in which soft tissue damage occurs beneath the skin and the skin is not broken.

Critical burn: Any burn that is potentially life-threatening, disabling, or disfiguring; a burn requiring medical attention.

Dressing: A pad placed directly over a wound to absorb blood and other body fluids and to prevent infection.

Full-thickness burn: A burn injury involving both layers of skin and underlying tissues; skin may be charred.

Open wound: A wound resulting in a break in the skin surface.

Partial-thickness burn: A burn injury involving both layers of skin; characterized by red, wet skin and blisters.

Soft tissue: Body structures that include the layers of skin, fat, and muscles.

Superficial burn: A burn injury involving only the top layer of skin, characterized by red, dry skin.

Wound: An injury to the soft tissues.

For Review

Before reading this chapter, you should have a basic understanding of the circulatory and integumentary systems and the interrelationship of the body systems (Chapter 2). You should also know how to control bleeding (Chapter 6) and how to care for shock (Chapter 7).

◆ Introduction

An infant falls and bruises his arm while learning to walk; a toddler scrapes her knee while learning to run; a child needs stitches in his chin after he falls off the "monkey bars" on the playground; an adolescent gets a black eye in a fist fight; a teenager suffers a sunburn as a result of a weekend at the beach; and an adult cuts a hand while working in a woodshop. What do these injuries have in common? They are all **soft tissue** injuries.

In the course of growing up and in our daily lives, soft tissue injuries occur often and in many different ways. Fortunately, most soft tissue injuries are minor, requiring little attention. Often only an adhesive bandage or ice and rest are needed. Some injuries, however, are more severe and require immediate medical attention. In this chapter, you will learn how to recognize and care for the most common types of injuries—soft tissue injuries.

◆ What Are Soft Tissues?

The soft tissues include the layers of skin, fat, and muscles that protect the underlying body structures (see Figure 8-1 on the next page). In Chapter 2, you learned that the skin is the largest single organ in the body and that without it the human body could not function. It provides a protective barrier for the body; it helps regulate the body's temperature; and it absorbs information about the environment by way of the nerves in the skin.

The skin has two layers. The outer layer of skin, the epidermis, provides a barrier to bacteria and other organisms that can cause infection. The deeper layer, called the dermis, contains the important structures of the nerves, the sweat and oil glands, and the blood vessels. Because the skin is well supplied with blood vessels and nerves, most soft tissue injuries are likely to bleed and be painful.

Beneath the skin layers lies a layer of fat. This layer helps insulate the body to help maintain body temperature. The fat layer also

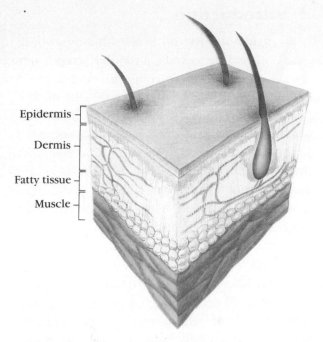

Epidermis —

Dermis —

Fatty tissue —

Muscle —

Figure 8-1 The soft tissues include the layers of skin, fat, and muscle.

stores energy. The amount of fat varies in different parts of the body and in each person.

The muscles lie beneath the fat layer and comprise the largest segment of the body's soft tissues. Most soft tissue injuries involve the outer layers of tissue. However, more violent forces, such as can occur with sharp or penetrating objects or deep burns, can involve all the soft tissue layers. Although the muscles are considered soft tissues, muscle injuries are discussed more thoroughly in the next chapter with other musculoskeletal injuries.

♦ Types of Soft Tissue Injuries

Any injury to the skin or soft tissues beneath threatens the body. Injuries causing breaks in the skin carry great risk of infection. Since the skin tends to collect microorganisms, injuries involving breaks in the skin can become infected unless properly cared for.

An injury to the soft tissues is called a **wound**. Soft tissue injuries are typically classified as either **closed wounds** or **open wounds**. A wound is closed when the soft tissue damage occurs beneath the surface of the skin, leaving the outer layer intact. A wound is open if there is a break in the skin's outer layer. Open wounds usually result in external bleeding.

Burns are a special kind of soft tissue injury. A burn injury occurs when intense heat, certain chemicals, electricity, or radiation contacts the skin or other body tissues. Burns are classified as superficial, partial-thickness, or full-thickness. **Superficial burns** affect only the outer layer of skin. **Partial-thickness burns** damage both layers of skin. **Full-thickness burns** penetrate the layers of skin and can affect other soft tissues and even bone. Burns are discussed in more detail later in this chapter.

Closed Wounds

Closed wounds are generally more common than open wounds. The simplest closed wound is a bruise, also called a contusion (Fig. 8-2). Bruises result when the body is subjected to force, such as when you bump your leg on a table or chair. This usually results in damage to soft tissue layers and vessels beneath the skin, causing internal bleeding. When blood and other fluids seep into the surrounding tissues, the area discolors and swells. The amount of discoloration and swelling varies depending on the severity of the injury. At first, the area may only appear red. Over time, more fluid leaks into the area, which turns dark red or purple. Violent forces can cause more severe soft tissue injuries involving larger blood vessels and the deeper layers of muscle tissue. These injuries can result in profuse bleeding beneath the skin.

Open Wounds

Open wounds are injuries that break the skin. These breaks can be as minor as a scrape of the surface layers or as severe as a deep pene-

Figure 8-2 The simplest closed wound is a bruise.

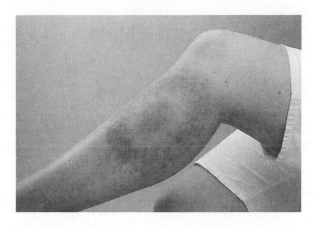

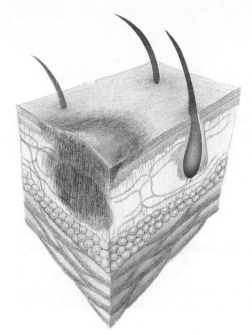

tration. The amount of bleeding depends on the severity of the injury. However, any break in the skin provides an entry point for disease-producing microorganisms.

There are four main types of open wounds:

* Abrasions
* Lacerations
* Avulsions
* Punctures

An abrasion is the most common type of open wound. It is characterized by skin that has been rubbed or scraped away (Fig. 8-3). This often occurs when a child falls and scrapes his or her hands or knees. An abrasion is sometimes called a rug burn, road rash, or strawberry. Because the scraping of the outer skin layers exposes sensitive nerve endings, an

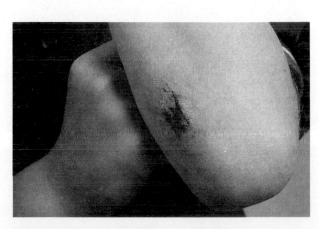

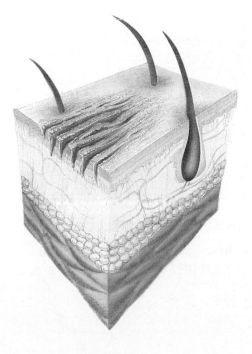

Figure 8-3 Abrasions can be painful, but bleeding is easily controlled.

Figure 8-4 A laceration may have jagged or smooth edges.

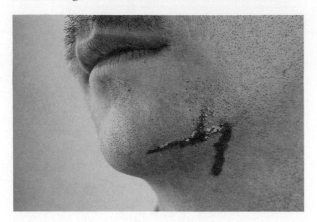

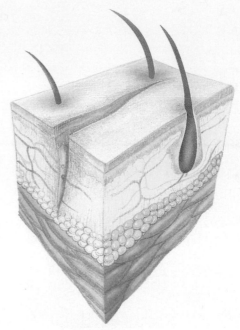

abrasion is usually painful. Bleeding is easily controlled and not severe, since only the small capillaries are affected. Because of the way the injury occurs, dirt and other matter can easily become embedded in the skin, making it especially important to clean the wound.

A laceration is a cut, usually from a sharp object. The cut may have either jagged or smooth edges (Fig. 8-4). Lacerations are commonly caused by sharp-edged objects such as knives, scissors, or broken glass. A laceration can also result when a blunt force splits the

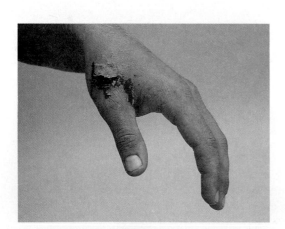

Figure 8-5 In an avulsion, part of the skin and other soft tissue is torn away.

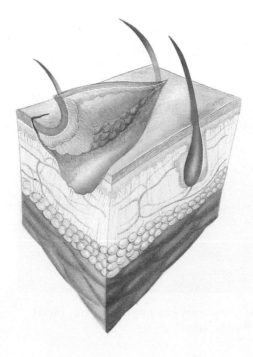

skin. This often occurs in areas where bone lies directly under the skin's surface, such as the chinbone. Deep lacerations can also affect the layers of fat and muscle, damaging both nerves and blood vessels. Lacerations usually bleed freely and, depending on the structures involved, can bleed profusely. Because the nerves may also be injured, lacerations are not always painful.

An avulsion is an injury in which a portion of the skin and sometimes other soft tissue is partially or completely torn away (Fig. 8-5). A partially avulsed piece of skin may remain attached but hangs like a flap. Bleeding is usually significant because avulsions often involve deeper soft tissue layers. Sometimes a force is so violent that a body part, such as a finger, may be severed (Fig. 8-6). Although damage to the tissue is severe, bleeding is usually not as bad as you might expect. The blood vessels usually constrict and retract (pull in) at the point of injury, slowing bleeding and making it relatively easy to control with direct pressure. In the past, a completely severed body part could not be successfully reattached. With today's technology, reattachment is often successful.

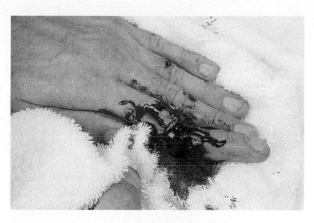

Figure 8-6 In a severe avulsion, a body part may be completely removed.

A puncture wound results when the skin is pierced with a pointed object such as a nail, a piece of glass, a splinter, or a knife (Fig. 8-7). A gunshot wound is also a puncture wound. Because the skin usually closes around the penetrating object, external bleeding is generally not severe. However, internal bleeding can be severe if the penetrating object damages major blood vessels or internal organs. An object that remains embedded in the open

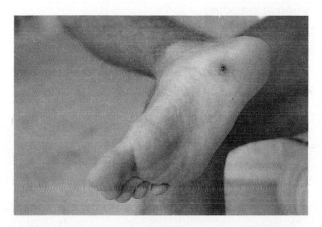

Figure 8-7 A puncture wound results when skin is pierced by a pointed object.

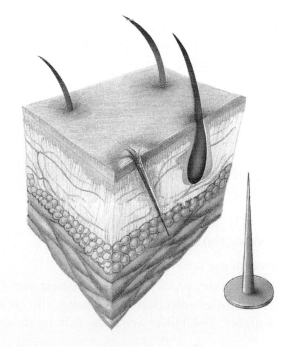

Figure 8-8 An impaled object is an object that remains embedded in a wound.

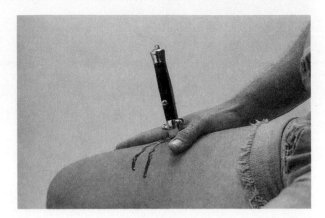

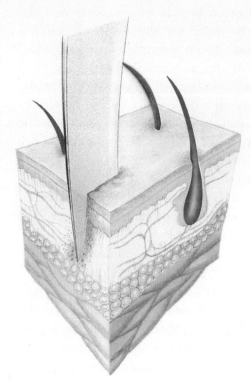

wound is called an impaled object (Fig. 8-8). An object may also pass completely through a body part, making two open wounds—one at the entry point and one at the exit point.

Although puncture wounds generally do not bleed profusely, they are potentially more dangerous than wounds that do because they more readily become infected. Objects penetrating the soft tissues carry microorganisms that cause infections. Of particular danger is the microorganism that causes tetanus, a severe infection. Tetanus is a bacteria that produces a powerful poison in the body. This poison enters the nervous system and affects specific muscles. For example, jaw muscles will contract, causing "lockjaw." Once tetanus reaches the nervous system, its effects are irreversible.

◆ Infection

Preventing Infection

When an injury breaks the skin, the best initial defense against infection is to cleanse the area thoroughly. For minor wounds, that is, those

that do not bleed severely, wash the area with soap and water. Most soaps are effective in removing harmful bacteria. Wounds that require medical attention because of more extensive tissue damage or bleeding need not be washed. These wounds will be cleaned thoroughly in the medical facility as a routine part of their care. It is more important for you to control bleeding.

Because infected wounds can cause serious

Table 8-1	Four Main Types of Open Wounds
Type	**Cause**
Abrasion	Rubbing or scraping away of the skin
Laceration	Usually a cut from a sharp object; may have either jagged or smooth edges
Avulsion	Complete or partial tearing away of the skin and/or other soft tissues
Puncture	Piercing of the skin by a pointed object

Figure 8-9 An infected wound may become swollen and may have a pus discharge.

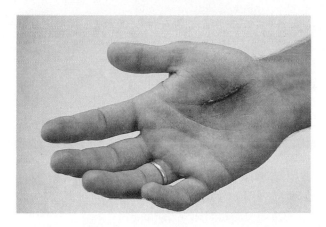

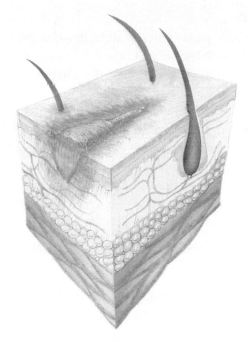

medical problems, it is important to maintain an up-to-date record of immunizations. These immunizations, which begin shortly after birth, help your immune system defend against invading microorganisms such as bacteria. Your immune system is the body system responsible for fighting off infection. Immunizations assist the natural function of the immune system by building up antibodies, disease-fighting proteins, which help protect the body against specific infections in the future.

One of these immunizations prevents tetanus. The best way to prevent tetanus is to receive a booster shot every 5 to 10 years or whenever a wound is contaminated by a dirty object such as a rusty nail. Because the effects of immunizations do not last a lifetime, booster shots help maintain the antibodies that protect against tetanus.

Signals of Infection

Sometimes, even the best care for a soft tissue injury is not enough to prevent infection. You can easily recognize the early signals of infection. The area around the wound be- comes swollen and red. The area may feel warm or throb with pain. Some wounds have a pus discharge (Fig. 8-9). More serious infections may cause a person to develop a fever and feel ill. Red streaks may develop that progress from the wound in the direction of the heart.

Caring for Infection

If you see these initial signals of infection, care for the wound by keeping the area clean, elevating the affected area, and applying warm, wet compresses and an antibiotic ointment such as Neosporin^R or Neomycin^R. Change coverings over the wound daily. If a fever or red streaks develop, the infection is worsening. If the infection persists or worsens, seek medical care without delay.

◆ Dressings and Bandages

All open wounds need some type of covering to help control bleeding and prevent infection. These coverings are commonly referred to as **dressings** and **bandages**. There are many different types of both.

Dressings

Dressings are pads placed directly on the wound to absorb blood and other fluids and to prevent infection. To minimize the chance of infection, dressings should be sterile. Most dressings are porous, allowing air to circulate to the wound to promote healing. Standard dressings include varying sizes of cotton gauze, commonly ranging from 2 to 4 inches square. Much larger dressings called universal dressings are used to cover very large wounds and multiple wounds in one body area (Fig. 8-10). Some dressings have nonstick surfaces to prevent the dressing from sticking to the wound.

A special type of dressing does not allow air to pass through. Sterile aluminum foil, plastic wrap, and petroleum jelly–soaked gauze are examples of this type of dressing (Fig. 8-11). These dressings are used for certain chest and abdominal injuries that are discussed in Chapter 11.

Bandages

A bandage is any material used to wrap or cover any part of the body. Bandages are used to hold dressings in place, to apply pressure to control bleeding, to protect a wound from dirt and infection, and to provide support to an injured limb or body part. Many different types of bandages are available commercially (Fig. 8-12). A bandage applied snugly to create pressure on a wound or injury is called a pressure bandage.

A common type of bandage is a commercially made adhesive compress such as a Band-Aid (Fig. 8-13). Available in assorted sizes, it consists of a small pad of nonstick gauze on a strip of adhesive tape that is applied directly to small injuries. Also available is the bandage compress. The bandage compress is a thick gauze dressing attached to a gauze bandage. This bandage can be tied in place. Because it is specially designed to help control severe bleeding, the bandage compress usually comes in a sterile package.

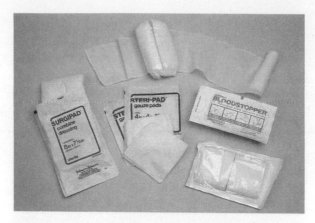

Figure 8-10 Dressings come in various sizes.

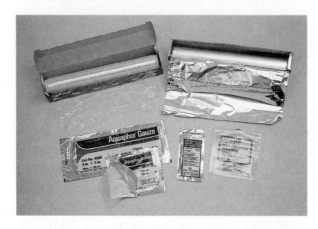

Figure 8-11 Airtight dressings are designed to prevent air from passing through.

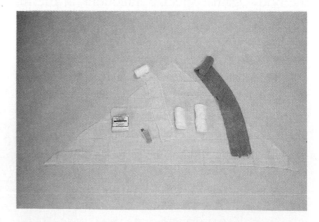

Figure 8-12 Different types of bandages are used to hold dressings in place, apply pressure to a wound, protect the wound from infection, and provide support to an injured area.

A Stitch in Time. . .

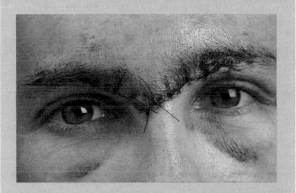

It can be difficult to judge when a wound should be seen by a doctor for stitches. A general rule of thumb is that stitches are needed when the edges of skin do not fall together or when any wound is more than an inch long. Stitches speed the healing process, lessen the chances of infection, and improve the look of scars. They should be placed within the first few hours following the injury. The following major injuries often require stitches:

* Bleeding from an artery or uncontrollable bleeding.
* Deep cuts or avulsions that show the muscle or bone, involve joints such as the elbows, gape widely, or involve the hands or feet.
* Large or deep punctures.
* Large or deeply embedded objects.
* Human and animal bites.
* Wounds that, if left unattended, could leave a conspicuous scar, such as those that involve the lip or eyebrow.

If you are caring for a wound and think it may need stitches, it probably does. Once applied, stitches are easily cared for by dabbing them with hydrogen peroxide once or twice a day. If the wound gets red or swollen or if pus begins to form, notify your doctor.

Stitches in the face are often removed in less than a week. In the joints, they are often removed in two weeks. Stitches on most other body parts require removal within 6 to 10 days. Some stitches dissolve naturally and do not require removal.

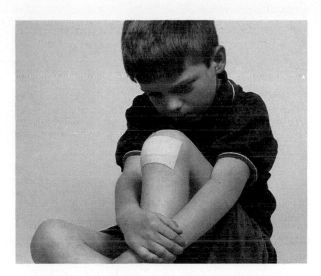

Figure 8-13 A common type of bandage is an adhesive compress.

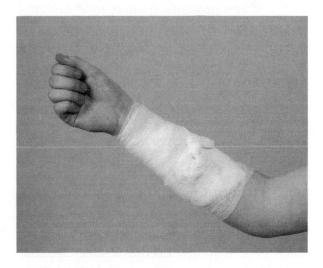

Figure 8-14 Roller bandages are usually made of gauze and are easy to apply.

A roller bandage is usually made of gauze or gauzelike material (Fig. 8-14). Roller bandages are available in assorted widths from ½ to 12 inches and lengths from 5 to 10 yards. A roller bandage is generally wrapped around the body part, over a dressing, using overlapping turns until the dressing is completely covered. It can be tied or taped in place. A roller bandage may also be used as a dressing or compress. In the next chapter, you will learn to

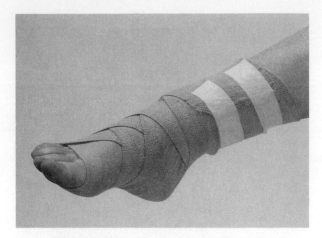

Figure 8-15 Elastic bandages can be applied to control swelling or support an injured limb.

use roller bandages to hold splints in place.

Elastic roller bandages are designed to keep continuous pressure on a body part (Fig. 8-15). When properly applied, they can effectively control swelling or support an injured limb. Elastic bandages are available in 2-, 3-, 4-, and 6-inch widths. Because of their versatility, elastic bandages are used in athletic environments, where injuries to muscles, bones, and joints are common.

Another commonly used bandage is the triangular bandage. It can be made easily by cutting a 40-inch square of muslin or similar cloth in half diagonally, making two triangular pieces (Fig. 8-16, *A*). Folded, it can hold a dressing or splint in place on most parts of the body (Fig. 8-16, *B*). Used as a sling, the triangular bandage can support an injured shoulder, arm, or hand (Fig. 8-17).

Applying a bandage

To apply a roller bandage, follow these general guidelines:

- If possible, elevate the injured body part above the level of the heart.
- Secure the end of the bandage in place. Wrap the bandage around the body part until the dressing is completely covered and

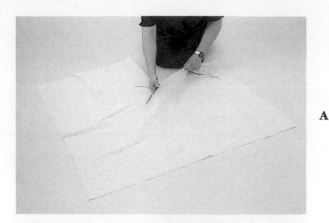

A

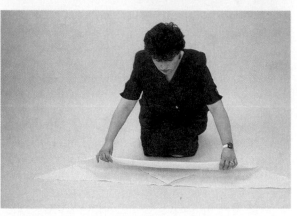

B

Figure 8-16 **A,** A triangular bandage can be made by cutting a 40-inch square of cloth in half diagonally. **B,** A cravat is made by folding the triangular bandage.

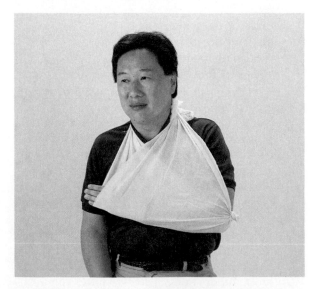

Figure 8-17 A triangular bandage is commonly used as a sling.

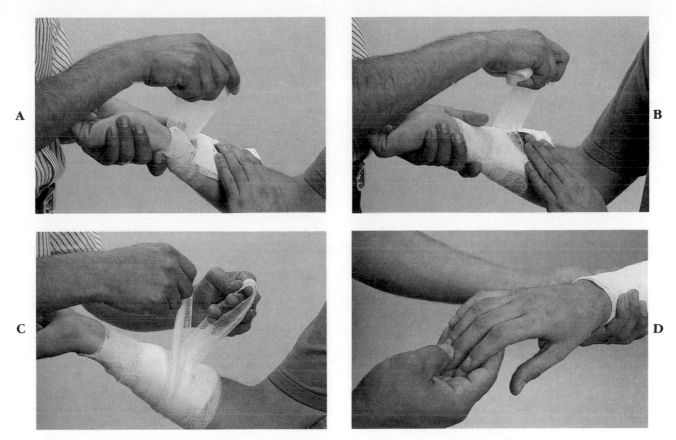

Figure 8-18   **A,** Start by securing a roller bandage over the dressing. **B,** Use overlapping turns to cover the dressing completely. **C,** Tie or tape the bandage in place. **D,** Check the fingers for warmth and color.

the bandage extends several inches beyond the dressing. Tie or tape the bandage in place (Fig. 8-18, *A-D*).

* Do not cover fingers or toes, if possible. By keeping these parts uncovered, you will be able to see if the bandage is too tight. If fingers or toes become cold or begin to turn pale or blue, the bandage is too tight and should be loosened slightly.
* If blood soaks through the bandage, apply additional dressings and another bandage. *Do not* remove the blood-soaked ones.

Elastic bandages, sometimes called Ace[R] bandages or elastic wraps, can easily restrict blood flow if not applied properly. Restricted blood flow is not only painful, but can cause

tissue damage if not corrected. Figure 8-19, *A-D,* on the next page shows some simple ways to ensure proper application of elastic bandages.

Q

1. Explain how elevation of an injured part helps reduce bleeding and swelling.

◆ Care for Wounds

First Aid for Closed Wounds

Most closed wounds do not require special medical care. Direct pressure on the area decreases bleeding. Elevating the injured part

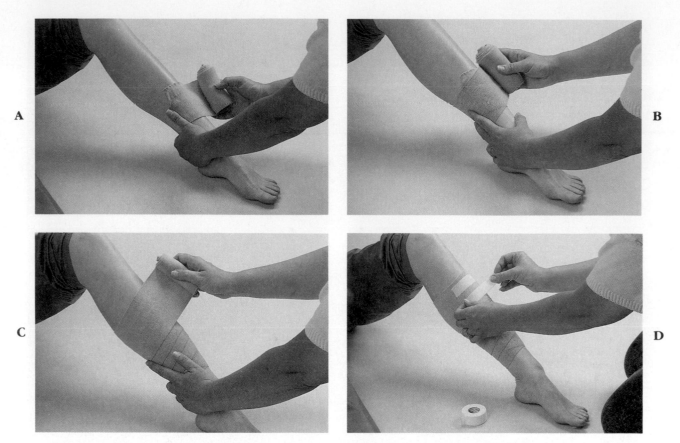

Figure 8-19   **A,** Start the elastic bandage at the point furthest from the heart. **B,** Anchor the bandage. **C,** Wrap the bandage using overlapping turns. **D,** Tape the end of the bandage in place.

helps reduce swelling. Cold can be effective in helping control both pain and swelling. When applying ice or a chemical cold pack, place a gauze pad, towel, or other cloth between the ice and the skin (Fig. 8-20).

Do not dismiss a closed wound as "just a bruise." Be aware of possible serious injuries to internal organs or other underlying structures such as the muscles. Take the time to evaluate whether more serious injuries could be present. If a person complains of severe pain or cannot move a body part without pain, or if you think the force that caused the injury was great enough to cause serious damage, seek medical attention immediately. Care for these injuries is described in later chapters.

First Aid for Major Open Wounds

A major open wound is one with severe bleeding, with a deep destruction of tissue, or with

a deeply embedded impaled object. To care for a major open wound, follow these general guidelines:

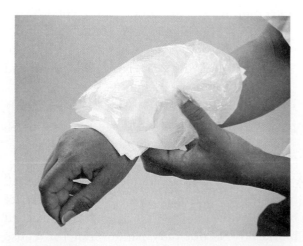

Figure 8-20   For a closed wound, apply ice to help control pain and swelling.

- *Do not* waste time trying to wash the wound.
- Quickly control bleeding using pressure and elevation. Apply direct pressure by placing a sterile dressing over the wound. If nothing sterile is available, use any clean covering such as a towel, tie, handkerchief, sock, disposable gloves, or plastic wrap. If you do not have a pad or cloth available, have the injured person use his or her hand. As a last resort, use your own bare hand.
- Apply a bandage over the dressings to maintain pressure on the wound.
- Wash your hands immediately after completing care.
- Seek medical attention (call EMS personnel or transport the victim to a medical facility).
- Recommend to the victim that he or she get a tetanus booster shot if he or she has not had one within the last 5 to 10 years.

If the victim has an avulsion in which a body part has been completely severed, try to retrieve the severed body part. Wrap the part in sterile gauze, if any is available, or in any clean material such as a washcloth. Place the wrapped part in a plastic bag. If possible, keep the part cool by placing the bag on ice (Fig. 8-21). Make sure the part is transported to the medical facility with the victim.

If the victim has an impaled object in the wound, follow these additional guidelines:

- *Do not* remove the object.
- Use bulky dressings to stabilize it. Any movement of the object can result in further tissue damage (Fig. 8-22, *A*).
- Control bleeding by bandaging the dressings in place around the object (Fig. 8-22, *B*).

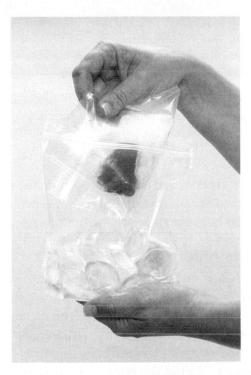

Figure 8-21 Wrap a severed body part in sterile gauze, put it in a plastic bag, and put the bag on ice.

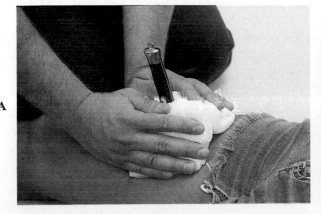 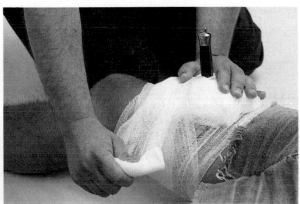

A   B

Figure 8-22 **A,** Use a bulky dressing to support an impaled object. **B,** Use bandages over the dressing to control bleeding.

First Aid for Minor Open Wounds

A minor wound is one, such as an abrasion, in which damage is only superficial and bleeding is minimal. To care for a minor wound, follow these general guidelines:

- Wash the wound thoroughly with soap and water.
- Place a sterile dressing over the wound.
- Apply direct pressure for a few minutes to control any bleeding.
- Once bleeding is controlled, remove the dressing and apply an antibiotic ointment.
- Apply a new sterile dressing.
- Hold the dressing in place with a bandage (tape can also be used, or a Band-Aid-type bandage) (Fig. 8-23).

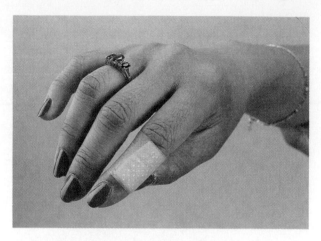

Figure 8-23 Minor wounds should be washed and then bandaged to prevent infection.

◆ Burns

Burns are another type of soft tissue injury, caused primarily by heat. Burns can also occur when the body is exposed to certain chemicals, electricity, or solar or other forms of radiation.

When burns occur, they first destroy the epidermis, the top layer of skin. If the burn progresses, the dermis, the second layer, is injured or destroyed. Burns break the skin and thus can cause infection, fluid loss, and loss of temperature control. Deep burns can damage underlying tissues. Burns can also damage the respiratory system and the eyes.

The severity of a burn depends on—

- The temperature of the object or gas causing the burn.
- The length of exposure to the source.
- The location of the burn.
- The extent of the burn.
- The victim's age and medical condition.

In general, people over age 60 have thinner skin than younger people and often burn more severely. Children under age five also may burn more severely. People with chronic medical problems also tend to have more severe burns, especially if they are not well-nourished, have heart or kidney problems, or are exposed to the burn source for a prolonged period because they are unable to escape.

Types of Burns

Burns are classified by their source, such as heat, chemicals, electricity, or radiation. They are also classified by depth. The deeper the burn, the more severe it is. Generally, there are three depth classifications: superficial (first degree), partial-thickness (second degree), and full-thickness (third degree).

Superficial burns (first degree)

A superficial burn involves only the top layer of skin (Fig. 8-24). The skin is red and dry, and the burn is usually painful. The area may swell. Most sunburns are superficial burns. Superficial burns generally heal in five to six days without permanent scarring.

Partial-thickness burns (second degree)

A partial-thickness burn involves both the epidermis and the dermis (Fig. 8-25). These injuries are also red and have blisters that may open and weep clear fluid, making the skin appear wet. The burned skin may look mottled. These burns are usually painful, and the area

Figure 8-24 A superficial burn

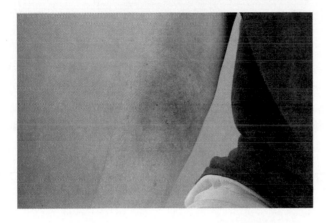

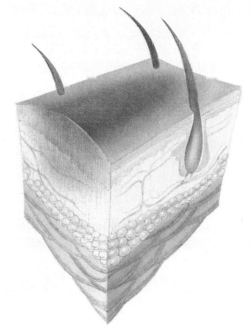

often swells. The burn usually heals in three or four weeks. Scarring may occur.

Full-thickness burns (third degree)

A full-thickness burn destroys both layers of skin, as well as any or all of the underlying structures—fat, muscles, bones, and nerves (Fig. 8-26). These burns look brown or charred (black), with the tissues underneath sometimes appearing white. They can be either extremely painful or relatively painless if the burn destroyed nerve endings in the skin.

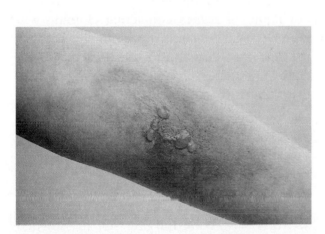

Figure 8-25 A partial-thickness burn

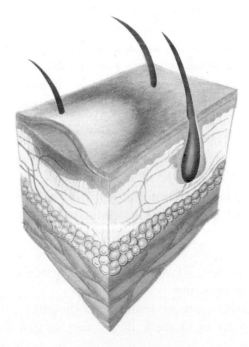

Figure 8-26 A full-thickness burn

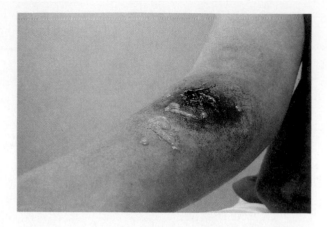

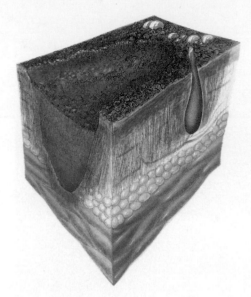

Full-thickness burns are life-threatening. Because the burns are open, the body loses fluid, and shock is likely to occur. These burns also make the body highly prone to infection. Scarring occurs and may be severe. Many burn sites eventually require skin grafts.

Identifying Critical Burns

A **critical burn** is one that requires the attention of medical professionals. Critical burns are potentially life-threatening, disfiguring, or disabling. Knowing whether you should activate the EMS system for a burn injury is often hard. It is not always easy or possible to assess the severity of a burn immediately after injury. Even superficial burns to large areas of the body or to certain body parts can be critical. You cannot judge severity by the pain the victim feels because nerve endings may be destroyed. Call EMS personnel immediately for assistance for the following burns:

- Burns whose victims are experiencing breathing difficulty
- Burns covering more than one body part
- Burns to the head, neck, hands, feet, or genitals
- Any partial-thickness or full-thickness burn to a child or an elderly person
- Burns resulting from chemicals, explosions, or electricity

Expect that burns caused by flames or hot grease will require medical attention, especially if the victim is under 5 or over 65 years of age. Hot grease is slow to cool and difficult to remove from the skin. Burns that involve hot liquid or flames contacting clothing will also be serious, since the clothing prolongs the heat contact with the skin. Some synthetic fabrics melt and stick to the body. They may take longer to cool than the soft tissues. Although these burns may appear minor at first, they can continue to worsen for a short time.

♦ Care for Burns

As you approach the victim, decide if the scene is safe. Look for fire, smoke, downed electrical wires, and warning signs for chemicals or radiation. If the scene is unsafe, call your emergency number and wait for fire or EMS personnel to arrive.

If the scene is safe, approach cautiously. Do

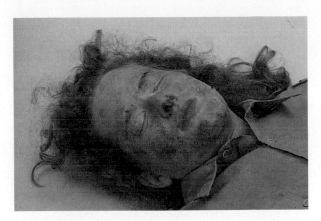

Figure 8-27 Facial burns may signal that air passages or lungs have been burned.

a primary survey. Call EMS personnel. Pay close attention to the victim's airway. Note burns around the mouth or nose or the rest of the face that may signal that air passages or lungs have been burned (Fig. 8-27). If you suspect a burned airway or burned lungs, continually monitor breathing. Air passages may swell, impairing or stopping breathing.

As you do a secondary survey, look for additional signals of burn injuries. Look also for other injuries, especially if there was an explosion or electric shock.

If burns are present, follow these four basic care steps:

◆ Cool the burned area.
◆ Cover the burned area.
◆ Prevent infection.
◆ Minimize shock.

Even after the source of heat has been removed, soft tissue will continue to burn for minutes afterwards, causing more damage. Therefore, it is essential to cool any burned areas immediately with large amounts of cool water (Fig. 8-28, A). Do not use ice or ice water other than on small superficial burns. Ice causes critical body heat loss. Use whatever resources are available—a tub, shower, or garden hose is often handy. You can apply soaked towels, sheets, or other wet cloths to a burned face or other area that cannot be im-

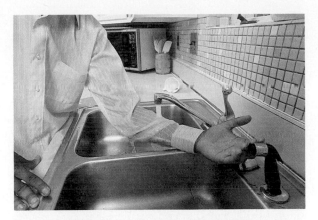

A

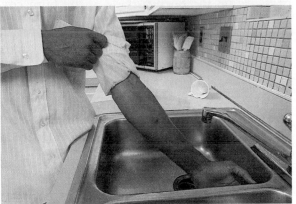

B

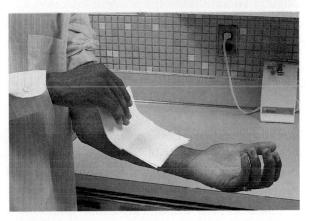

C

Figure 8-28 **A,** Large amounts of cool water are essential to cool burned areas. **B,** Remove any clothing covering the burned area. **C,** Cover the burned area.

mersed. Be sure to keep these compresses cool by adding more water. Otherwise, they will quickly absorb the heat from the skin's surface.

Allow plenty of time for the burned area to cool. If pain continues or if the edges of the burned area are still warm to the touch when the area is removed from the water, continue cooling. When the burn is cool, remove all clothing from the area by carefully pulling or cutting material away (Fig. 8-28, *B*). Do not try to remove any clothing that is sticking to skin.

Burns often expose sensitive nerve endings. Cover the burned area to keep out air and help reduce pain (Fig. 8-28, *C*). Use dry, sterile dressings if possible, and loosely bandage them in place. The bandage should not put pressure on the burn surface. If the burn covers a large area of the body, cover it with clean, dry sheets or other cloth.

Covering the burn also helps to prevent infection. Do not put ointments, butter, oil, or other commercial or home remedies on blisters or full-thickness burns or on any burn that will receive medical attention. Oils and ointments seal in heat and do not relieve pain well. Other home remedies can contaminate open skin areas, causing infection. Do not break blisters. Intact skin helps prevent infection.

For small superficial burns and burns with open blisters that are not sufficiently severe or extensive to require medical attention, care for the burned area as an open wound. Wash the area with soap and water and keep the area clean. Apply an antibiotic ointment and watch for signals of infection. Your pharmacist or doctor may be able to recommend products that are effective in caring for superficial burns such as sunburn.

Full-thickness burns can cause shock as a result of pain and loss of body fluids. Lay the victim down unless he or she is having difficulty breathing. Elevate burned areas above the level of the heart, if possible. Burn victims have a tendency to chill. Help the victim maintain body temperature by protecting him or her from drafts.

Special Situations
Chemical burns

Chemical burns are common in industrial settings, but also occur in the home. Cleaning

---

Table 8-2 Dos and Don'ts of Burn Care

Dos

- Do cool burns by flushing with cool water.
- Do cover the burn with a dry, sterile dressing.
- Do take steps to minimize shock.

Don'ts

- Don't apply ice directly to partial- or full-thickness burns.
- Don't touch burns with anything except sterile or clean dressings; do not use absorbent cotton or pull clothes over any burned area.
- Don't remove pieces of cloth that stick to a burned area.
- Don't try to clean a full-thickness burn.
- Don't break blisters.
- Don't use any kind of grease or ointment on severe burns.

---

solutions, such as household bleach, drain cleaners, toilet bowl cleaners; paint strippers; and lawn or garden chemicals are common sources of caustic chemicals. Caustic chemicals destroy tissues. Typically, burn injuries result from chemicals that are strong acids or alkalis. These substances can quickly injure the skin. As with heat burns, the stronger the chemical and the longer the contact, the more severe the burn. The chemical will continue to burn as long as it is on the skin. You must remove the chemical from the body as quickly as possible and call EMS personnel.

Flush the burn with large amounts of cool, running water (Fig. 8-29). Continue flushing until EMS personnel arrive. Do not use a forceful flow of water from a hose; the force may further damage burned skin. Have the victim remove contaminated clothes, if possible. Take steps to minimize shock. Do not forget the eyes. If an eye is burned by a chemical,

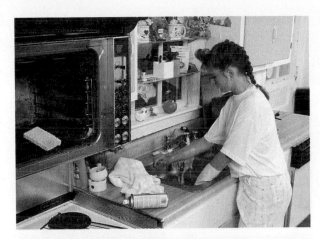

Figure 8-29 Flush a chemical burn with cool running water.

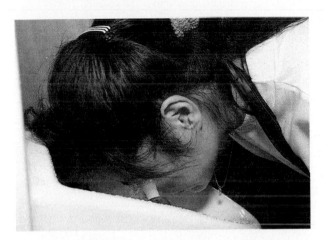

Figure 8-30 Flush the affected eye with cool water in the case of a chemical burn to the eye. Some facilities may have special eyewash stations.

flush the affected eye until EMS personnel arrive (Fig. 8-30).

Electrical burns

The human body is a good conductor of electricity. When someone comes in contact with an electrical source, such as a power line, a malfunctioning household appliance, or lightning, he or she conducts the electricity through the body. Some body parts, such as the skin, resist the electrical current. Resistance produces heat, which can cause burn injuries (Fig. 8-31). The severity of an electrical

burn depends on the type and amount of contact, the current's path through the body, and how long the contact lasted. Electrical burns are often deep. The victim will have both an entrance and an exit wound. Although these wounds may look superficial, the tissues below may be severely damaged.

Electrical injuries cause problems in addition to burns. Electricity can make the heart beat erratically or even stop. Respiratory arrest may occur. Suspect a possible electrical injury if you hear a sudden loud pop or bang and/or see an unexpected flash.

The signals of electrical injury include—

- Unconsciousness.
- Dazed, confused behavior.
- Obvious burns on the skin surface.
- Breathing difficulty.
- Weak, irregular, or absent pulse.
- Burns both where the current entered and where it exited, often on the hand or foot.

Never approach a victim of an electrical injury until you are sure the power is turned off. If there is a downed power line, *wait for the fire department and the power company*. If people are in a car with a downed wire across it, tell them to stay in the vehicle.

To care for a victim of an electrical injury, make sure the scene is safe. Call EMS person-

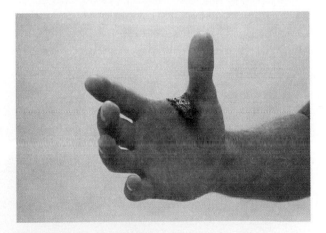

Figure 8-31 An electrical burn may severely damage underlying tissues.

Striking Distance

In medieval times, people believed that ringing church bells would dissipate lightning during thunderstorms. It was an unfortunate superstition for the bell ringers. Over 33 years, lightning struck 386 church steeples and 103 bell ringers died.[1]

Church bell ringers have dropped off the list of people most likely to be struck during a thunderstorm, but lightning strikes remain extremely dangerous. Lightning causes more deaths annually in the United States than any other weather hazard, including blizzards, hurricanes, floods, tornadoes, earthquakes, and volcanic eruptions. The National Weather Service estimates that lightning kills nearly 100 people annually and injures about 300 others. Lightning occurs when particles of water, ice, and air moving inside storm clouds lose electrons. Eventually, the cloud becomes divided into layers of positive and negative particles. Most electrical currents run between the layers inside the cloud. However, occasionally, the negative charge flashes toward the ground, which has a positive charge. An electrical current snakes back and forth between the ground and the cloud many times in the seconds that we see a flash crackle down from the sky. Anything tall—a tower, a tree, or a person—becomes a path for the electrical current.

Traveling at speeds up to 300 miles per second, a lightning strike can hurl a person through the air, burn his or her clothes off, and sometimes cause the heart to stop beating. The most severe lightning strikes carry up to 50 million volts of electricity, enough to keep 13,000 homes running. Lightning can "flash" over a person's body, or, in its more dangerous path, it can travel through blood vessels and nerves to reach the ground.

Besides burns, lightning can also cause neurologic damage, fractures, and loss of hearing or eyesight. The victim sometimes acts confused and amnesiac and may describe the episode as getting hit on the head or hearing an explosion.

Use common sense around thunderstorms. If you see a storm approaching in the distance, do not wait until you are drenched to seek shelter.

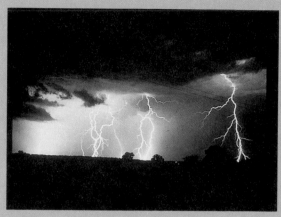

From National Oceanic and Atmospheric Adminstration (NOAA).

If a thunderstorm threatens, the National Weather Service advises you to—

♦ Go inside a large building or home.
♦ Get inside a car and roll up the windows.
♦ Stop swimming or boating as soon as you see or hear a storm. Water conducts electricity.
♦ Stay away from the telephone, except in an emergency.
♦ Stay away from telephone poles and tall trees if you are caught outside.
♦ Stay off hilltops; try to crouch down in a ravine or valley.
♦ Stay away from farm equipment and small metal vehicles such as motorcycles, bicycles, and golf carts.
♦ Avoid wire fences, clotheslines, metal pipes and rails, and other conductors.
♦ Stay several yards apart if you are in a group.

REFERENCES
1. Kessler, Edwin. *The Thunderstorm in Human Affairs*, Norman, Oklahoma: University of Oklahoma, 1983.
2. Randall, Teri. "50 million volts may crash through a lightning victim," *The Chicago Tribune*, Section 2D, August 13, 1989, p. 1.

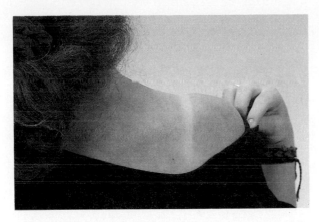

Figure 8-32 Solar radiation burns can be painful.

nel immediately. Do a primary survey. The victim may have breathing difficulties or be in cardiac arrest. Give care for any life-threatening conditions.

In the secondary survey, look for two burn sites. Cover any burn injuries with a dry, sterile dressing, and give care for shock.

With a victim of lightning, look for life-threatening conditions such as respiratory or cardiac arrest. The victim may also have fractures, including spinal fracture, so do not move him or her. Any burns are a lesser problem.

Radiation burns

Both the solar radiation of the sun and other types of radiation can cause burns. Solar burns are similar to heat burns. Usually they are mild but can be painful (Fig. 8-32). They may blister, involving more than one layer of skin. Care for sunburns as you would any other burn. Cool the burn and protect the burned area from further damage by staying out of the sun. People are rarely exposed to other types of radiation unless working in special settings such as certain medical, industrial, or research settings. If you work in such set-

tings, you will be informed and will be required to take precautions to prevent overexposure. Training is also provided to teach you how to prevent and respond to such emergencies.

◆ Summary

Caring for wounds does not require a high degree of skill. You need only follow the basic guidelines to control bleeding and minimize the risk of infection. Remember that with minor wounds your primary concern is to cleanse the wound to prevent infection. With major wounds, you should control the bleeding quickly and seek medical attention. Dressings and bandages, when correctly applied, help control bleeding, reduce pain, and can minimize the danger of infection.

Burn injuries damage the layers of the skin and sometimes the internal structures as well. Heat, chemicals, electricity, and radiation all cause burns. When caring for a burn victim, always first ensure your personal safety. When the scene is safe, approach the victim and do a primary survey and a secondary survey if necessary. Follow the four steps for burn care: (1) Cool the burned area with water to minimize additional tissue destruction. (2) Keep air away from the burned area by covering it with dry, sterile dressings. Cover extensive burns with dry, clean sheets or other cloth. (3) Take appropriate measures to prevent infection. (4) Maintain the victim's body temperature to minimize shock. In addition, always check for inhalation injury if the person has a heat or chemical burn. With electrical burns, check carefully for additional problems such as breathing difficulty, cardiac problems, and fractures.

In the next chapter, you will learn how to provide care for injuries involving muscles and bones.

Answer to Application Question

1. Swelling occurs when blood vessels and tissues are damaged, causing blood and other fluids to leak into the damaged area. Elevation raises the injured part above the level of the heart. Blood flow to the area slows as blood tries to flow against the force of gravity. This reduces bleeding and swelling in the injured area.

Study Questions

1. Match each term with the correct definition.

a. Soft tissue   d. Open wound
b. Critical burn   e. Bandages
c. Closed wound   f. Full-thickness burn

_____ Any burn that is potentially life-threatening, disabling, or disfiguring.
_____ A burn that destroys skin and underlying tissues.
_____ The layers of the skin, fat, and muscles.
_____ Wrappings that hold dressings in place.
_____ Injury resulting in tissue damage beneath the skin's surface, while the skin remains intact.
_____ Injury resulting in blood loss and tissue damage through a break in the skin.

2. Match each type of injury to its example.

a. Abrasion   _____ Torn earlobe
b. Avulsion   _____ Black eye
c. Puncture   _____ Scraped knee
d. Bruise   _____ Gunshot wound

3. Match each type of wound with the appropriate care.

a. A major open wound
b. A major open wound with an impaled object
c. A minor open wound
d. A severed body part

_____ Cover with dressing and pressure bandage.
_____ Wash the wound thoroughly with soap and water.
_____ Wrap and place on ice.
_____ Use bulky dressings to stabilize.

4. List four signals of infection.

5. List two purposes of bandaging.

6. List and describe four types of open wounds.

7. List four causes of burn injury.

8. List three types of burn injury.

In questions 9 through 23, circle the letter of the correct answer.

9. To protect a minor open wound from infection—

    a. Wash the area with soap and water.
    b. Apply a clean covering.
    c. Apply an antibiotic ointment.
    d. b and c
    e. a, b, and c

10. Signals of infection include—

    a. Swelling or reddening around the wound.
    b. A throbbing pain.
    c. A cool sensation.
    d. a and b
    e. a, b, and c

11. Caring for an infected wound includes—

    a. Keeping the area clean.
    b. Seeking medical help if the infection persists.
    c. Applying warm, wet compresses.
    d. Applying an antibiotic ointment.
    e. All of the above

12. Closed wounds—

    a. Can result from force exerted on the body by a blunt object.
    b. Are at a high risk for infection.
    c. Often produce swelling and discoloration of the area.
    d. a and c
    e. a, b, and c

13. The differences that distinguish major open wounds from minor open wounds
are —

    a. The severity of bleeding.
    b. The depth of tissue damage.
    c. The amount of pain that the victim is experiencing.
    d. a and b
    e. a, b, and c

14. In caring for major open wounds, you should—

    a. Apply a dressing and control bleeding.
    b. Wash the wound.
    c. Recommend to the victim that he or she get a tetanus booster shot, if necessary.
    d. a and c
    e. a, b, and c

15. When caring for an injury in which the body part has been completely severed, you should—

    a. Place the part directly on ice.
    b. Seek medical assistance and make sure the part is transported with the victim.
    c. Wash the body part thoroughly with soap and water.
    d. b and c
    e. a, b, and c

16. Immunizations—

    a. Provide lifetime protection against all threats of infection.
    b. Prepare your body to defend against certain infections.
    c. Stimulate the body to produce more blood.
    d. a and c
    e. a, b, and c

17. When caring for an injury with an impaled object, you should—

a. Remove the object.
b. Allow the area to bleed freely.
c. Stabilize the object in the position you find it.
d. b and c
e. a, b, and c

18. When applying bandages—

a. Cover the dressing completely.
b. Cover fingers or toes.
c. Remove any blood-soaked bandages and apply new ones.
d. a and c
e. a, b, and c

19. Swelling and discoloration may signal—

a. A closed wound.
b. Damage to underlying structures.
c. Internal bleeding.
d. Infection.
e. All of the above

20. Care for closed wounds includes—

a. Using a warm compress to control pain and swelling.
b. Applying cold and elevating the injured area.
c. Keeping the injured area below the level of the heart.
d. a and b
e. None of the above

21. In caring for an electrical burn injury, you must first—

a. Remove the victim from the power source.
b. Do a primary survey.
c. Make sure the power source is turned off.
d. Look for two burn sites.

22. Burns that require professional medical attention—

   a. Cover more than one body part.
   b. Are those resulting from electricity, explosions, or chemicals.
   c. Are burns whose victims are having difficulty breathing.
   d. a and c
   e. a, b, and c

23. The chemist at the lab table near you spills a corrosive chemical on his arm. You should first—

   a. Remove the chemical with a clean cloth.
   b. Put a sterile dressing over the burn site.
   c. Flush the burn with water.
   d. Have the victim remove contaminated clothes.

Answers are in Appendix A.

PRACTICE SESSION: *Caring for a Major Open Wound (Forearm)*

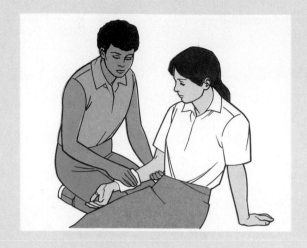

☐ **Apply direct pressure**
* Place sterile dressing or clean cloth over wound.
* Press firmly against wound with your hand.

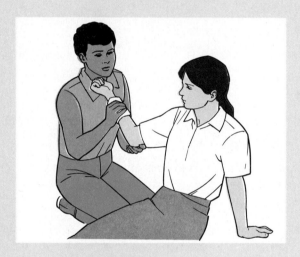

☐ **Elevate body part**
* Raise wound above level of heart, if possible.

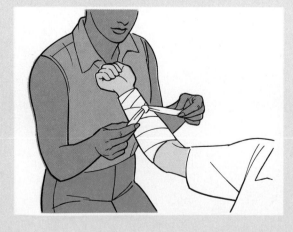

☐ **Apply a pressure bandage**
* Using a roller bandage, cover dressing completely, using overlapping turns.
* Tie or tape bandage in place.
* If blood soaks through the bandage, place additional dressings and bandage over the wound.

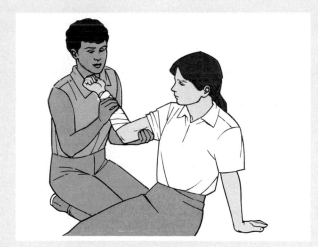

☐ Apply pressure to a pressure point

- Maintain direct pressure and elevation.
- Locate brachial artery.
- Apply pressure to brachial artery by squeezing artery against underlying bone.

☐ Take steps to minimize shock

- Maintain direct pressure, elevation, and pressure point.
- Position person on back.
- Monitor ABCs.
- Maintain normal body temperature.
- Apply additional dressings and/or bandages as necessary.

PRACTICE SESSION: *Caring for a Major Open Wound (Leg)*

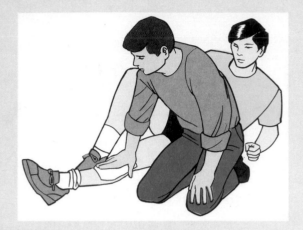

☐ Apply direct pressure

- Place sterile dressing or clean cloth over wound.
- Press firmly against wound with your hand.

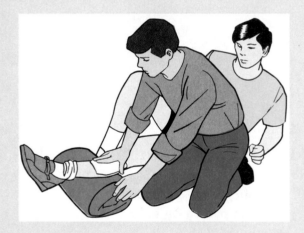

☐ Elevate body part

- Raise wound above level of heart, if possible.

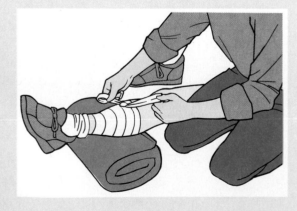

☐ Apply a pressure bandage

- Using a roller bandage, cover dressing completely, using overlapping turns.
- Tie or tape bandage in place.
- If blood soaks through the bandage, place additional dressings and bandage over the wound.

If bleeding stops. . .
* Determine if further care is needed.

If bleeding does not stop. . .
* Send someone to call for an ambulance.

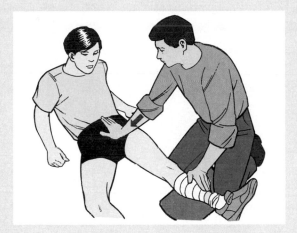

☐ Apply pressure to a pressure point

* Maintain direct pressure and elevation.
* Locate femoral artery.
* Apply pressure to femoral artery by squeezing artery against underlying bone.

☐ Take steps to minimize shock

* Maintain direct pressure, elevation, and pressure point.
* Position person on back.
* Monitor ABCs.
* Maintain normal body temperature.
* Apply additional dressings and/or bandages as necessary.

Musculoskeletal Injuries

For Review

Before reading this chapter, you should have a basic understanding of the anatomy of the musculoskeletal system and how the muscles, bones, and other tissues function to move the body (Chapter 2). You should understand how the musculoskeletal system interacts with the nervous system. You should also know how to perform a secondary survey (Chapter 3).

◆ Introduction

Injuries to the musculoskeletal system are common. Millions of people at home, at work, or at play, injure their **muscles, bones,** or **joints.** No age group is immune. A person may fall and bruise the muscles of the hip, making walking painful. Heavy machinery may fall on a worker and break ribs, making breathing difficult. A person who braces a hand against a dashboard in a car crash may injure the bones at the shoulder, disabling the arm. A person who falls while skiing may twist a leg, tearing the supportive tissues of a knee and making it impossible to stand or move.

Although musculoskeletal injuries are almost always painful, they are rarely life-threatening. However, when not recognized and taken care of properly, they can have serious consequences and even result in permanent disability. In this chapter, you will learn how to recognize and care for musculoskeletal injuries. Developing a better understanding of the structure and function of the body's framework will help you assess musculoskeletal injuries and give appropriate care.

◆ Musculoskeletal System

The musculoskeletal system is made up of muscles and bones that form the skeleton, and the connective tissues, the **tendons** and **ligaments**. Together, these structures give the body shape, form, and stability. Bones and muscles connect to form various body segments. They work together to provide body movements.

Muscles

Muscles are soft tissues. The body has over 600 muscles (see Figure 9-1 on the next page). Most are **skeletal muscles,** which attach to the bones. Skeletal muscles account for most of your lean body weight (body weight without excess fat).

Unlike the other soft tissues, muscles are able to contract (shorten) and relax (lengthen).

FRONT VIEW   **BACK VIEW**

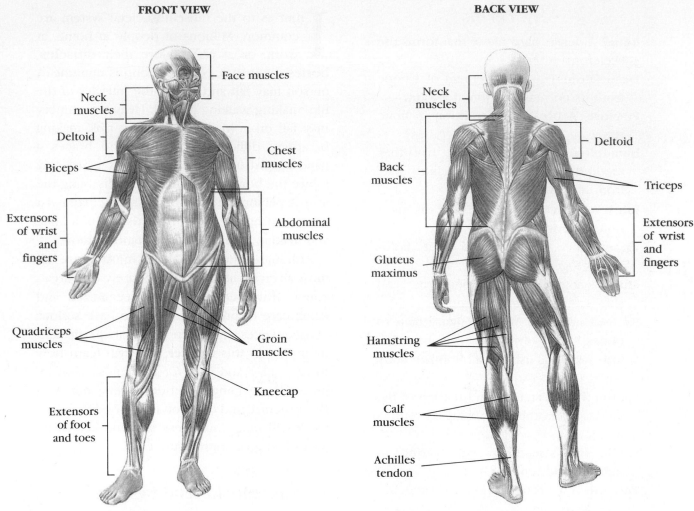

Figure 9-1   Skeletal muscles, muscles that attach to bones, comprise the majority of the body's muscles.

All body movements result from skeletal muscles contracting and relaxing. Through a pathway of nerves, the brain directs muscles to move. Skeletal muscle actions are under your conscious control. Because you move them voluntarily, skeletal muscles are also called voluntary muscles. Skeletal muscles also protect the bones, nerves, and blood vessels.

Most skeletal muscles are anchored to bone at each end by strong, cordlike tissues called tendons. Muscles and their adjoining tendons extend across joints. When the brain sends a command to move, electrical impulses travel through the spinal cord and nerve pathways to the individual muscles and stimulate the muscle fibers to contract. When a muscle contracts, the muscle fibers shorten, pulling the ends of the muscle closer together. The muscles pull the bones, causing motion at the joint.

Motion is usually caused by a group of muscles close together pulling at the same time. For instance, the "hamstring" muscles are a group of muscles at the back of the thigh. When the hamstrings contract, the leg bends at the knee. The "biceps" are a group of mus-

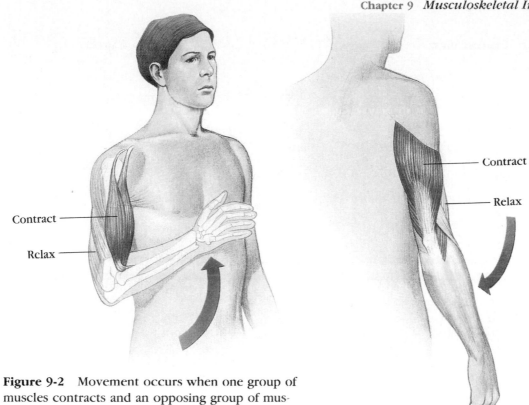

Figure 9-2 Movement occurs when one group of muscles contracts and an opposing group of muscles relaxes.

cles at the front of the arm. When the biceps contract, the arm bends at the elbow. Generally, when one group of muscles contracts, another group of muscles on the opposite side of the body part relaxes (Fig. 9-2). Even simple tasks, such as bending to pick up an object from the floor, involve a complex series of movements in which different muscle groups contract and relax.

Injuries to the brain, the spinal cord, or the nerves can affect muscle control. A loss of muscle control is called paralysis. Less serious or isolated muscle injuries may only affect strength because adjacent muscles can often assume the function of the injured muscle (Fig. 9-3).

Skeleton

The skeleton is formed by over 200 bones of various sizes and shapes (see Figure 9-4 on the next page). These bones shape the skeleton, giving each body part a unique form. The skeleton protects vital organs and other soft tis-

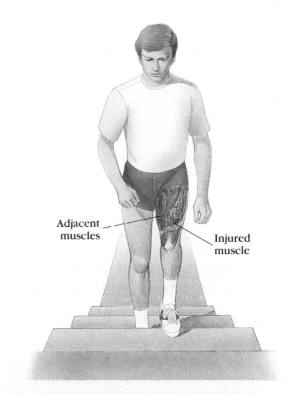

Figure 9-3 Adjacent muscles can often assume the function of an injured muscle.

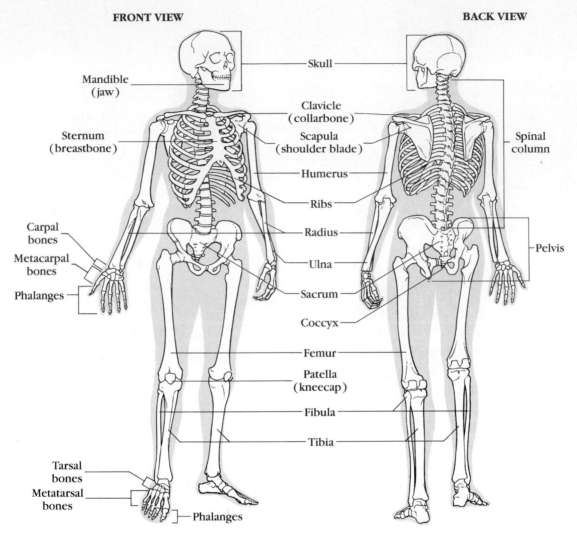

FRONT VIEW

BACK VIEW

Mandible (jaw)

Skull

Clavicle (collarbone)

Sternum (breastbone)

Scapula (shoulder blade)

Spinal column

Humerus

Ribs

Carpal bones

Radius

Metacarpal bones

Ulna

Pelvis

Phalanges

Sacrum

Coccyx

Femur

Patella (kneecap)

Fibula

Tibia

Tarsal bones

Metatarsal bones

Phalanges

Figure 9-4 The bones of the skeleton give the body its shape and protect vital organs.

sues. The skull protects the brain (Fig. 9-5, *A*). The ribs protect the heart and lungs (Fig. 9-5, *B*). The spinal cord is protected by the canal formed by the bones that form the spinal column (Fig. 9-5, *C*). Two or more bones come together to form joints. Ligaments, fibrous bands that hold bones together at joints, give the skeleton stability and, with the muscles, help maintain posture.

Bones

Bones are hard, dense tissues. Their strong, rigid structure helps them to withstand stresses that cause injuries. The shape of bones depends on what the bones do and the

stresses on them. For instance, the surfaces of bones at the joints are smooth (Fig. 9-6). Although similar to the bones of the arm, the bones of the legs are much larger and stronger because they carry the body's weight (Fig. 9-7).

Bones have a rich supply of blood and nerves. Some bones store and manufacture red blood cells and supply them to the circulating blood. Bone injuries can bleed and are usually painful. The bleeding can become life-threatening if not properly cared for. Bones heal by forming new bone cells. Bone is the only body tissue that can regenerate in this way.

Bones weaken with age. Bones in young

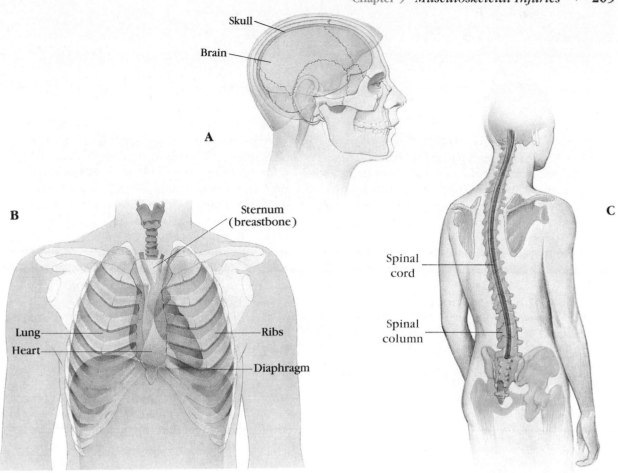

Figure 9-5 **A,** The immovable bones of the skull protect the brain. **B,** The rib cage protects the lungs and heart. **C,** The spinal cord is protected by the vertebrae.

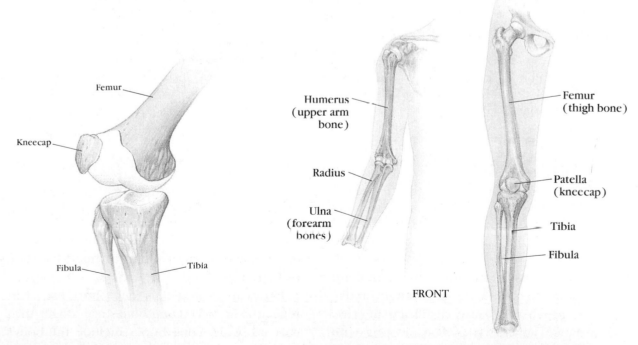

Figure 9-6 Bone surfaces at the joints are smooth.

Figure 9-7 Leg bones are larger and stronger than arm bones because they carry the body's weight.

The Breaking Point

Osteoporosis, a degenerative bone disorder usually discovered after the age of 60, affects 30 percent of people over age 65. It will affect one out of four American women and occur less frequently in men. Fair-skinned women with ancestors from northern Europe, the British Isles, Japan, or China are genetically predisposed to osteoporosis. Inactive people are more susceptible to osteoporosis.

Osteoporosis occurs when there is a decrease in the calcium content of bones. Normally, bones are hard, dense tissues that endure tremendous stresses. Bone-building cells constantly repair damage that occurs as a result of everyday stresses, keeping bones strong. Calcium is a key to bone growth, development, and repair. When the calcium content of bones decreases, bones become frail, less dense, and less able to repair the normal damage they incur.

This loss of density and strength leaves bones more susceptible to fractures. Where once tremendous force was necessary, fractures may now occur with little or no aggravation, especially to hips, vertebrae, and wrists. Spontaneous fractures are those that occur without trauma. The victim may be taking a walk or washing dishes when the fracture occurs. Some hip fractures thought to be caused by falls are actually spontaneous fractures that caused the victim's fall.

Osteoporosis can begin as early as age 30 to 35. The amount of calcium absorbed from the diet naturally declines with age, making calcium intake increasingly important. When calcium in the diet is inadequate, calcium in bones is withdrawn and used by the body to meet its other needs, leaving bones weakened.

Building strong bones before age 35 is the key to preventing osteoporosis. Calcium and exercise are necessary to bone building. The United States Recommended Daily Allowance (U.S. RDA) is currently 800 milligrams of calcium each day for adults. Many physicians recommend 1,000 milligrams for women age 19 and over. Three to four daily servings of low-fat dairy products should provide adequate calcium. Vitamin D is also necessary because it aids in absorption of calcium. Exposure to sunshine enables the body to make vitamin D. Fifteen minutes of sunshine on the hands and face of a young, light-skinned individual are enough to supply the RDA of 5 to 10 micrograms of vitamin D per day. Dark-skinned and elderly people need more sun exposure. People who do not receive adequate sun exposure need to consume vitamin D. The best sources are vitamin-fortified milk and fatty fish such as tuna, salmon, and eel.

Calcium supplements combined with vitamin D are available for those who do not take in adequate calcium. However, before taking a calcium supplement, consult a physician. Many highly advertised calcium supplements are ineffective because they do not dissolve in the body.

Exercise seems to increase bone density and the activity of bone-building cells. Regular exercise may reduce the rate of bone loss by promoting new bone formation and also stimulate the skeletal system to repair itself. An effective exercise program, such as aerobics, jogging, or walking, involves the weight-bearing muscles of the legs.

If you have any questions regarding your health and osteoporosis, consult your physician. Take care of your bones and don't let osteoporosis get you down.

---

children are more flexible than adults' bones, so they are less likely to break. In contrast, elderly people have more brittle bones that are more likely to give way to even everyday stresses, which can cause significant injuries. For instance, an elderly person pivoting with the weight on one leg can break the strongest bone in the body, the thigh bone. This gradual, progressive weakening of bone is called osteoporosis.

Bones are classified as long, short, flat, or irregular (Fig. 9-8). Long bones are longer than they are wide. Long bones include the bones of the upper arm (humerus), the forearm (ra-

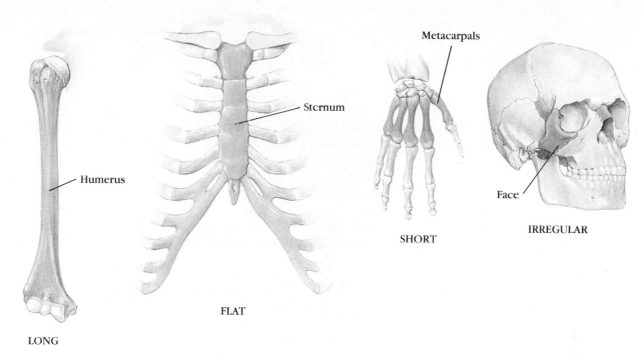

Figure 9-8 Bones vary in shape and size. Bones are weakest at the points where they change shape and usually fracture at these points.

dius, ulna), the thigh (femur), and lower leg (tibia, fibula). Short bones are about as wide as they are long. Short bones include the small bones of the hand (metacarpals) and feet (metatarsals). Flat bones have a relatively thin, flat shape. Flat bones include the breastbone (sternum), the ribs, the shoulder blade (scapula), and some of the bones that make up the skull. Bones that do not fit in the other categories are called irregular bones. Irregular bones include the vertebrae and the bones of the face. Bones are weakest at the points where they change shape and usually fracture at these points.

Joints

A joint is a structure formed by the ends of two or more bones coming together at one place. Most joints allow motion. However, the bone ends at some joints are fused together, which restricts motion. Fused bones, such as the bones of the skull, form solid structures that protect their contents (Fig. 9-9).

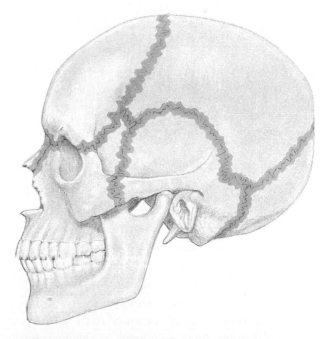

Figure 9-9 Fused bones, such as the bones of the skull, form solid structures that protect their contents.

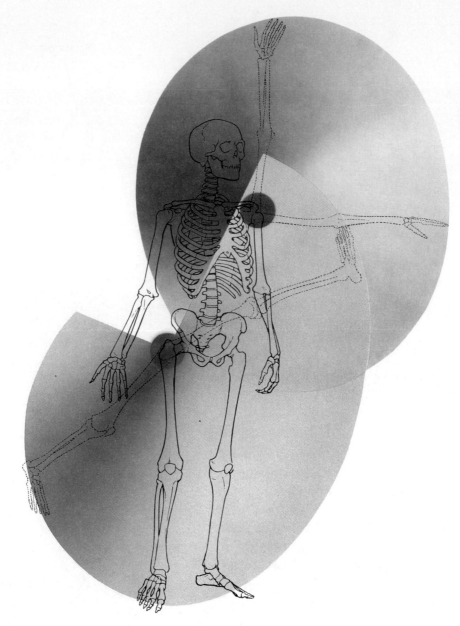

Figure 9-10   The shoulder joint, which has few ligaments, allows greater range of motion than the hip joint, although their structure is similar.

Joints are held together by tough, fibrous connective tissues called ligaments. Ligaments resist joint movement. Joints surrounded by ligaments have restricted movement; joints that have few ligaments move more freely. For instance, the shoulder joint, with few ligaments, allows greater motion than the hip joint, although their structure is similar (Fig. 9-10). Joint motion also depends on the bone structure.

Joints that move more freely have less nat-ural support and are therefore more prone to injury. However, all joints have a normal range of movement. When a joint is forced be-yond its normal range, ligaments stretch and tear. Stretched and torn ligaments permit too much motion, making the joint unstable. Un-stable joints can be disabling, particularly when they are weight-bearing, such as the knee or ankle. Unstable joints are also prone to reinjury and often develop arthritis in later years.

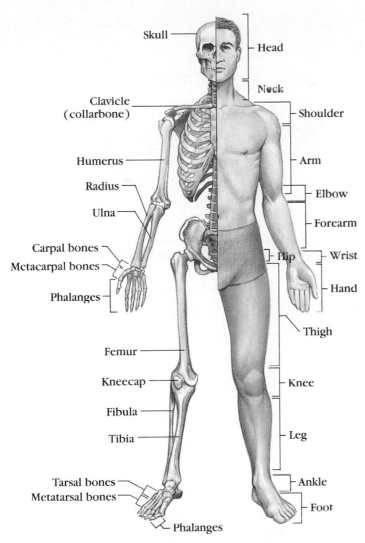

Figure 9-11 Bones that can be seen and felt beneath the skin provide landmarks for locating parts of the body.

Parts of the skeleton

The bony structures that form the skeleton define the parts of the body. For example, the head is defined by the bones that form the skull, and the chest is defined by the bones that form the rib cage. Prominent bones, bones that can be seen or felt beneath the skin, provide landmarks for locating parts of the body, as illustrated in Figure 9-11.

◆ Injuries to the Musculoskeletal System

Injuries to the musculoskeletal system occur in a variety of ways. They are more commonly

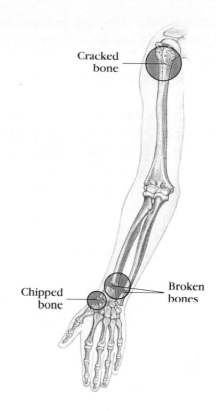

Figure 9-12 Fractures include chipped or cracked bones and bones broken all the way through.

caused by forces generated by mechanical forms of energy but can also occur from heat, chemical, or electrical forms of energy.

Types of Musculoskeletal Injuries

The four basic types of musculoskeletal injuries are—**fracture, dislocation, sprain,** and **strain.** Injuries to the musculoskeletal system can be classified according to the body structures that are damaged. Some injuries may involve more than one type of injury. For example, a direct blow to the knee may injure both ligaments and bones. Injuries are also classified by the nature and extent of the damage.

Fracture

A fracture is a break or disruption in bone tissue. Fractures include chipped or cracked bones, as well as bones that are broken all the way through (Fig. 9-12). Fractures are commonly caused by direct and indirect forces.

However, if strong enough, twisting forces and strong muscle contractions can cause a fracture.

Fractures are classified as open or closed. An open fracture involves an open wound. Open fractures often occur when the limb is severely angulated or bent, causing bone ends to tear the skin and surrounding soft tissues, or when an object penetrates the skin and breaks the bone. Bone ends do not have to be visible for a fracture to be classified as open. Closed fractures leave the skin unbroken and are more common than open fractures. Open fractures are more serious than closed fractures because of the risks of infection and severe blood loss. Although fractures are rarely an immediate threat to life, any fracture involving a large bone can cause severe shock because bones and soft tissue may bleed heavily.

Fractures are not always obvious unless there is a telltale sign such as an open wound with protruding bone ends or a severely deformed body part. But the way in which the injury occurred is often enough to suggest a possible fracture.

Dislocation

A dislocation is a displacement or separation of a bone from its normal position at a joint (Fig. 9-13). Dislocations are usually caused by severe forces. Some joints, such as the shoulder or fingers, dislocate easily because their bones and ligaments do not provide adequate protection. Others, such as the elbow or the joints of the spine, are well protected and therefore dislocate less easily.

When bone ends are forced far enough beyond their normal position, ligaments stretch and tear. Subsequent dislocations are then more likely to occur. A force violent enough to cause a dislocation can also cause a fracture and can damage nearby nerves and blood vessels.

Dislocations are generally more obvious than fractures because the joint appears de-

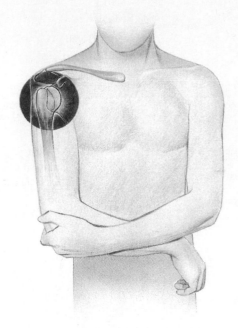

Figure 9-13 A dislocation is a displacement of a bone from its normal position at a joint.

formed (Fig. 9-14). The displaced bone end often causes an abnormal lump, ridge, or depression, sometimes making dislocations easier to identify than other musculoskeletal injuries.

Sprain

A sprain is the partial or complete tearing of ligaments and other tissues at a joint. A sprain usually results when the bones that form a joint are forced beyond their normal range of motion (Fig. 9-15). The more ligaments that are torn, the more severe the injury. The sudden, violent forcing of a joint beyond its limit can completely rupture ligaments and dislocate the bones. Severe sprains may also involve a fracture of the bones that form the joint. Ligaments may pull bone away from its point of attachment.

Mild sprains, which only stretch ligament fibers, generally heal quickly. The victim may

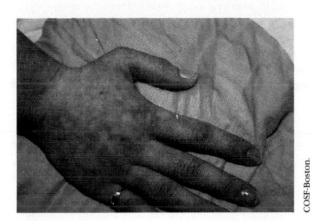

Figure 9-14 Because of deformity, dislocations are generally more obvious than fractures.

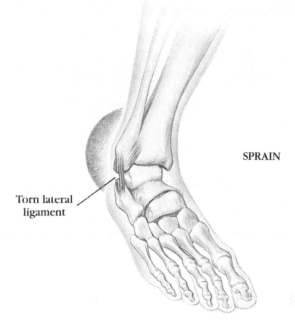

SPRAIN

Torn lateral ligament

Figure 9-15 A sprain results when bones that form a joint are forced beyond their normal range of motion.

have only a brief period of pain or discomfort and quickly return to activity with little or no soreness. For this reason, people often neglect sprains and the joint is often reinjured. Severe sprains or strains that involve a fracture usually cause pain when the joint is moved or used. The weight-bearing joints of the ankle and knee and the joints of the fingers and wrist are those most commonly sprained.

Generally, a sprain is more disabling than a fracture. When fractures heal, they usually leave the bone as strong as it was before, or stronger, thus decreasing the likelihood that a repeat break would occur at the same spot. On the other hand, ligaments cannot regenerate. Once ligaments become stretched or torn, if not repaired, they render the joint less stable, making the injured area more susceptible to repeated injury.

Strains

A strain is a stretching and tearing of muscle or tendon fibers. It is sometimes called a "muscle pull" or "tear." Because tendons are tougher and stronger than muscles, tears usually occur in the muscle itself or where the muscle attaches to the tendon. Strains are often the result of overexertion, such as lifting something too heavy or working a muscle too hard. They can also result from sudden or uncoordinated movement. Strains commonly involve the muscles in the neck or back, the front or back of the thigh, or the back of the lower leg. Strains of the neck and lower back can be particularly painful and therefore disabling.

Like sprains, strains are often neglected, which commonly leads to reinjury. Strains sometimes reoccur chronically, especially to the muscles of the neck, lower back, and the

Sprains and Strains

Spring is the season of flowers, trees, strains, and sprains. Almost as soon as armchair athletes come out of hibernation to become intramural heroes, emergency clinics see an increase in sprained ankles, twisted knees, and strained backs. So what do you do when you attempt the first slide of the softball season and wind up injured? Should you apply heat or apply cold?

The answer is both. First cold, then heat. And it does not matter whether it is a strain or sprain!

How cold helps initially

When a person twists an ankle or strains his or her back, the tissues underneath the skin are injured. Blood and fluids seep out from the torn blood vessels and cause swelling to occur at the site of the injury. By keeping the injured area cool, you can help control internal bleeding and reduce pain. Cold causes the broken blood vessels to constrict, limiting the blood and fluid that seep out. Cold also reduces muscle spasms and numbs the nerve endings.

How heat helps repair the tissue

A physician will most likely advise applying ice to the injury periodically for about 72 hours or until the swelling goes away. After that, applying heat is appropriate. Heat speeds up chemical reactions needed to repair the tissue. White blood cells move in to rid the body of infections, and other cells begin the repair process. This process enhances proper healing of the injury. If you are unsure whether to use cold or heat on an injured area, always apply cold until you can consult your physician.

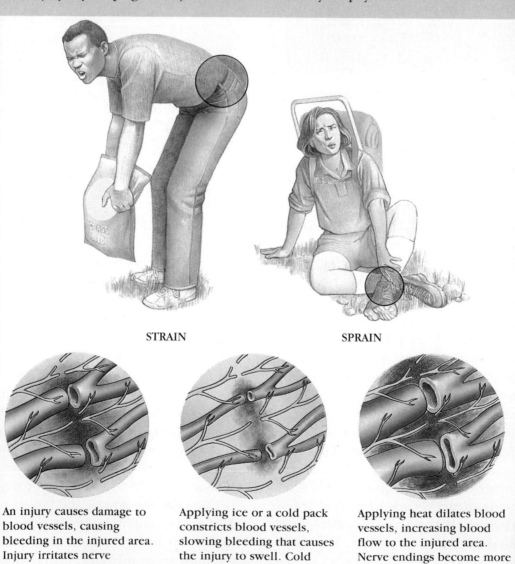

STRAIN

SPRAIN

An injury causes damage to blood vessels, causing bleeding in the injured area. Injury irritates nerve endings, causing pain.

Applying ice or a cold pack constricts blood vessels, slowing bleeding that causes the injury to swell. Cold deadens nerve endings relieving pain.

Applying heat dilates blood vessels, increasing blood flow to the injured area. Nerve endings become more sensitive.

back of the thigh. Neck and back problems are two of the leading causes of absenteeism from work, accounting for more than 15 billion dollars in workman's compensation claims and lost productivity annually.

Q

1. Which do you think is more severe, a strain or sprain? Why?

Signals of Musculoskeletal Injuries

You identify and care for injuries to the musculoskeletal system during the secondary survey. Because they appear similar, it may be difficult for you to determine exactly what type of injury has occurred. As you do the secondary survey, think about how the body normally looks and feels. Ask how the injury happened and if there are any areas that are painful. Visually inspect the entire body, beginning with the head. Then, check each body part by asking if the victim can move without pain or discomfort. Start with the neck, followed by the shoulders, the chest, and so on. As you conduct the secondary survey, look and listen for clues that may indicate a musculoskeletal injury.

Common signals of musculoskeletal injuries

Five common signals associated with musculoskeletal injuries are—

* Pain.
* Swelling.
* Deformity.
* Discoloration of the skin.
* Inability to use the affected part normally.

Pain, swelling, and discoloration of the skin commonly occur with any significant injury. Irritation to nerve endings that supply the injured area causes pain. Pain is the body's signal that something is wrong. The injured area may be painful to touch and to move. Swelling

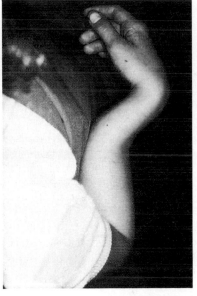

Figure 9-16 Deformity may be obvious when an injured part is compared to an uninjured part.

is caused by bleeding from damaged blood vessels and tissues in the injured area. However, swelling is often deceiving. It may appear rapidly at the site of injury, may develop gradually, or may not appear at all. Swelling by itself, therefore, is not a reliable signal of the severity of an injury or of the structures involved. Bleeding may discolor the skin in surrounding tissues. At first, the skin may only look red. As blood seeps to the skin's surface, the area begins to look bruised.

Deformity is also a signal of significant injury. Swelling, abnormal lumps, ridges, depressions, or unusual bends or angles in body parts are types of deformities. Marked deformity is often a sign of fracture or dislocation. Comparing the injured part to an uninjured part may help you detect deformity (Fig. 9-16).

A victim's inability to move or use an injured part may also indicate a significant injury. The victim may tell you he or she is un-

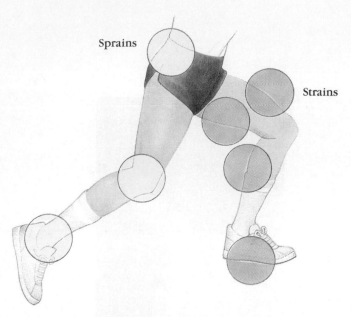

Sprains

Strains

Figure 9-17 Sprains involve the soft tissues at a joint. Strains involve the soft tissue structures that, for the most part, stretch between joints.

able to move, or that it is simply too painful to move. Moving or using injured parts can disturb tissues, further irritating nerve endings, which causes or increases pain. Often, the muscles of an affected area contract in an attempt to hold the injured part in place. This helps to reduce pain and prevent additional damage.

Similarly, a victim often supports the injury in the most comfortable position. To manage musculoskeletal injuries, try to avoid causing pain. Avoid any motion or use of an injured body part that causes pain.

Specific signals of musculoskeletal injuries

In the secondary survey, you may notice certain telltale signals that help you determine the type of injury. Often, what the victim feels or can recall from the moment of injury provides important clues.

Sprains or strains are fairly easy to tell apart. Because a sprain involves the soft tissues at a joint, pain, swelling, and deformity are generally confined to the joint area. Strains involve the soft tissue structures that, for the most

part, stretch between joints. In most strains, pain, swelling, and any deformity are generally in the areas between the joints (Fig. 9-17).

However, it is not always easy to determine if an injury involves a fracture or dislocation. Sometimes, the only reliable way to determine the nature of the injury is by x-ray. Always suspect a serious injury when the following signals are present:

* Significant deformity
* Moderate or severe swelling and discoloration
* Inability to move or use the affected body part
* Bone fragments protruding from a wound
* Victim feels bones grating, or felt or heard a snap or pop at the time of injury
* Loss of circulation in an extremity
* Cause of the injury suggests the injury may be severe

◆ Care for Musculoskeletal Injuries

Some musculoskeletal injuries are obvious because they involve severe deformities such as protruding bones or bleeding. The victim may also be in much pain. Do not be distracted. Such injuries are rarely life-threatening. Complete the primary survey and care first for any life-threatening conditions. Then do the secondary survey and care for any other injuries. When you find a musculoskeletal injury, call EMS personnel if—

* The injury involves the head, neck, or back.
* The injury impairs walking or breathing.
* You see or suspect multiple musculoskeletal injuries.

General Care

The general care for all musculoskeletal injuries is similar. Just remember, rest, ice, and elevation (Fig. 9-18).

Rest

Avoid any movements or activities that cause pain. Help the victim find the most com-

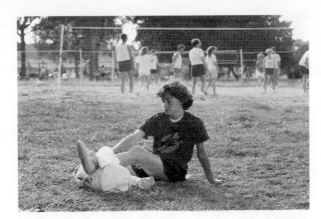

Figure 9-18 General care for all musculoskeletal injuries is similar. Remember rest, ice, and elevation.

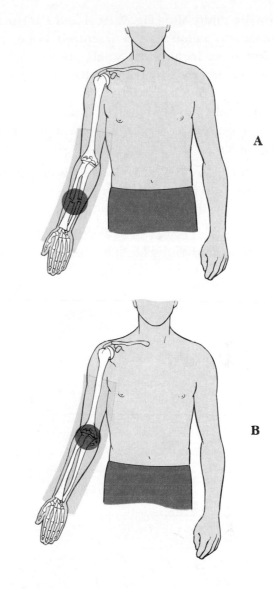

Figure 9-19 **A,** To immobilize a bone, splint the joints above and below the fracture. **B,** To immobilize a joint, splint the bones above and below the injured joint.

fortable position. If you suspect head, neck, or back injuries, leave the victim lying flat.

Ice

Regardless of whether the injury is a closed fracture, dislocation, sprain, or strain, apply ice or a cold pack. Cold helps reduce swelling and eases pain and discomfort. Place a layer of gauze or cloth between the source of cold and the skin to prevent damage to the skin. You can make an ice pack by placing ice in a plastic bag and wrapping it with a towel or cloth. Do not apply a cold pack to an open fracture because doing so would require you to put pressure on the open fracture site and could cause discomfort to the victim.

Elevation

Elevating the injured area helps slow the flow of blood, reducing swelling. If possible, elevate the injured area above the level of the heart. Do not attempt to elevate a part you suspect is fractured until it has been splinted.

Immobilization

If you suspect a serious musculoskeletal injury, you must immobilize the injured part before giving additional care such as applying ice or elevating the injured part.

The purposes of **immobilizing** an injury are to—

- Lessen pain.
- Prevent further damage to soft tissues.
- Reduce the risk of serious bleeding.
- Reduce the possibility of loss of circulation to the injured part.
- Prevent closed fractures from becoming open fractures.

You can immobilize an injured part by applying a **splint,** sling, or bandages to keep the injured body part from moving. A splint is a device that maintains an injured part in place. An effective splint must extend above and below the injury site (Fig. 9-19, *A* and *B).* For instance, to immobilize a fractured bone, the splint must include the joints above and below the fracture. To immobilize a sprain or dislocation, the splint must include the bones above and below the injured joint.

When using a splint, follow these four basic principles:

- Splint only if you can do it without causing more pain and discomfort to the victim.
- Splint an injury in the position you find it.
- Splint the injured area and the joints above and below the injury site.
- Check for proper circulation before and after splinting.

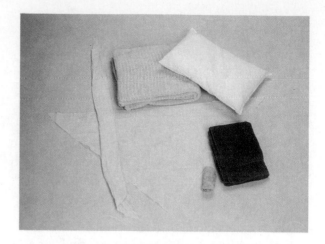

Figure 9-20 Soft splints include a folded blanket, a towel, a pillow, and a sling or cravat.

A
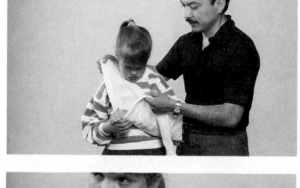

B
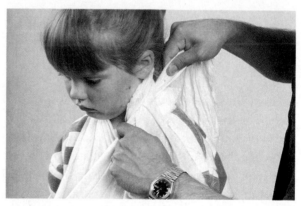

C
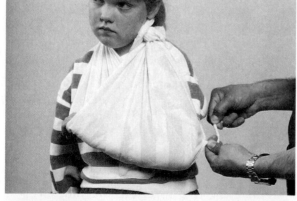

D
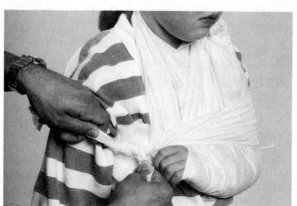

E
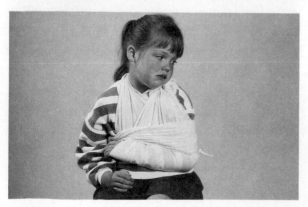

Figure 9-21 Triangular bandages can be tied to support the arm. **A,** While the victim supports her arm, position the bandage. **B,** Tie both ends at the side of the neck. Pad the knot. **C,** Secure the bandage at the elbow. **D,** Use a cravat to hold the arm in place against the chest. **E,** A finished sling will support the injured arm.

Types of Splints

Splints, whether commercially made or improvised, are of three types—soft, rigid, and anatomic. Soft splints include folded blankets, towels, pillows, and a sling or cravats (Fig. 9-20). A sling is a triangular bandage tied to support an arm, wrist, or hand (Fig. 9-21, *A-E*). A cravat is a folded triangular bandage used to hold dressings or splints in place. A wad of cloth and bandages can serve as effective splints for small body parts such as the hand or fingers (Fig. 9-22).

Rigid splints include boards, metal strips, and folded magazines or newspapers (Fig. 9-23). Anatomic splints refer to the use of the body as a splint. You may not ordinarily think of the body as a splint, but it works very well. For example, an arm can be splinted to the chest. An injured leg can be splinted to the uninjured leg (Fig. 9-24).

As a citizen responder, you are unlikely to have commercial splints immediately available to you. If they are available, however, you should become familiar with them before you have to use them. Commercial splints include

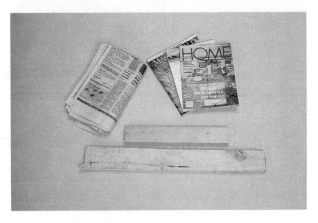

Figure 9-23 Rigid splints include boards, metal strips, and folded magazines or newspapers.

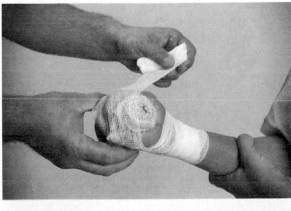

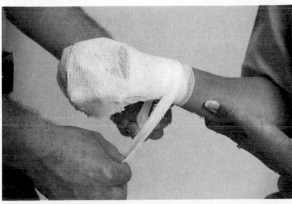

Figure 9-22 A wad of cloth and bandages can effectively splint small body parts.

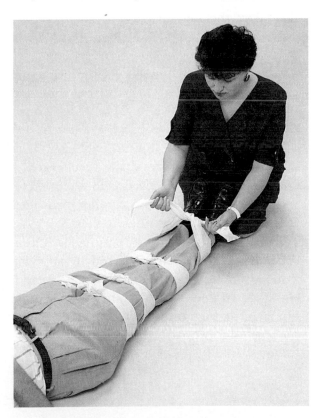

Figure 9-24 An injured leg can be splinted to the uninjured leg.

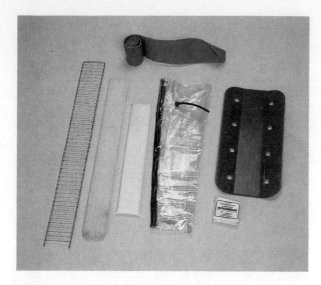

Figure 9-25 Commercial splints.

padded board splints, air splints, and specially designed flexible splints (Fig. 9-25).

To splint an injured body part—

1. Support the injured part. If possible, have the victim or a bystander help you (Fig. 9-26, *A)*.
2. Cover any open wounds with a dressing and bandage to help control bleeding and prevent infection.
3. If using a rigid splint, pad the splint so that it is shaped to the injured part (Fig. 9-26, *B)*. This will help prevent further injury.
4. Secure the splint in place with folded triangular bandages (cravats), roller bandages, or other wide strips of cloth (Fig. 9-26, *C)*.
5. Check fingers or toes to ensure that circulation has not been restricted by applying the splint too tightly. Loosen the splint if the victim complains of numbness, or if the fingers or toes discolor (turn blue) or become cold.
6. Elevate the splinted part, if possible.

After the injury has been immobilized, recheck the ABCs. Help the victim rest in the most comfortable position, apply ice or a cold pack, maintain normal body temperature, and reassure him or her. Determine what additional care is needed and whether to call EMS personnel for an ambulance. Continue to monitor the victim's level of consciousness, breathing, and skin color. Be alert for signals, such as shock, that may indicate the victim's condition is worsening.

◆ Considerations for Transporting a Victim

Some musculoskeletal injuries are obviously minor and do not require professional medical care. Others are obviously more serious and may require you to call EMS personnel. If you discover a life-threatening emergency or think it likely one might develop, call EMS personnel and wait for help. Always call EMS personnel for any injury involving severe bleeding, injuries to the head, neck, or back, and possible broken bones that may be difficult to transport properly, such as the hip and legs. Fractures of large bones can bleed a lot and are likely to cause shock.

Some injuries are not serious enough for you to call EMS personnel but still require professional medical care. If you decide to transport the victim yourself to a medical facility, follow the general rule: "When in doubt, splint." Always splint the injury before moving the victim. If possible, have someone drive you so you can continue to provide care.

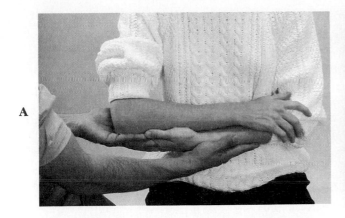

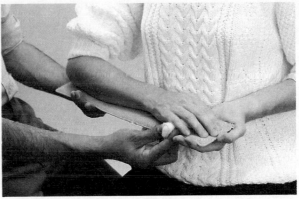

Figure 9-26 A, Support the arm above and below the injury site. The victim can help you. **B,** Pad a rigid splint to conform to the injured body part. **C,** Then secure the splint in place.

◆ Summary

Sometimes it is difficult to tell whether an injury is a fracture, dislocation, sprain, or strain. Since you cannot be sure which of these a victim might have, always care for the injury as if it is serious. If EMS personnel are on the way, do not move the victim. Control any bleeding first. Take steps to minimize shock and monitor the ABCs. If you are going to transport the victim to a medical facility, be sure to first immobilize the injury before moving the victim.

Chapters 10 through 12 discuss recognition and care for injuries, starting with the head and progressing downward, much like the sequence of the secondary survey.

Answer to Application Question

1. Neither injury is inherently more severe than the other. Both injuries can range from mild, with slight stretching of the muscle, tendon, or ligament, to severe, involving torn muscles or ligaments that require surgery. Both injuries can be disabling.

Study Questions

1. Match each term with the correct definition.

    a. Bone
    b. Dislocation
    c. Fracture
    d. Joint
    e. Ligaments
    f. Muscle
    g. Skeletal muscles
    h. Splint
    i. Sprain
    j. Strain
    k. Tendon

    _____ Device used to keep body parts from moving.
    _____ Displacement of a bone from its normal position at a joint.
    _____ Tissue that lengthens and shortens to create movement.
    _____ Broken bone.
    _____ Dense, hard tissue that forms the skeleton.
    _____ Injury that stretches and tears ligaments and other soft tissues at joints.
    _____ Fibrous band attaching muscle to bone.
    _____ Structure formed where two or more bones meet.
    _____ Injury that stretches and tears muscles and tendons.
    _____ Muscles that attach to bones.
    _____ Fibrous bands holding bones together at joints.

2. List three common signals of musculoskeletal injuries.

3. List four principles of splinting.

4. List three types of splints.

In questions 5 through 8, circle the letter of the correct answer.

5. When caring for an injured joint, you should—

   a. Control external bleeding.
   b. Straighten the fracture or dislocation before splinting.
   c. Splint the fracture or dislocation in the position found.
   d. a and c
   e. a, b, and c

6. You would suspect a fracture or dislocation if—

   a. You saw severe swelling and discoloration.
   b. The area was significantly deformed.
   c. The victim heard a snap at the time of the injury.
   d. a, b, and c

7. You find a person lying at the foot of a steep cliff. Her right leg is twisted at an unusual angle and you can see protruding bones and blood. What do you do first?

   a. Straighten the leg.
   b. Do a primary survey.
   c. Use direct pressure to stop the bleeding.
   d. Look for material to use as a splint.

8. You should immobilize a musculoskeletal injury in order to—

   a. Prevent further soft tissue damage.
   b. Lessen pain.
   c. Lessen the danger of infection.
   d. a and c
   e. a and b

Answers are in Appendix A.

PRACTICE SESSION: *Applying an Anatomic Splint*

You are doing a secondary survey and suspect that the victim may have a serious leg injury. You decide to use an anatomic splint.

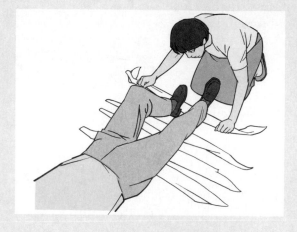

☐ **Secure injured limb to uninjured limb**
- Thread 4 or 5 cravats under legs at ankles, at lower legs, and at thighs.
- Do not thread cravat at injury site.

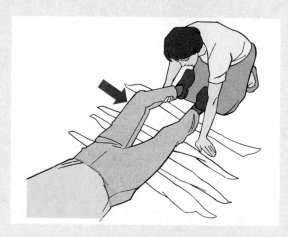

- Slide uninjured leg next to injured leg.

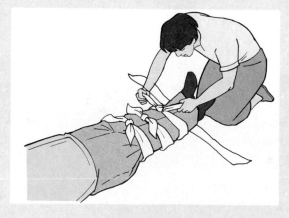

☐ **Tie the ends**
- Tie ends of each cravat together, with knots on uninjured leg.
- Check to see that cravats are snug but not too tight.
- If more than 1 finger fits under cravats, tighten cravats.

PRACTICE SESSION: *Applying a Soft Splint*

You are doing a secondary survey and suspect that the victim may have an ankle injury. You decide to use a soft splint to immobilize the injured area.

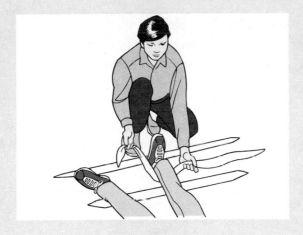

☐ **Apply the splint**
- Leave footwear in place (sock or shoe).
- Thread 3 cravats: 1 each at heel, under ankle, and under lower leg.

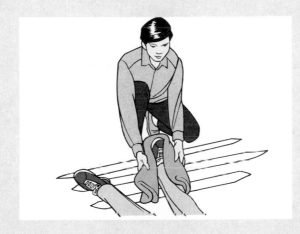

- Fold or wrap blanket or pillow gently around ankle.

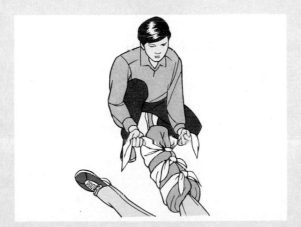

☐ **Secure the splint in place**
- Secure blanket or pillow around ankle and lower leg.
- Tie third cravat around foot, from heel to front of ankle.
- If more than 1 finger fits under cravats, tighten cravats.

PRACTICE SESSION: *Applying a Rigid Splint*

You are doing a secondary survey and suspect that the victim may have a serious forearm injury. You decide to use a rigid splint to immobilize the injury.

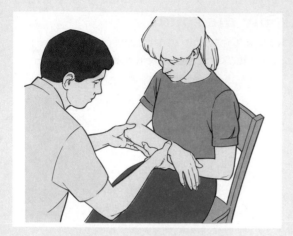

☐ Support the limb

- ◆ Support the arm above and below the injury. If possible, have victim or bystander help you.

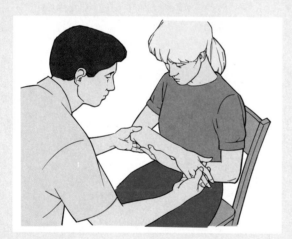

☐ Check circulation

- ◆ Check the fingers for color and warmth.

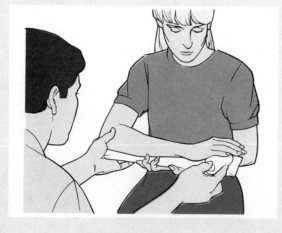

☐ Apply a rigid splint

- ◆ Place padded splint under injured forearm.
- ◆ Have victim or bystander hold splint in place.
- ◆ Place a soft object in palm of victim's hand to keep it in a natural position.

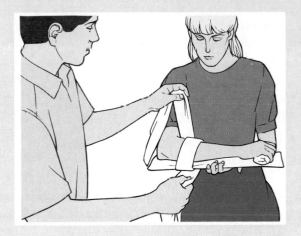

☐ Secure the splint in place

- Secure the splint above and below the injury with cravats or roller bandage.

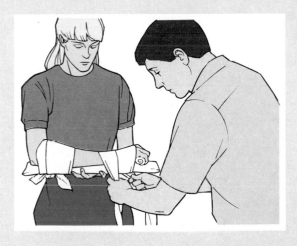

- If cravats are used, tie ends together on underside of splint, leaving fractured area uncovered.

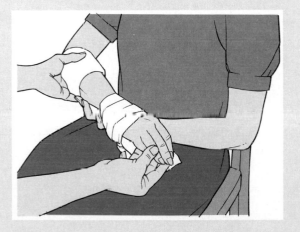

☐ Check circulation

- Check fingers for color and warmth.
- Splint should fit snugly but not so tightly that blood flow to hand is impaired.
- If fingers are bluish or cool, loosen splint.

PRACTICE SESSION: *Applying a Sling and Binder*

You are doing a secondary survey and suspect that the victim has an injured arm. You decide to apply a sling and binder. (A sling and binder can be used whether or not a rigid splint has been applied.)

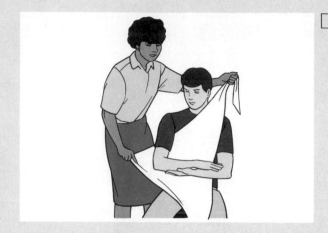

☐ Position the triangular bandage
- Have victim or bystander support injured arm.
- Thread one end of bandage under injured arm, across chest, and over uninjured shoulder.
- Position point of bandage at elbow.

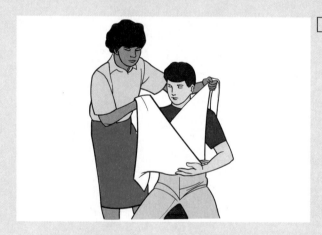

☐ Tie the ends
- Bring other end across chest and over opposite shoulder.

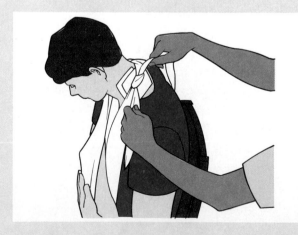

- Tie ends at side of neck opposite injury.
- Place a pad under the knot.

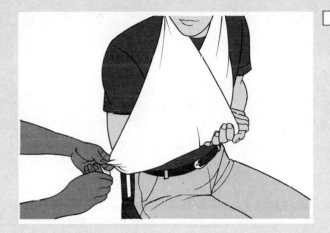

☐ Secure bandage at elbow

- Tie or pin the point of sling at elbow, if possible.

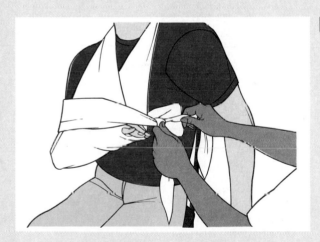

☐ Secure arm to chest

- Place cravat over injured arm.
- Tie ends on opposite side under uninjured arm.
- Place pad under knot.

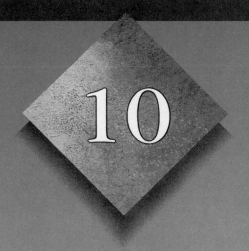

Injuries to the Head and Spine

Objectives

After reading this chapter, you should be able to—

1. Name the most common cause of head and spine injuries.

2. List at least five situations that might indicate serious head and spine injuries.

3. List at least six signals of head and spine injuries.

4. Describe how to minimize movement of the victim's head and spine.

5. Describe how to care for specific injuries to the head, face, and neck.

6. List at least five ways to prevent head and spine injuries.

7. Define the key terms for this chapter.

After reading this chapter and completing the class activities, you should be able to—

1. Make appropriate decisions regarding care when given an example of an emergency situation in which injuries to the head and spine are likely to have occurred.

Key Terms

Concussion (kon KUSH un): A temporary impairment of brain function, usually without permanent damage to the brain.

In-line stabilization: A technique used to minimize movement of the victim's head and neck while providing care.

Spinal column: The column of vertebrae extending from the base of the skull to the tip of the tailbone (coccyx).

Spinal cord: A bundle of nerves extending from the base of the skull to the lower back, protected by the spinal column.

Vertebrae (VER tĕ bra): The 33 bones of the spinal column.

For Review

Before reading this chapter, you should have a basic understanding of the interrelationship of different body systems (Chapter 2), how to care for soft tissue injuries (Chapter 8), and how to care for musculoskeletal injuries (Chapter 9).

◆ Introduction

Spring break at the beach. High school and college students are having fun in the sun. The weather is great, the water refreshing. The day is perfect for a game of touch football on the beach.

Later in the day, the tide comes in, and the game becomes more aggressive. Players lunge into the surf to catch passes and fleet-footed runners. As the game is about to end, the quarterback throws a long pass. The receiver has the chance to score the winning touchdown, or the defender can intercept the pass to guarantee victory. They both run into the surf and dive headfirst at the ball. As they strike the water, a wave crashes over them, *forcing them underwater and into a sandbar. Both players strike their heads on the sandy bottom. The result? Both are pulled from the surf by their friends. One player is lucky and escapes with only a concussion. The other, not so lucky, suffers a broken neck and is paralyzed for life.*

◆ Head and Spine Injuries

Although injuries to the head and spine account for a small percentage of all injuries, they cause more than half the fatalities. Each year, nearly 2 million Americans suffer a head or spine injury. Most of these victims are males between ages 15 and 30.

Motor vehicle collisions account for about half of all head and spine injuries. Other causes include falls, sports and recreational activities, and violent acts such as assault. Figure 10-1 on the next page shows the causes of spinal injuries.

In addition to the victims who die each year in America, nearly 80,000 victims are permanently disabled. Today there are hundreds of thousands of permanently disabled victims of head or spine injury in the United States. These survivors have a wide range of physical and mental impairments, including paralysis, speech and memory problems, and behavioral disorders.

Fortunately, prompt, appropriate care can often prevent most head and spine injuries from resulting in death or disability. In this chapter, you will learn how to recognize when a head or spine injury may be serious. You will also learn how to provide appropriate care to minimize injuries to the head and spine.

◆ Recognizing Serious Head and Spine Injuries

Injuries to the head or spine often damage both bone and soft tissue, including brain tissue and the **spinal cord.** It is usually difficult

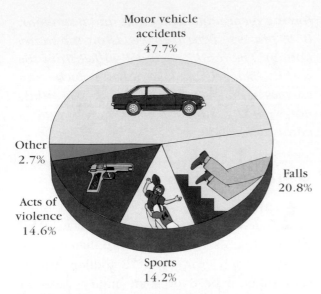

Figure 10-1 Motor vehicle collisions account for about half of all spinal injuries. (Data from *Spinal Cord Injury: the Facts and Figures,* 1986.)

ports the head and the trunk and encases and protects the spinal cord. The spine consists of small bones, **vertebrae,** with circular openings. The vertebrae are separated from each other by cushions of cartilage called disks (Fig. 10-3, *A).* This cartilage acts as a shock absorber when a person is walking, running, or jumping. The spinal cord, a bundle of nerves, runs through the hollow part of the vertebrae. Nerve branches extend to various parts of the body through openings on the sides of the vertebrae.

The spine is divided into five regions: the cervical or neck region, the thoracic or midback region, the lumbar or lower back region, the sacrum, and the coccyx, the small triangular bone at the lower end of the **spinal column** (Fig. 10-3, *B).* Injuries to the spinal column include fractures and dislocations of the vertebrae, sprained ligaments, and compres-

to determine the extent of damage in head and spine injuries. In most cases, the only way to assess the damage is by having x-rays taken in an emergency department. Since you cannot know how severe an injury is, always provide initial care as if the injury is serious.

The Brain

Injuries to the head can affect the brain. Blood from a ruptured vessel in the brain can accumulate within the skull (Fig. 10-2). Because there is very little free space in the skull, bleeding can build up pressure that can cause further damage to brain tissue.

Bleeding within the skull can occur rapidly or slowly over a period of days. This bleeding will affect the brain, resulting in changes in consciousness. Altered consciousness is often the first and most important signal of a serious head injury.

The Spine

The spine is a strong, flexible column that sup-

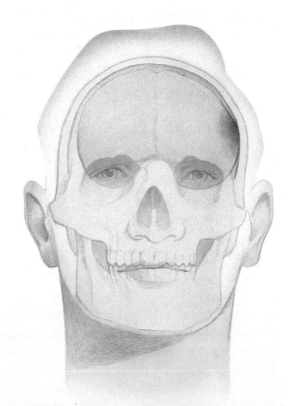

Figure 10-2 Injuries to the head can rupture blood vessels in the brain. Pressure builds within the skull as blood accumulates, causing brain damage.

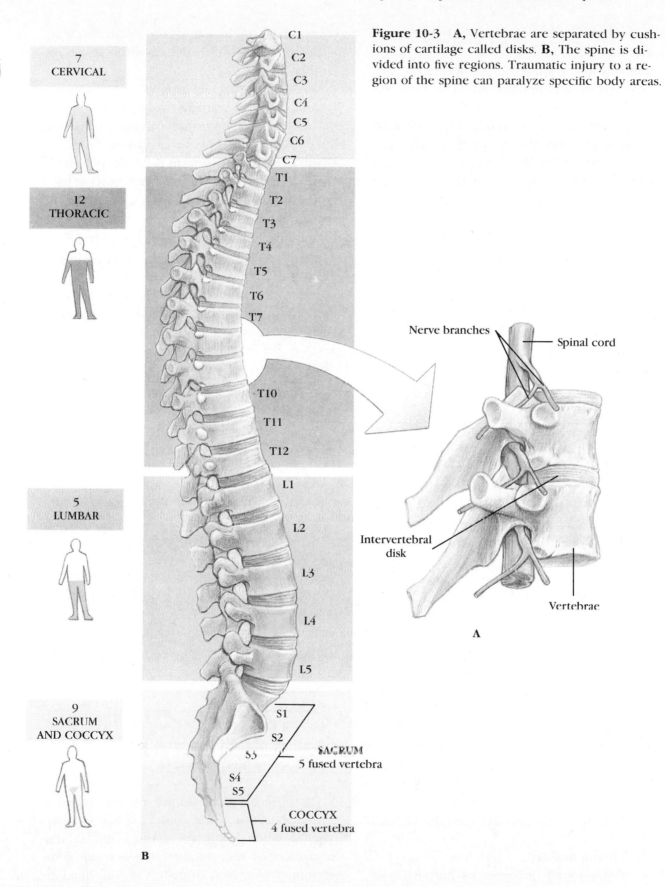

Figure 10-3 A, Vertebrae are separated by cushions of cartilage called disks. **B,** The spine is divided into five regions. Traumatic injury to a region of the spine can paralyze specific body areas.

7
CERVICAL

12
THORACIC

5
LUMBAR

9
SACRUM
AND COCCYX

C1
C2
C3
C4
C5
C6
C7
T1
T2
T3
T4
T5
T6
T7
T10
T11
T12
L1
L2
L3
L4
L5
S1
S2
S3
S4
S5

SACRUM
5 fused vertebra

COCCYX
4 fused vertebra

Nerve branches
Spinal cord

Intervertebral
disk

Vertebrae

A

B

sion or displacement of the disks between the vertebrae.

Injuries to the spine often fracture the vertebrae and sprain the ligaments. These injuries usually heal without problems. With severe injuries, however, the vertebrae may shift and compress or sever the spinal cord. This can cause temporary or permanent paralysis, even death. The extent of the paralysis depends on which area of the spinal cord is damaged. See Figure 10-3, *B.*

Q

1. How may compression or severing of the spinal cord cause death?

Causes of Injury

Consider the cause of the injury to help you determine when a head or spine injury may be serious. The cause often is the best initial measure of an injury's severity. Survey the scene and think about the forces involved in the injury. Strong forces are likely to cause severe injury to the head and spine. For example, a driver whose head breaks a car windshield in a crash may have a potentially serious head and spine injury. Similarly, a diver who hits his or her head on the bottom of a swimming pool may also have a serious injury. Evaluate the scene for clues as to whether a head and spine injury is potentially serious.

Injury Situations

Head injuries are often minor. However, you should consider the possibility of a serious head and/or spine injury in several situations. These include—

- A fall from a height greater than the victim's height.
- Any diving mishap.
- A person found unconscious for unknown reasons.

- Any injury involving severe blunt force to the head or trunk, such as from a car or other vehicle.
- Any injury that penetrates the head or trunk, such as a gunshot wound.
- A motor vehicle crash involving a driver or passengers not wearing safety belts.
- Any person thrown from a motor vehicle.
- Any injury in which a victim's helmet is broken, including a motorcycle, football, or industrial helmet.
- Any incident involving a lightning strike.

Signals of Head and Spine Injuries

You may also notice certain physical signals that indicate a serious head or spine injury. These signals may be obvious at first or may develop later. These physical signals include—

- Changes in the level of consciousness.
- Severe pain or pressure in the head, neck, or back.
- Tingling or loss of sensation in the extremities.
- Partial or complete loss of movement of any body part.
- Unusual bumps or depressions on the head or spine.
- Blood or other fluids in the ears or nose.
- Profuse external bleeding of the head, neck, or back.
- Seizures.
- Impaired breathing or vision as a result of injury.
- Nausea or vomiting.
- Persistent headache.
- Loss of balance.
- Bruising of the head, especially around the eyes and behind the ears.

These signals alone do not always suggest a serious head or spine injury, but they may when combined with the cause of the injury. Regardless of the situation, always call EMS personnel when you suspect a serious head or spine injury.

A Call From the Beach

When Liz Linton scanned the beach from one of the lifeguard towers at Newport Beach, she saw a man bobbing awkwardly in the water. As she swam through the surf toward the victim, she felt an uneasy sense of déjà vu. As a lifeguard for two summers, Linton had already saved one victim of spinal cord injury from drowning. The memory reminded her of how quickly a serious injury can occur.

As she swam, she marked the victim's position, fearful he would sink before she could reach him. Fortunately, she was able to get to him in time. He told her his head and shoulders had hit the bottom when he dove through a wave. She held him carefully to protect his neck and back from movement and began moving toward shore. He was partially paralyzed.

The man rescued by Liz Linton was lucky. After many months of rehabilitation, he regained full use of his body. Others are not so lucky. Each year, approximately 1,000 people suffer permanent damage to their spinal cords from diving mishaps. Statisticians describe the typical victim with grim accuracy. He is a single, white male between 15 and 30, an active person who loves sports and the outdoors.

Bill Brooks fits that description. The 29-year-old Davidsonville, Maryland, man was diving through an inner tube into a pool on a Sunday afternoon when his neck hit the tube. As he floated in the water, he remembers being aware of everything, yet powerless to move.

At the hospital, doctors told Brooks he was a "C5" quadraplegic, which described the area of the neck that he had damaged. In college, Brooks had played baseball, and after college he had taken up slow-pitch softball. In one afternoon, Brooks lost control of his legs, chest, and arms. He lost the ability to dress himself, feed himself, go to the bathroom by himself, or even hold a softball in his hand.

Months of rehabilitation have improved Brooks' life. Although his right hand remains paralyzed, with his left hand, Brooks can grasp a telephone and control a computer mouse. With the computer mouse, he is learning to design the sprinkler systems he once installed as the foreman for a sprinkler company. Brooks is learning to survive with his injury, but his spinal nerves will never regenerate, so there is little

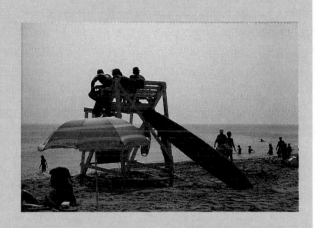

hope that he will ever walk again. Many states and private organizations have begun education and prevention campaigns to reduce the high rate of diving injuries. The American Red Cross offers the following water safety tips:

- Check for adequate water depth. When you first enter the water, enter feet first. Even at the edge of a pool or dock, diving into water less than nine feet deep is potentially dangerous. There is always the possibility of injury if you strike the bottom.
- For diving off a one-meter diving board, the water depth should be a minimum of 10 feet. This depth should extend 16 feet in front of the diver. The higher the board, the deeper the water should be. Pools at homes, motels, or hotels may not have an adequate area for safe diving.
- Never dive into an above-ground pool.
- Starting blocks should be used only by trained swimmers under the supervision of a qualified coach.
- Always swim with a buddy.
- Never drink and dive.
- Before you dive, check for objects hidden below the surface, such as logs or pilings.
- Running into the water and then diving head-first into the waves is dangerous.
- If you are bodysurfing, always keep your arms out in front of you to protect your head and neck.

◆ General Care for Head and Spine Injuries

Head and spine injuries can become life-threatening emergencies. A serious injury can cause a victim to stop breathing. Providing care for serious head and spine injuries involves supporting the respiratory, circulatory, and nervous systems. Always give the following care while waiting for EMS personnel to arrive:

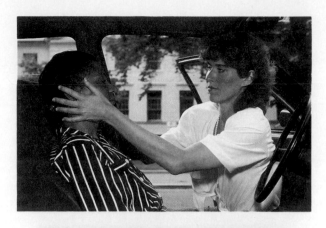

* Minimize movement of the head and spine.
* Maintain an open airway.
* Monitor consciousness and breathing.
* Control any external bleeding.
* Maintain normal body temperature.

Minimize Movement

Caring for a head or spine injury is similar to caring for any soft tissue or musculoskeletal injury. You should immobilize the injured area and control any bleeding. Because excessive movement of the head and spine can damage the spinal cord irreversibly, keep the victim as still as possible until you can obtain advanced care. To minimize movement of the head and neck, use the technique called **in-line stabilization.**

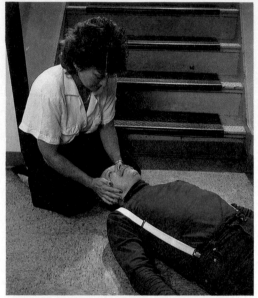

With this technique, you place your hands on both sides of the victim's head, position it gently, if necessary, in line with the body, and support it in that position until EMS personnel arrive. You can do this in various ways, depending on how you find the victim (Fig. 10-4). This is a simple skill to perform, but it is important to the victim's outcome. Keeping the head in this anatomically normal position helps prevent further damage to the spinal column.

However, some circumstances require that you do not move the victim's head in-line with the body. These include—

* When the victim's head is severely angled to one side.

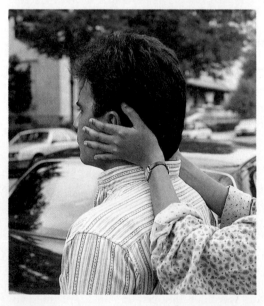

Figure 10-4 Support the victim's head in line with the body in the position in which you find the victim, using in-line stabilization.

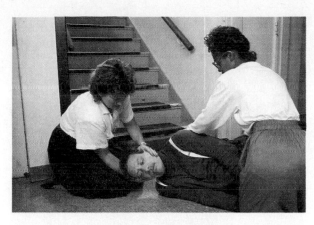

Figure 10-5 Maintain in-line stabilization while rolling the victim's body.

* When the victim complains of pain, pressure, or muscle spasms on initial movement of the head.
* When the rescuer feels resistance when attempting to move the head.

In these circumstances, support the victim's head in the position in which it was found.

Maintain an Open Airway

As you learned in Chapter 3, you do not always have to roll the victim onto his or her back to check breathing. A cry of pain, chest movement, or the sound of breathing tells you the victim is breathing. If the victim is breathing, support the victim in the position in which you found him or her. If the victim begins to vomit, position the victim onto one side to keep the airway clear. This is more easily done by two people. Ask another rescuer to help move the victim's body while you maintain in-line stabilization (Fig. 10-5).

Monitor Consciousness and Breathing

While stabilizing the head and neck, observe the victim's level of consciousness and breathing. A serious injury will result in changes in consciousness. The victim may give inappropriate responses to name, time, place, or what happened. He or she may speak incoherently. The victim may be drowsy, appear to lapse into sleep, and then suddenly awaken or lose consciousness completely. Breathing may become rapid or irregular. Because injury to the head or spine can paralyze chest nerves and muscles, breathing can stop. If this happens, perform rescue breathing.

Control External Bleeding

Some head and neck injuries include soft tissue damage. Because there are many blood vessels in the head and two major arteries (the carotid arteries) in the neck, the victim can lose much blood quickly. If there is external bleeding, control it promptly with dressings, direct pressure, and bandages.

Maintain Normal Body Temperature

A serious injury to the head or spine can result in a disruption of the body's normal heating or cooling mechanism. When this happens, the person is more susceptible to shock. For example, a person suffering a serious head or spine injury while outside on a cold day will be more likely to become hypothermic, because the normal shivering response to rewarm the body may not work. For this reason, it is important to minimize shock by maintaining normal body temperature.

Q

2. The two goals of care for victims of head and spine injuries are to maintain an open airway and minimize movement. Is one more important than the other? Why?

◆ Care for Specific Head Injuries

The head is easily injured because it lacks the padding of muscle and fat in other areas of the body. You can feel bone just beneath the surface of the skin over most of the head, includ-

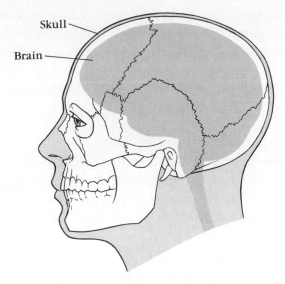

Figure 10-6 The head is easily injured because it lacks the padding of muscle and fat found in other areas of the body.

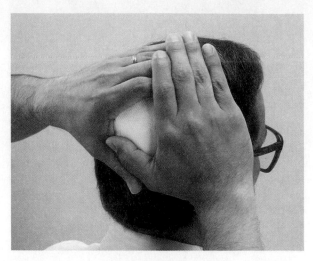

Figure 10-7 To avoid putting direct pressure on a deep scalp wound, apply pressure with your hands to the area around the wound.

ing the chin, cheekbones, and scalp (Fig. 10-6).

Concussion

Any significant force to the head can cause a **concussion.** A concussion is a temporary impairment of brain function. It usually does not result in permanent physical damage to brain tissue. In most cases, the victim loses consciousness for only an instant and may say that he or she "blacked out" or "saw stars." A concussion sometimes results in a loss of consciousness for longer periods of time. Other times, a victim may be confused or have amnesia (loss of memory). Anyone suspected of having a concussion should be examined by a physician.

Scalp Injury

Scalp bleeding can be minor or severe. The bleeding is usually easily controlled with direct pressure. But because the skull may be fractured, be careful to press gently at first. If you feel a depression, a spongy area, or bone fragments, do not put direct pressure on the wound. Call EMS personnel. Attempt to control bleeding with pressure on the area around

the wound (Fig. 10-7). Examine the injured area carefully because the victim's hair may hide part of the wound. If you are unsure about the extent of a scalp injury, call your local emergency number. EMS personnel will be better able to evaluate the injury.

If the victim has only an open wound, control the bleeding with direct pressure. Apply several dressings and hold them in place with your hand. Secure the dressings with a roller-type or a triangular bandage (Fig. 10-8, *A* and *B*).

Cheek Injury

Injury to the cheek usually involves only soft tissue. Control bleeding from the cheek in the same manner as other soft tissue bleeding. The only difference is that you may have to control bleeding on either the outside or the inside of the cheek. Begin by examining both the outside and inside of the cheek. Bleeding inside the cheek may result from a blow that caused the teeth to cut the cheek inside or from a laceration or puncture wound outside the cheek. To control bleeding, place several dressings, folded or rolled, inside the mouth,

A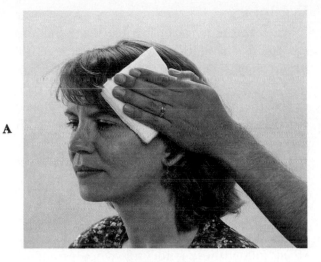

B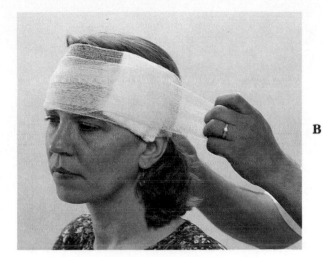

Figure 10-8 A, Apply pressure to control bleeding from a scalp wound. **B,** Then secure dressings with a bandage.

against the cheek. If possible, have the victim hold them in place. If external bleeding is also present, place dressings on the outside of the cheek and apply direct pressure (Fig. 10-9).

If an object passes completely through the cheek and becomes impaled, it may have to be removed to control bleeding. This circumstance is the only exception to the general rule not to remove impaled objects from the body. An impaled object in the cheek cannot be easily stabilized, makes control of bleeding more difficult, and may become dislodged and obstruct the airway. You can remove the object by pulling it out the same way it entered. If doing this is difficult or painful to the victim, leave the object in place, and stabilize it with bulky dressings.

Once the object is removed, fold or roll several dressings and place them inside the mouth. Be sure not to obstruct the airway. Apply dressings to the outside of the cheek as well. The victim may be able to hold these in place, or you may have to hold them. Bleeding inside the cheek can result in the victim swallowing blood. If the victim swallows enough blood, nausea or vomiting can result, which would complicate the situation. Place the victim in a seated position leaning slightly for-

ward so that blood will not drain into the throat. As with any serious bleeding or impaled object, call EMS personnel.

Nose Injury

Nose injuries are usually caused by a blow from a blunt object. The result is often a nosebleed. High blood pressure or changes in altitude can also cause nosebleeds. In most cases, you can control bleeding by having the victim

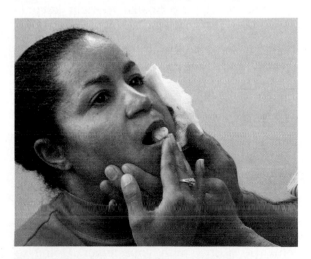

Figure 10-9 To control bleeding inside the cheek, place folded dressings inside the mouth against the wound. To control external bleeding, use dressings to apply pressure directly to the wound.

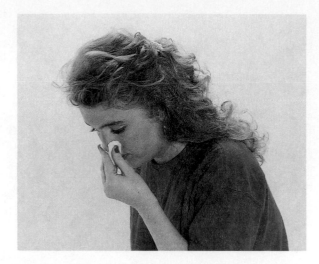

Figure 10-10 To control a nosebleed, have the victim lean forward and pinch the nostrils together until bleeding stops.

apply pressure rt. under nose
helps also

sit with the head slightly forward while pinching the nostrils together (Fig. 10-10). Other methods of controlling bleeding include applying an ice pack to the bridge of the nose or putting pressure on the upper lip just beneath the nose.

Once you have controlled the bleeding, tell the victim to avoid rubbing, blowing, or picking the nose, since this could restart the bleeding. Later, you may apply a little petroleum jelly inside the nostril to help keep it moist.

You should seek additional medical care if the nosebleed continues after you use the techniques described, if bleeding recurs, or if the victim says the bleeding is the result of high blood pressure. If the victim loses consciousness, place the victim on his or her side to allow blood to drain from the nose. Contact EMS personnel immediately.

If you think an object is in the nostril, look into the nostril. If you see the object and can easily grasp it, then do so. However, do not probe the nostril with your finger. Doing so may push the object farther into the nose and cause bleeding or make it more difficult to remove later. If the object cannot be removed easily, the victim should receive medical care.

Eye Injury

Injuries to the eye can involve the bone and soft tissue surrounding the eye, or the eyeball. Blunt objects like a fist or a baseball may injure the eye area, or a smaller object may penetrate the eyeball. Care for open or closed wounds *around* the eyeball as you would for any other soft tissue injury.

Injury to the eyeball itself requires different care. Injuries that penetrate the eyeball or cause the eye to be removed from its socket are very serious and can cause blindness. Never put direct pressure on the eyeball. Instead, follow these guidelines when providing care for an eye in which an object has been impaled:

1. Place the victim on his or her back.
2. Do not attempt to remove any object impaled in the eye.
3. Place a sterile dressing around the object (Fig. 10-11, *A*).
4. Stabilize any impaled object in place as best you can. You can do this by placing a paper cup to support the object (Fig. 10-11, *B*).
5. Apply a bandage (Fig. 10-11, *C*).

Foreign bodies that get in the eye, such as dirt, sand, or slivers of wood or metal, are irritating and can cause significant damage. The eye produces tears immediately in an attempt to flush out such objects. Pain from the irritation is often severe. The victim may have difficulty opening the eye because light further irritates it.

First, try to remove the foreign body by telling the victim to blink several times. Then try gently flushing the eye with water. If the object remains, the victim should receive professional medical attention.

Flushing the eye with water is also appropriate if the victim has any chemical in his or her eye (Fig. 10-12). The eye should be continuously flushed until EMS personnel arrive.

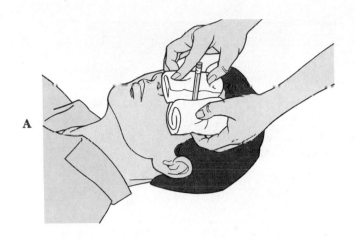

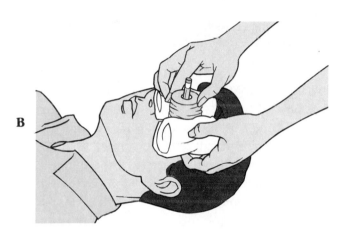

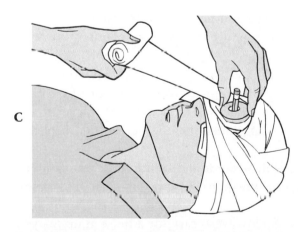

Figure 10-11 A, Do not remove an object impaled in the eye. Place sterile dressings around the object. **B,** Support the object with a paper cup. **C,** Carefully bandage the cup in place.

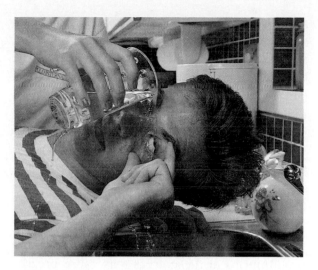

Figure 10-12 If chemicals enter the eye, flush the eye continuously with water.

Ear Injury

Ear injuries are common. Either the soft tissue of the ear or the eardrum within the ear may be injured. Open wounds, such as lacerations or abrasions, can result from recreational injuries, for example, being struck by a racquetball or falling off a bike. An avulsion of the ear may occur when a pierced earring catches on something and tears away from the ear. You can control bleeding from the soft tissues of the ear by applying direct pressure to the affected area.

If the victim has a serious head or spine injury, blood or other fluid may be in the ear canal or be draining from the ear. *Do not* attempt to stop this drainage with direct pressure. Instead, just cover the ear lightly with a sterile dressing. Call EMS personnel.

The ear can also be injured internally. A direct blow to the head may rupture the eardrum. Sudden pressure changes, such as those caused by an explosion or a deep-water dive, can also injure the ear internally. The victim may lose hearing or balance or experience inner ear pain. These injuries require professional medical care.

A foreign object, such as dirt, an insect, or cotton, can easily become lodged in the ear canal. If you can easily see and grasp the object, remove it. But do not try to remove any object by using a pin, toothpick, or a similar sharp item. You could force the object farther back or puncture the eardrum. Sometimes you can remove the object if you pull down on the earlobe, tilt the head to the side, and shake or gently strike the head on the affected side. If you cannot easily remove the object, seek professional medical assistance.

Mouth, Jaw, and Neck Injuries

Your primary concern for any injury to the mouth, jaw, or neck is to ensure an open airway. Injuries in these areas may cause breathing problems if blood or loose teeth obstruct the airway. A swollen or fractured trachea may also obstruct breathing.

If you do not suspect a serious head or spine injury, place the victim in a seated position with the head tilted slightly forward to allow any blood to drain. If this position is not possible, place the victim on his or her side to allow blood to drain from the mouth.

For injuries that penetrate the lip, place a rolled dressing between the lip and the gum. You can place another dressing on the outer surface of the lip. If the tongue is bleeding, apply a dressing and direct pressure. Applying cold to the lips or tongue can help reduce swelling and ease pain. If the bleeding cannot be controlled easily, the victim should seek additional medical attention.

If the injury knocked out one or more of the victim's teeth, control the bleeding and save the tooth for replantation. To control the bleeding, roll a sterile dressing and insert it into the space left by the missing tooth. Have the victim bite down to maintain pressure (Fig. 10-13).

There are varying opinions as to how the tooth should be saved. One thought is to place the dislodged tooth or teeth in the injured person's mouth. This, however, is not always the best approach, since a crying child could aspirate the tooth. The tooth could also be swallowed with blood or saliva. In addition, there may be a need to control serious bleed-

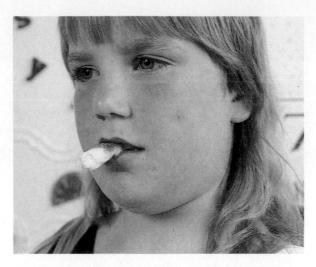

Figure 10-13 If a tooth is knocked out, place a sterile dressing directly in the space left by the tooth. Tell the victim to bite down.

ing in the mouth. Because of these concerns, it is best to simply place it in a cup of milk or water, if milk is not available. If the injury is severe enough to call EMS personnel, give the tooth to them when they arrive. If the injury is not severe enough to contact EMS personnel, the victim should immediately seek a dentist who can replant the tooth. For the tooth to be successfully replanted, time is critical. Ideally, the tooth should be replanted within an hour after the injury.

Injuries serious enough to fracture or dislocate the jaw can also cause other head or spine injuries. Be sure to maintain an adequate airway. Check inside the mouth for bleeding. Control bleeding as you would for other head injuries. Minimize movement of the head and neck. Call EMS personnel for an injury of this type.

A soft tissue injury of the neck can produce severe bleeding and swelling that may result in airway obstruction. Because the spine may also be involved, care for a neck injury as you would a possible serious spine injury. If the victim has struck his or her neck on a steering wheel or ran into a clothesline, the injury can be devastating. The trachea may be fractured, causing an airway obstruction that requires immediate medical attention. While waiting

Now Smile

Enamel
(chewing edge)

Nerves and
blood vessels

Root

A tooth must be replanted so the periodontal fibers will reattach.

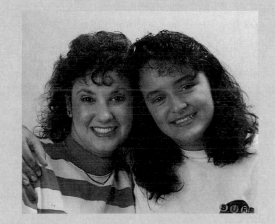

Now smile!

Knocked-out teeth no longer spell doom for pearly whites. Most dentists can successfully replant a knocked-out tooth if they can do so quickly, and if the tooth is properly cared for.

Replanting a tooth is similar to replanting a tree. On each tooth, tiny root fibers called periodontal fibers attach to the jawbone to hold the tooth in place. Inside the tooth, a canal filled with bundles of blood and nerves runs from the tooth into the jawbone and surrounding tissues.

When these fibers and tissues are torn from the socket, it is important that they be replaced within an hour. Generally, the sooner the tooth is replanted, the greater the chance it will survive. The knocked-out tooth must be handled carefully to protect the fragile tissues. Be careful to pick up the tooth by the chewing edge (crown), not the root. Do not rub or handle the root part of the tooth. It is best to preserve the tooth by placing it in a closed container of cool, fresh milk until it reaches the dentist. Because milk is not always available at an injury scene, water may be substituted.

A dentist or emergency room doctor will clean the tooth, taking care not to damage the root fibers. The tooth is then placed back into the socket and secured with special splinting devices. The devices keep the tooth stable for two to three weeks while the fibers reattach to the jawbone. The bundles of blood vessels and nerves grow back within six weeks.

REFERENCES

Bogert, John, DDS, Executive Director, American
   Academy of Pediatric Dentists. Interview April 1990.
Medford, Houck, DDS: Acute Care of An Avulsed Tooth.
   Annals of Emergency Medicine 11:559-61, 1982.

for EMS personnel, try to keep the victim from moving, and encourage him or her to breathe slowly. Control any external bleeding with direct pressure. Be careful not to apply pressure that constricts both carotid arteries.

Q

3. To control bleeding in the neck, you should apply direct pressure to only one of the carotid arteries. Why?

◆ Preventing Head and Spine Injuries

Injuries to the head and spine are a major cause of death, disability, and disfigurement. However, many such injuries can be prevented. By using safety practices in all areas of your life, you can help reduce risks to yourself and to others around you.

Safety practices that can help prevent injuries to the head and spine include—

• Wearing safety belts.
• When appropriate, wearing approved helmets, eyewear, faceguards and mouthguards.
• Preventing falls.
• Obeying rules in sports and recreational activities.
• Avoiding inappropriate use of drugs.
• Inspecting work and recreational equipment periodically.
• Thinking and talking about safety.

Wearing Safety Belts

Always wear safety belts, including shoulder restraints, when driving or riding in an automobile. Be sure all passengers also wear them. Airbags, available in some cars, provide additional protection. All small children riding in a car must be in approved safety seats correct for the child's age and weight (Fig. 10-14). Infants weighing under 20 pounds should ride in a safety seat facing the rear of the vehicle to protect the infant's head and neck.

Wearing Helmets and Eyewear

Helmets can prevent many needless injuries to the head and spine. They are designed for different purposes, with varying degrees of protection, and offer protection only for their intended use (Fig. 10-15). For example, the industrial work helmet called a "hard hat" provides adequate protection against falling debris but does not offer the proper protection for riding a motorcycle.

Any open form of transportation, such as a motorcycle, a moped, an all-terrain vehicle,

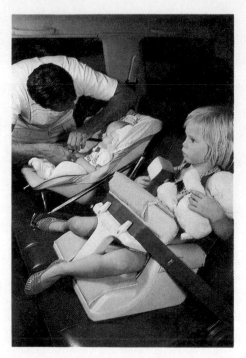

Figure 10-14 Children in cars must ride in approved safety seats.

and even a bicycle, exposes the head and spine to injury. Wearing a helmet can help reduce such injuries. The ideal helmet, sometimes called a "full-face helmet," protects the lower face and jaw and has a large, clear or tinted face shield. Bicycle riders should wear helmets appropriate for the type of riding. In all cases, the helmet should be the correct size and fit comfortably and securely.

Eyewear can help prevent many needless injuries that result in loss of sight. Anytime you operate machinery or perform an activity that may involve flying particles or a splash of chemicals, you should wear protective eyewear such as goggles.

Safeguarding Against Falls

Most falls occur around the home. Young children and the elderly are frequently victims. You can take precautions to prevent falls. Floors should be of a nonslip type. Stairs should have nonslip tread and handrails. Rugs should be secured to the floor with double-sided tape. If moisture accumulates and causes

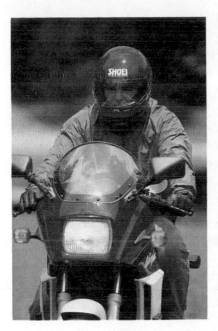
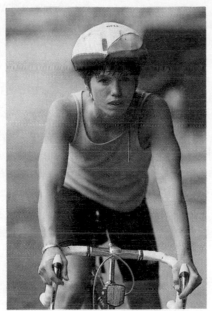
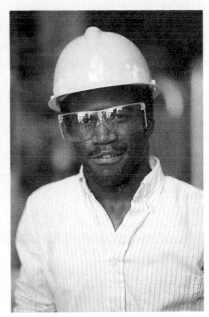

Figure 10-15 Wearing a helmet helps protect against head and spine injuries.

damp spots, correct the cause of the problem. Clean up any spills promptly. The bathroom should be safe for all those using it. If necessary, install handrails by the bathtub and toilet (Fig. 10-16).

Taking Safety Precautions in Sports and Recreation

Participants in sports or recreational activities should know their own physical limitations. Proper protective equipment is necessary for any activity in which serious injury may occur. In all sports involving physical contact, participants should wear mouthpieces. Most important, everyone must know and follow the rules. Rules not only make the activity fair, they also help prevent injuries. The coach or a more experienced participant may impose additional rules for the safety of newcomers. Never participate in a new activity until you know the rules and risks involved.

Not Using Drugs

Alcohol and other drugs used inappropriately cause or contribute to many serious motor vehicle collisions and water-related injuries that

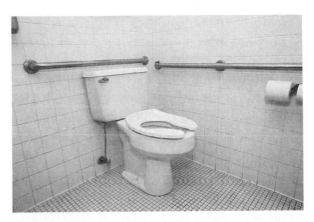

Figure 10-16 Bathroom handrails help to protect against falls.

result in head and spine injuries. Drugs impair judgment and reflexes, causing your body to respond abnormally. Drugs can give the user a feeling of false confidence. Under the influence of drugs, a person might not brake the car quickly enough or might dive into shallow water. Prescription and common drugstore medications can also have side effects, such as drowsiness, that can make driving or operating machinery dangerous. Always follow your physician's directions and the directions on medication labels.

Inspecting Equipment

Inspect mechanical equipment and ladders periodically to ensure good working order. Check for worn or loose parts that could break and cause a mishap. Before climbing a ladder, place its legs on a firm, flat surface and have someone anchor it while you climb.

Thinking and Talking Safety

People too often neglect thinking about safety in their daily lives; yet we are most vulnerable to injury at work, during recreational activities, or while traveling. Take the time to inspect and think about your daily environment. Evaluate your habits. Answer the following questions:

- Are there things that you could do in your home or workplace to help prevent injuries to yourself or others?
- Are you taking unnecessary risks in any activities?
- Do you follow rules meant for your safety?
- Do you frequently check the tires on your car, truck, motor bike, or bicycle?
- Do you ever attempt any activity without being in physical condition to do it without injury?

Talk with others about preventing injuries at work, at home, and in recreational activities. Make sure children know about safety. They need guidance to help prevent injuries that could permanently affect their lives. Talk to them about safety on bikes, on the playground, and at home. Their future may depend on your experience and advice.

◆ Summary

In this chapter, you have learned how to recognize and care for serious head and spine injuries and specific injuries to the head and neck. To decide whether an injury is serious, you must consider its cause. Often the cause is the best indicator of whether an injury to the head or spine should be considered serious. If you have any doubts about the seriousness of an injury, call EMS personnel.

Like injuries elsewhere on the body, injuries to the head and spine often involve both soft tissues and bone. Control bleeding as necessary, usually with direct pressure on the wound. With scalp injuries, be careful not to apply pressure to a possible skull fracture. Similarly, with eye injuries, remember not to apply pressure on the eyeball.

If you suspect that the victim may have a fracture of the skull or spine, minimize movement of the injured area when providing care. This is best accomplished by using in-line stabilization.

As you read the next chapter about how to care for injuries to the chest and abdomen, remember the principles of care for head and spine injuries. Serious injuries of the chest and abdomen often also affect the spine.

Answers to Application Questions

1. The spinal cord is a bundle of nerves that branch out to communicate with all parts of the body. Some nerves are responsible for controlling breathing. If these nerves are damaged by compression or severing of the spinal cord, death may result.
2. Both are important, but maintaining an open airway is more important. A person who is not breathing will quickly die, at which point other injuries cease to be important. It is highly unlikely that you would cause any damage by opening the airway carefully.
3. The carotid arteries supply oxygen-rich blood to the brain. If blood flow through both arteries is reduced, the brain does not receive enough oxygen-rich blood to function.

Study Questions

1 Match each term with the correct definition.

a. Concussion

d. Spinal cord

b. In-line stabilization

e. Vertebrae

c. Spinal column

_____ Technique used to minimize movement of the victim's head and neck while providing care.

_____ Head injury that usually does not permanently damage the brain.

_____ Column of vertebrae extending from the base of the skull to the tip of the tailbone.

_____ The 33 bones of the spinal column.

_____ A bundle of nerves extending from the base of the skull to the lower back, protected by the spinal column.

2. List at least five situations that might result in serious head and/or spine injuries.

3. List at least six signals of head or spine injuries.

4. List at least five ways to prevent head and spine injuries.

5. List the steps of care for an eye injury in which the eyeball has been penetrated.

In questions 6 through 13, circle the letter of the correct answer.

6. The most common causes of head or spine injury are—

a. Diving mishaps.

b. Motor vehicle collisions.

c. Falls.

d. Assaults.

7. Serious injuries to the head or spine damage—

   a. Soft tissues.
   b. Nerve tissues.
   c. Bones.
   d. a and b
   e. a, b, and c

8. When determining the severity of a head or spine injury, you should consider—

   a. The cause of the injury.
   b. The physical signals present.
   c. What bystanders who saw the injury occur can tell you.
   d. a, b, and c

9. When caring for a victim of head injury, you should—

   a. Stabilize the head and spine.
   b. Stop the flow of fluids from the ears.
   c. Remove any impaled object.
   d. Apply direct pressure to control all scalp bleeding.

10. At the scene of a car crash, a victim has blood seeping from his ears. You should—

   a. Loosely cover the ears with a sterile dressing.
   b. Do nothing; this is a normal finding in a head injury.
   c. Collect the fluid in a sterile container for analysis.
   d. Pack the ears with sterile dressings to prevent further fluid loss.

11. Your primary concern when caring for an injury to the mouth or neck is—

   a. Infection.
   b. An open airway.
   c. Swelling.
   d. None of the above.

12. Caring for an injury to the eyeball includes—

  a. Not putting direct pressure on the eyeball.
  b. Removing objects penetrating the eye.
  c. Covering the unaffected eye.
  d. a and c
  e. a, b, and c

13. An internal ear injury may be signaled by—

  a. Hearing loss.
  b. Loss of balance.
  c. Inner ear pain.
  d. a and c
  e. a, b, and c

---

14. As you begin to apply direct pressure to control bleeding for a scalp injury, you notice a depression of the skull in the area of the bleeding. How should you alter care?

15. What should you do for a victim of suspected head and spine injury whom you find lying on his side, moaning in pain?

Answers are in Appendix A.

Injuries to the Chest, Abdomen, and Pelvis

Objectives

After reading this chapter, you should be able to—

1. Explain why injuries to the chest, abdomen, and pelvis can be fatal.

2. List the five steps of care for these injuries.

3. List at least four signals of chest injury.

4. Describe the care for rib fractures.

5. Describe the care for a sucking chest wound.

6. List at least four signals of serious abdominal and pelvic injury.

7. Describe the care for open and closed abdominal and pelvic injuries.

8. Describe the care for injuries to the genitals.

9. Define the key terms for this chapter.

After reading this chapter and completing the class activities, you should be able to—

1. Make appropriate decisions regarding care when given an example of an emergency situation in which chest, abdominal, or pelvic injuries have occurred.

◆ Introduction

Most injuries to the **chest** and **abdomen** involve only soft tissues. Often these injuries, like those that occur elsewhere on the body, are only minor cuts, scrapes, and bruises. Occasionally, severe injuries occur such as fractures or injuries to organs that cause severe bleeding or impair breathing. Fractures and lacerations often occur in motor vehicle collisions to occupants not wearing seat belts. Falls, sports mishaps, and other forms of trauma may also cause such injuries.

Injuries to the **pelvis** may be minor soft tissue injuries or serious injuries to bone and internal structures. The pelvis includes a group of large bones that form a protective girdle around the organs inside. A great force is required to cause serious injury to the pelvis.

Because the chest, abdomen, and pelvis contain many organs important to life, injury to these areas can be fatal. You may recall from the previous chapter that a force capable of causing severe injury in these areas may also cause injury to the spine.

Care for these injuries includes—

- Calling EMS personnel.
- Monitoring the ABCs.
- Controlling bleeding.
- Minimizing shock.
- Limiting movement.

This chapter describes the signals of and care for different injuries to the chest, abdomen, and pelvis. In all cases, follow the emergency action principles. Care for all life-threatening injuries first. *All injuries described in this chapter are serious enough that you should always call EMS personnel immediately for advanced medical care.*

◆ Injuries to the Chest

The chest is the upper part of the trunk. It is formed by 12 pairs of ribs that attach to the **sternum** (breastbone) in front and the spine in back. The **rib cage** protects vital organs such as the heart, major blood vessels, and the lungs (see Figure 11-1 on the next page). Also in the chest are the esophagus, the trachea, and the muscles of respiration.

Chest injuries are the second leading cause of trauma deaths each year. Approximately 35 percent of all traffic fatalities in the United States involve chest injuries. Injuries to the chest may result from a wide variety of other causes such as falls, sports mishaps, and crushing or penetrating forces (see Figure 11-2 on the next page).

Chest wounds are either open or closed. Open chest wounds occur when an object, such as a knife or bullet, penetrates the chest wall. Fractured ribs may break through the

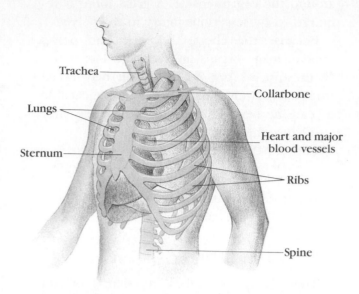

Figure 11-1   The rib cage surrounds and protects many vital organs.

skin to cause an open chest injury. A chest wound is closed if the skin is not broken. Closed chest wounds are generally caused by a blunt object such as a steering wheel.

Signals of Chest Injury

You should know the signals of serious chest injury. These may occur with both open and closed wounds. You will recognize some of these signals from Chapter 4 on breathing emergencies. They include—

* Difficulty breathing.
* Severe pain at the site of the injury.
* Flushed, pale, or bluish discoloration of the skin.
* Obvious deformity such as caused by a fracture.
* Coughing up blood.

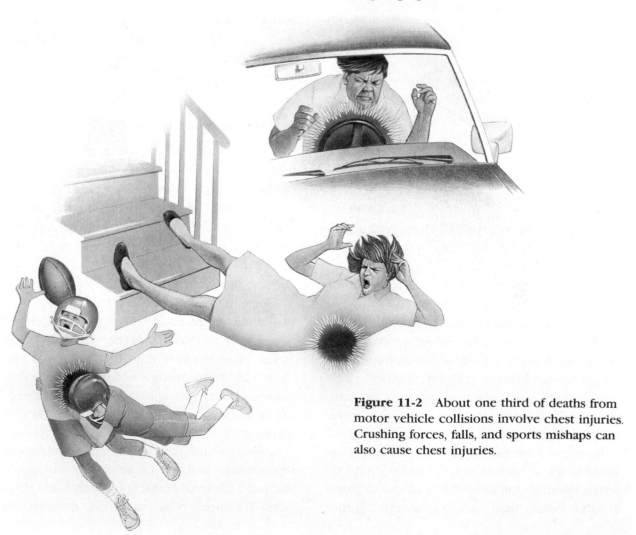

Figure 11-2   About one third of deaths from motor vehicle collisions involve chest injuries. Crushing forces, falls, and sports mishaps can also cause chest injuries.

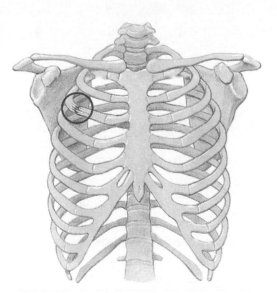

Figure 11-3   A simple rib fracture is painful but rarely life-threatening.

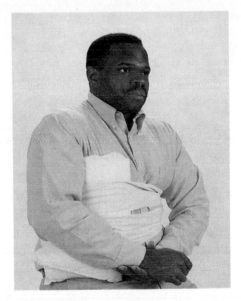

Figure 11-4   For a fractured rib, use a pillow to support and immobilize the injured area.

and pulse carefully and take steps to minimize shock.

Q

1. What does coughing up blood tell you about a chest injury?

Specific Types of Chest Injuries
Rib fractures

Rib fractures are usually caused by direct force to the chest. Although painful, a simple rib fracture is rarely life-threatening (Fig. 11-3). A victim with a fractured rib generally remains calm and breathes shallowly because normal or deep breathing is painful. The victim will usually attempt to ease the pain by supporting the injured area with a hand or arm. Therefore, shallow breathing and holding the area are both signals of possible rib fracture. If you suspect a fractured rib, have the victim rest in a position that will make breathing easier. Binding the victim's arm to the chest on the injured side will help support the injured area and make breathing more comfortable. You can use an object such as a pillow or rolled blanket to support and immobilize the area (Fig. 11-4). Monitor breathing

Q

2. How would you care for an open rib fracture?

Puncture injuries

Puncture wounds to the chest range from minor to life-threatening. Stab and gunshot wounds are examples of puncture injuries. A forceful puncture may penetrate the rib cage and allow air to enter the chest through the wound (see Figure 11-5 on the next page). This does not allow the lungs to function normally. The penetrating object can injure any structure within the chest including the lungs.

Puncture wounds cause varying degrees of internal or external bleeding. A puncture wound is a life-threatening injury. If the injury penetrates the rib cage, air can pass freely in and out of the chest cavity, and the victim cannot breathe normally. With each breath

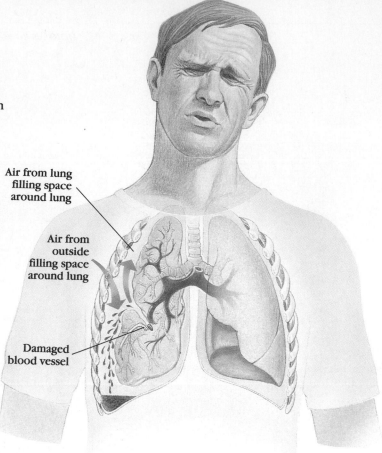

Figure 11-5 A puncture wound that penetrates the lung or the chest cavity surrounding the lung allows air to go in and out of the cavity.

Air from lung filling space around lung

Air from outside filling space around lung

Damaged blood vessel

the victim takes, you hear a sucking sound coming from the wound. This is the primary signal of a penetrating chest injury called a sucking chest wound.

Without proper care, the victim's condition will worsen. The affected lung or lungs will fail to function, and breathing will become more difficult. Your main concern is the breathing problem. To care for a sucking chest wound, cover the wound with a dressing that does not allow air to pass through it. If it is available, a piece of plastic wrap, a plastic bag, or aluminum foil folded several times and placed over the wound makes an effective dressing. Tape the dressing in place, except for one corner that remains loose (Fig. 11-6).

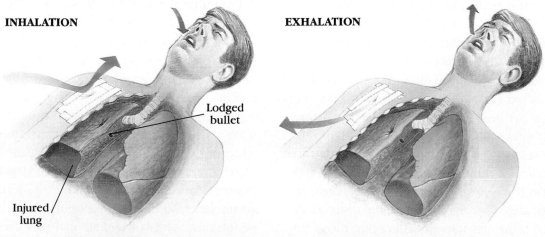

INHALATION

EXHALATION

Lodged bullet

Injured lung

Figure 11-6 A special dressing with one loose corner keeps air from the wound during inhalation and allows air to escape during exhalation.

FRONT VIEW

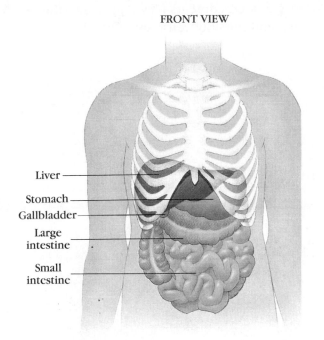

Liver

Stomach

Gallbladder

Large
intestine

Small
intestine

BACK VIEW

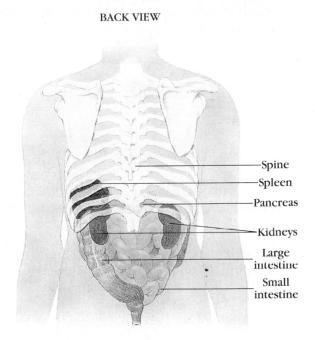

Spine

Spleen

Pancreas

Kidneys

Large
intestine

Small
intestine

Figure 11-7   Unlike the organs of the chest or pelvis, organs in the abdominal cavity are relatively unprotected by bones.

This keeps air from entering the wound during inhalation but allows it to escape during exhalation. If none of these materials are available, use a folded cloth or, as a last resort, your hand.

> *Q*
> **3.** Why is it best to use a special dressing to care for a sucking chest wound?

◆ Injuries to the Abdomen

The abdomen is the area immediately under the chest and above the pelvis. It is easily injured because it is not surrounded by bones. The upper abdomen is partially protected in front by the lower ribs. It is protected at the back by the spine. The muscles of the back and abdomen also help protect the internal or-

gans, many of which are vital (Fig. 11-7). Most important are the organs that are easily injured or tend to bleed profusely when injured, such as the liver, spleen, and stomach.

The liver is very rich in blood. Located in the upper abdomen, this organ is protected somewhat by the lower ribs. However, it is delicate and can be torn by blows from blunt objects or penetrated by a fractured rib. The resulting bleeding can be severe and can quickly be fatal. A liver, when injured, can also leak bile into the abdomen, which can cause severe infection.

The spleen is behind the stomach and is protected somewhat by the lower left ribs. Like the liver, this organ is easily damaged. The spleen may rupture when the abdomen is struck forcefully by a blunt object. Since the spleen stores blood, an injury can cause a severe loss of blood in a short time and can be life-threatening.

The stomach is one of the main digestive organs. The upper part of the stomach changes shape depending on its contents, the stage of digestion, and the size and strength of the stomach muscles. It is lined with many blood vessels and nerves. It can bleed severely when injured, and food contents may empty into the abdomen and possibly cause infection.

Surgical Lifeline

Teresa Smith never planned to make medical history, but the Texas schoolteacher did plan to see her 21-month-old daughter Alyssa grow up. She accomplished the first feat in 1989 when she donated part of her liver for her dying child, and, because of the transplant, she has given her daughter an excellent chance of growing up.

Because the liver is divided into lobes, it is perfectly suited for transplanting, but transplanting a liver from a living donor had never been attempted before in the United States. Doctors traditionally used organs from recently deceased donors, but there were many more patients than organs. Without a new liver, doctors estimated Alyssa would die within a year. She was one of 150 young children waiting for a liver in the United States—as many as a third to a half of those candidates were expected to die on that waiting list.

Dr. Christoph Broelsch, a pioneer in liver transplantation, had begun splitting cadaver livers in 1988 to provide two small livers from the liver of a deceased adult. He saw the living donor as a next step. To his colleagues, he outlined the advantages. By receiving her mother's liver, Alyssa would receive a better match, and her chances of survival would be increased. The liver's unique ability to regenerate would allow Teresa's liver to grow back to its normal size and Alyssa's liver to grow as she did.

Not all doctors were convinced. Many questioned the ethical aspects of asking a healthy parent to take such a grave risk. They criticized the procedure as too dangerous. But Teresa believed the experiment was worth the risk.

Dr. Broelsch and a team of surgeons attempted the transplant. The surgical team tied

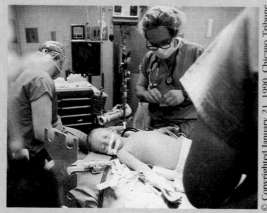

off blood vessels to Teresa's liver and removed her gallbladder to make it easier to reach the liver. Broelsch then sliced off nearly half of the liver and placed it in a chilled preserving solution. As one set of doctors removed Alyssa's impaired liver, another set trimmed Teresa's liver to fit into the child's body. Finally, they carefully reattached the blood vessels. The operation was not without mishaps. Teresa lost her spleen when an instrument nicked her, and the rush to take out the liver caused bruising on Alyssa's new liver, but the doctors were satisfied with the results of the operation.

Teresa was thrilled with the results. Before Alyssa received the transplant, Teresa had to watch her daughter carefully for infections. Now she's a healthy two-year-old who is learning to ride a tricycle. She takes an antirejection drug and one other medicine. Her body has responded well to her mother's donated liver.

"I was going to seek the best treatment for Alyssa," says Teresa, who is glad she underwent the surgery for her daughter. "You do what you have to for your children."

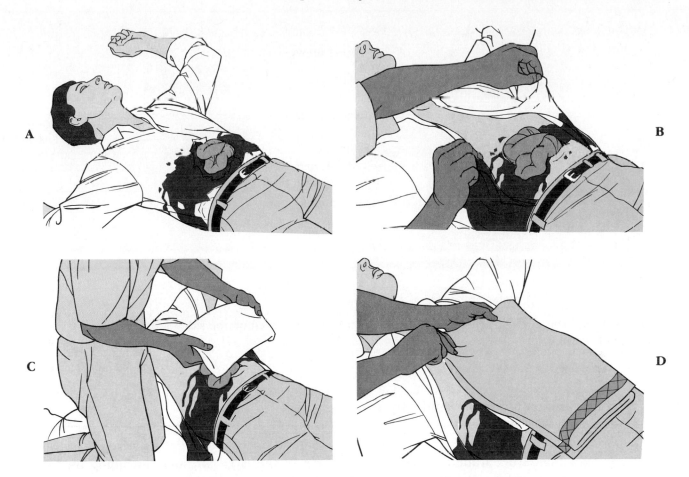

Figure 11-8 **A,** Severe open injuries to the abdominal cavity can result in protruding organs. **B,** Carefully remove clothing from around the wound. **C,** Apply a large, moist, sterile dressing over the wound and cover it loosely with plastic wrap. **D,** Place a folded towel or other cloth over the dressing to maintain warmth.

Signals of Abdominal Injury

The signals of serious abdominal injury include—

- Severe pain.
- Bruising.
- External bleeding.
- Nausea.
- Vomiting (sometimes vomit containing blood).
- Weakness.
- Thirst.
- Pain, tenderness, or a tight feeling in the abdomen.
- Organs possibly protruding from the abdomen.

Care for Abdominal Injuries

Like a chest injury, an injury to the abdomen is either open or closed. Even with a closed wound, the rupture of an organ can cause serious internal bleeding that results in shock. Injuries to the abdomen can be very painful. Serious reactions can occur if organs leak blood or other contents into the abdomen.

With a severe open injury, abdominal organs sometimes protrude through the wound (Fig. 11-8, *A*). To care for an open wound in the abdomen, follow these steps (Fig. 11-8, *B-D*):

FRONT VIEW

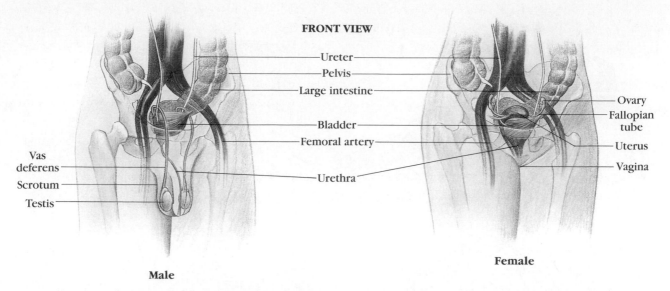

Male

Female

Figure 11-9 The internal structures of the pelvis are well protected on the sides and back, but not in front.

- Carefully position the victim on the back.
- *Do not* apply direct pressure.
- *Do not* push organs back in.
- Remove clothing from around wound.
- Apply moist, sterile dressings loosely over wound. (Warm tap water can be used.)
- Cover dressings loosely with plastic wrap, if available.
- Cover dressings lightly with a folded towel to maintain warmth.

To care for a closed abdominal injury—

- Carefully position the victim on the back.
- Bend the victim's knees slightly. This allows the muscles of the abdomen to relax. If the movement of the victim's legs causes pain, leave the legs straight.
- Place rolled-up blankets or pillows under the victim's knees.

Shock is likely to occur with a serious abdominal injury. Call EMS personnel immediately and take steps to minimize shock. Remember to maintain normal body temperature and monitor the ABCs until EMS personnel arrive.

◆ Injuries to the Pelvis

The pelvis is the lower part of the trunk and contains the bladder, reproductive organs, and part of the large intestine, including the rectum. Major arteries (the femoral arteries) and nerves pass through the pelvis. The organs within the pelvis are well protected on the sides and back but not in front (Fig. 11-9). Injuries to the pelvis may include fractures to the pelvic bone and damage to structures within. Fractured bones may puncture or lacerate them, or they can be injured when struck forceful blows by blunt or penetrating objects.

Signals of Pelvic Injury

Signals of injury to the pelvis are the same as those for an abdominal injury. Certain pelvic injuries may also cause loss of sensation in the legs or inability to move them. This may indicate an injury to the lower spine.

Care for Pelvic Injuries

Care for pelvic injuries is the same as that for abdominal injuries. Do not move the victim unless necessary. If possible, try to keep the victim İying flat. If not, help him or her become comfortable. Control any external bleeding and cover any protruding organs. If you suspect a spinal injury, do not move the victim. Always call EMS personnel and take steps to minimize shock.

An injury to the pelvis sometimes involves the **genitals,** the external reproductive organs. Genital injuries are either closed wounds, such as a bruise, or open wounds, such as an avulsion or laceration. Any injury to the genitals is extremely painful. Care for a closed wound as you would for any closed wound. If the injury is an open wound, apply a sterile dressing and direct pressure with your hand or the victim's hand. If any parts are avulsed, wrap them appropriately and make sure they are transported with the victim. Injuries to the genital area can be embarrassing for both the victim and the rescuer. Explain briefly what you are going to do, and do it. Do not act in a timid or hesitant manner. This will only make the situation more difficult for you and the victim.

♦ Summary

Injuries to the chest, abdomen, or pelvis can be serious. They can damage soft tissues,

bones, and internal organs. Although many injuries are immediately obvious, some may be detected only as the victim's condition worsens over time. Watch for the signals of serious injuries that require medical attention.

Care for any life-threatening condition, then give any additional care needed for specific injuries. For open wounds to the chest, abdomen, or pelvis, control bleeding. If you suspect fracture, immobilize the injured part. Use special dressings for sucking chest wounds and open abdominal wounds when these materials are available. Always call EMS personnel as soon as possible. This gives the victim of a serious injury the best chance for survival and full recovery.

In the next chapter, you will learn about injuries to the extremities, which, like injuries described in this chapter, are often caused by trauma.

Q

4. If injuries are not immediately obvious, what signals should alert you that the victim's condition is deteriorating?

Answers to Application Questions

1. Coughing up blood signals bleeding in the chest. This indicates that blood vessels, chest muscles, and other tissues are damaged. For instance, a lung may be punctured. More important, coughing up blood indicates that blood is entering and to some degree obstructing the airway, which may make breathing more difficult. Coughing up blood is also a warning sign that, if the victim becomes unconscious, there is a high probability that blood will be aspirated into the lungs.

2. In caring for an open rib fracture, be careful not to apply direct pressure to the fracture. Apply pressure around the fracture to control bleeding. Immobilize the area. If it

is necessary to splint the area, be careful not to put pressure on the fracture site.

3. When air enters the chest through a wound, one or more lungs may fail to function. A special dressing, one that does not allow air to enter, prevents air from being sucked into the chest when the victim inhales, helping the victim to breathe more easily.

4. Any signals of shock or internal bleeding should alert you that the victim's condition is deteriorating. Changes in breathing, heartbeat, or level of consciousness are very important. Call EMS personnel for help.

Study Questions

1. Match each term with the correct definition.

    a. Abdomen
    b. Chest
    c. Genitals
    d. Pelvis
    e. Sternum

       _____ External reproductive organs
       _____ The middle part of the trunk containing organs such as the stomach, liver, and spleen
       _____ The upper part of the trunk containing the heart, major blood vessels, and lungs
       _____ Long, flat bone in the middle of the front of the rib cage, also called the breastbone
       _____ The lower part of the trunk containing the intestines, bladder, and reproductive organs

2. List five steps of care for injuries to the chest, abdomen, and pelvis.

3. List at least four signals of chest injury.

4. List at least two signals of rib fractures.

5. Name the primary signal of a sucking chest wound.

6. List at least four signals of abdominal and pelvic injury.

Circle the letter of the correct answer.

7. Care for injuries to the chest, abdomen, and pelvis includes—

    a. Monitoring the ABCs and limiting movement.
    b. Controlling bleeding.
    c. Taking steps to minimize shock.
    d. a and b
    e. a, b, and c

You arrive at the local convenience store late Saturday night to satisfy your ice cream craving. As you enter, you notice drops of blood on the floor. A robbery has just occurred—the store clerk appears to have been beaten and stabbed. He is conscious, but in considerable pain and having difficulty breathing. You hear an abnormal sucking sound when he breathes.

8. List the signals of chest injury you find in the scenario.

9. Least at least four things you can do to provide care for the store clerk.

Answers are in Appendix A.

Injuries to the Extremities

Objectives

After reading this chapter, you should be able to—

1. List at least three signals that suggest a serious extremity injury.

2. Describe how to care for injuries to the shoulder, arm, and elbow.

3. Describe how to care for injuries to the forearm, wrist, and hand.

4. List at least two specific signals of a fractured thigh bone.

5. Describe how to care for injuries to the thigh, leg, and knee.

6. Describe how to care for injuries to the ankle and foot.

7. Define the key terms for this chapter.

After reading this chapter and completing the class activities, you should be able to—

1. Make appropriate decisions regarding care when given an example of an emergency situation involving injuries to the extremities.

Key Terms

Arm: The entire upper extremity from the shoulder to the hand.

Bandage: Material used to wrap or cover a part of the body; commonly used to hold a dressing or splint in place.

Extremities: The arms and legs, hands and feet.

Forearm: The upper extremity from the elbow to the wrist.

Immobilization: The use of a splint or other method to keep an injured body part from moving.

Leg: The entire lower extremity from the pelvis to the foot.

Lower leg: The lower extremity between the knee and the ankle.

Splint: A device used to immobilize body parts.

Thigh: The lower extremity between the pelvis and the knee.

Upper arm: The upper extremity from the shoulder to the elbow.

For Review

Before reading this chapter, you should have a basic understanding of how to control bleeding (Chapter 6) and how to care for musculoskeletal injuries (Chapter 9).

◆ Introduction

Injuries to the **extremities**, the **arms** and **legs,** hands and feet, are quite common. They range from a simple bruise to a critical injury with severe bleeding, such as a fracture of the thighbone. With any injury to the extremities, the prompt care you give can help prevent further pain and damage.

As you will learn in this chapter, care for soft tissue and musculoskeletal injuries involving the extremities is like the care for other parts of the body. In general, control bleeding first. Then rest the injured body part, apply ice or a cold pack, and elevate the area if possible or if it does not cause pain. If you suspect a serious injury, always immobilize the injured body part first and determine what further care is needed. If necessary, call EMS personnel and continue to monitor the ABCs until medical professionals arrive. To minimize shock, maintain normal body temperature and help the victim into the most comfortable position.

◆ Signals of Serious Extremity Injury

The extremities consist of bones, soft tissues, blood vessels, and nerves. They are subject to various kinds of injury. Injury can affect the soft tissues, resulting in open or closed wounds. Injury can also affect the musculoskeletal system, resulting in sprains, strains, fractures, or dislocations. Signals of a serious extremity injury include—

- Pain.
- Tenderness.
- Swelling.
- Discoloration.
- Deformity of the limb.
- Inability to use the limb.
- Severe external bleeding.

◆ Upper Extremity Injuries

The upper extremities are the arms and hands. The bones of each upper extremity include the collarbone (clavicle), shoulder blade (scapula), bones of the **upper arm** (humerus) and **forearm** (radius and ulna), and bones of the hand (carpals and metacarpals) and fingers (phalanges). Figure 12-1 on the next page shows the major structures of the upper extremities. In addition to damaging bones and muscles, injuries may damage blood vessels, nerves, and other soft tissues.

The upper extremities are the most com-

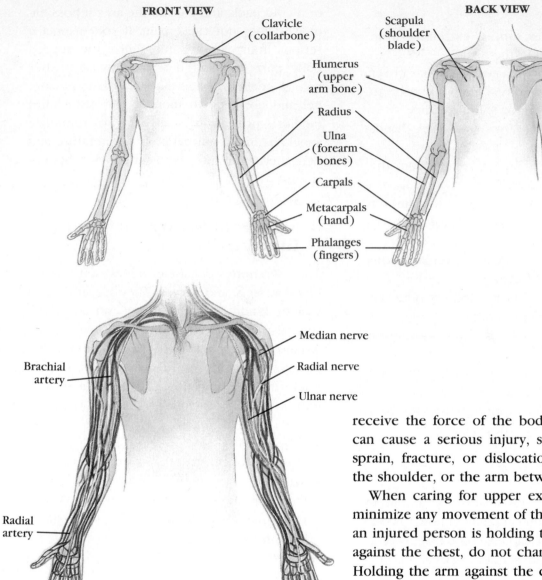

FRONT VIEW

Clavicle
(collarbone)

Humerus
(upper
arm bone)

Radius

Ulna
(forearm
bones)

Carpals

Metacarpals
(hand)

Phalanges
(fingers)

BACK VIEW

Scapula
(shoulder
blade)

Median nerve

Radial nerve

Ulnar nerve

Brachial
artery

Radial
artery

Figure 12-1   The upper extremities include the bones of the arms and hands, nerves, and blood vessels.

monly injured area of the body. These injuries may occur in many different ways. The most frequent cause is falling on a hand of an outstretched arm. Since the hands are rarely protected, abrasions occur easily. Because a falling person instinctively tries to break the fall by extending the arms and hands, these areas

receive the force of the body's weight. This can cause a serious injury, such as a severe sprain, fracture, or dislocation, of the hand, the shoulder, or the arm between.

When caring for upper extremity injuries, minimize any movement of the injured part. If an injured person is holding the arm securely against the chest, do not change the position. Holding the arm against the chest is an effective method of **immobilization.** Instead, help the person support the arm by binding it to the chest. Caring for a victim with an upper extremity injury does not require special equipment.

Specific Injuries of the Upper Extremities

Shoulder injuries

The shoulder consists of three bones that meet to form the shoulder joint. These bones are the clavicle, scapula, and humerus. The most common shoulder injuries are sprains. However, injuries of the shoulder may also in-

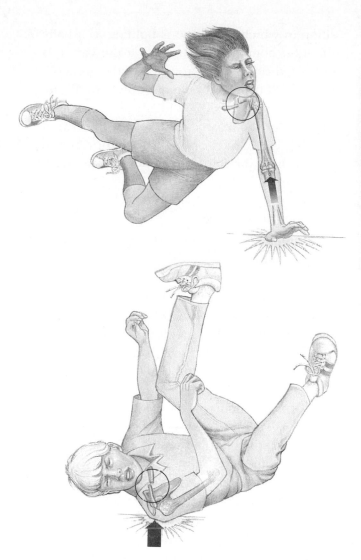

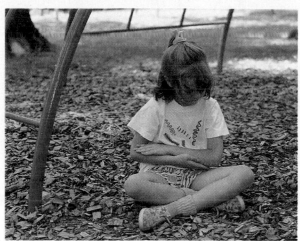

Figure 12-3 Someone with a fractured collarbone will usually support the arm on the injured side.

Figure 12-2 A collarbone fracture is commonly caused by a fall.

volve a fracture or dislocation of one or more of these bones.

The most frequently injured bone of the shoulder is the clavicle, more commonly injured in children than adults. Typically, the clavicle is fractured as a result of a fall (Fig. 12-2). The victim usually feels pain in the shoulder area. The pain may radiate down the arm. A person with a fractured clavicle usually attempts to ease the pain by holding the arm against the chest (Fig. 12-3). Since the clavicle lies directly over major blood vessels and

nerves to the arm, it is important to immobilize the injured area to prevent injury to these structures.

Scapula fractures are not common. A fracture of the scapula typically results from violent force. The signals of a fractured scapula are the same as for any other extremity fracture, although you are less likely to see deformity of the scapula. The most significant signals are extreme pain and the inability to move the arm.

Because it takes great force to break the scapula, consider that the force may have been great enough also to injure the chest cavity. If the chest cavity is injured, the victim with a fractured scapula may have difficulty breathing.

A dislocation, often called a shoulder separation, is another common type of shoulder injury. Like fractures, dislocations often result from falls. This happens frequently in sports such as football and rugby when a player attempts to break a fall with an outstretched arm or lands on the point of the shoulder. The impact can force the arm against the joint

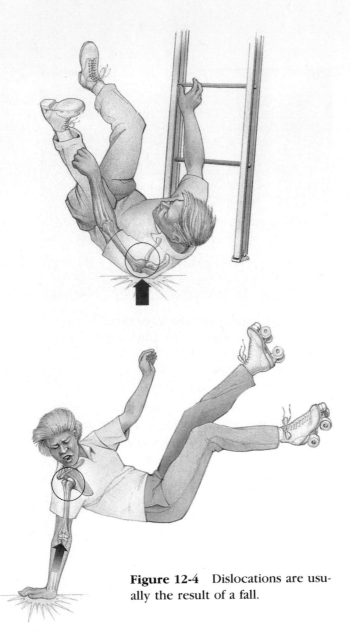

Figure 12-4 Dislocations are usually the result of a fall.

formed by the scapula and clavicle (Fig. 12-4). This can result in ligaments tearing, allowing bones to displace.

Shoulder dislocations are painful and can often be identified by the deformity present. As with other shoulder injuries, the victim often tries to minimize the pain by holding the arm in the most comfortable position.

First aid for shoulder injuries. To care for shoulder injuries, first control any external bleeding with direct pressure. Allow the victim to continue to support the arm in the position in which he or she is holding it, usually the most comfortable position. If the victim is holding the arm away from the body, use a pillow, rolled blanket, or similar object to fill the gap between the arm and chest to provide support for the injured area. **Splint** the arm in place (Fig. 12-5). Apply cold to the injured area to help minimize pain and reduce swelling.

Upper arm injuries

The bone of the upper arm is the humerus. It is the largest bone in the arm. This bone can be fractured at any point, although it is usually fractured at the upper end near the shoulder or in the middle of the bone. The upper end of the humerus often fractures in the elderly and in young children as a result of a fall. Breaks in the middle of the bone mostly occur in young adults.

When the humerus is fractured, there is danger of damage to the blood vessels and nerves supplying the entire arm. Most humerus fractures are very painful and will not permit the victim to use the arm. A fracture can also cause considerable arm deformity.

First aid for upper arm injuries. To care for a serious upper arm injury, immobilize the upper arm from the shoulder to the elbow. Care for the arm in the same way as for shoulder injuries. Control any external bleeding with direct pressure. Place the arm in a sling and bind it to the chest with cravats. Apply ice in the best way possible. You can use a short splint, if one is available, to give more support to the upper arm (Fig. 12-6).

Elbow injuries

Injuries to the elbow can cause permanent disability, since all the nerves and blood vessels to the forearm and hand go through the elbow. Therefore, take elbow injuries seriously. Like other joints, the elbow can be sprained, fractured, or dislocated. Injuries to a joint like the elbow can be made worse by

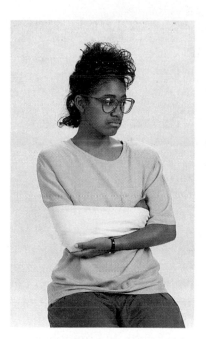
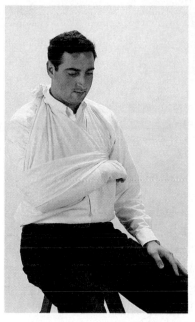
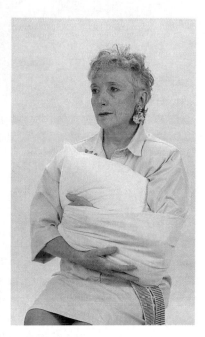

Figure 12-5 Splint the arm against the chest in the position in which the victim is holding it. Use cravats, a sling, and a small pillow or a rolled blanket, if necessary.

movement. If the victim says that he or she cannot move the elbow, do not try to move it. Support the arm and immobilize it in the position in which you find it. Call EMS personnel immediately.

First aid for elbow injuries. To provide care, first control any external bleeding with direct pressure. Next, immobilize the arm from the shoulder to the wrist in the best way possible. Place the arm in a sling and secure it to the chest as shown in Figure 12-5. If this is not possible, immobilize the elbow with a splint and two cravats. If the elbow is bent, apply the splint diagonally across the underside

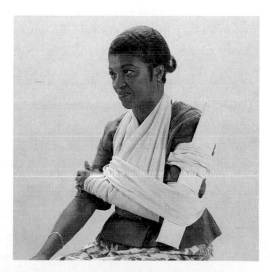

Figure 12-6 A short splint can provide additional support for a fractured upper arm.

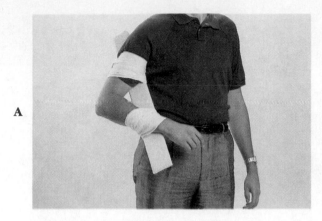

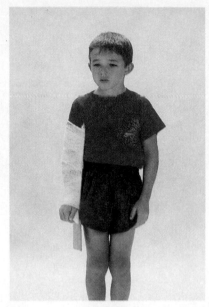

Figure 12-7 **A,** If the elbow is bent, apply the splint diagonally across the underside of the arm. **B,** If the arm is straight, apply the splint along the underside of the arm.

of the arm (Fig. 12-7, *A).* The splint should extend several inches beyond both the upper arm and the wrist. If the elbow is straight, apply the splint along the arm. Secure the splint at the wrist and upper arm with cravats or roller **bandages** (Fig. 12-7, *B).* Apply ice or a cold pack.

Forearm, wrist, and hand injuries

Fractures of the two forearm bones, the radius and ulna, are more common in children than adults. If a person falls on an outstretched arm, both bones may break, but not always in the same place. With forearm fractures, the arm may look s-shaped (Fig. 12-8). Because the radial artery and nerve are near the bones, a fracture may cause severe bleeding or a loss of movement in the wrist and hand.

The wrist is a common site of sprains and fractures. It is often difficult to tell the extent of the injury. Therefore, care for wrist injuries in the same way as forearm injuries.

Because the hands are used in so many daily activities, they are very susceptible to injury. Most injuries to the hands and fingers involve only minor soft tissue damage. However, a serious injury may damage nerves, blood

vessels, and bones. Home, recreational, and industrial mishaps often produce lacerations, avulsions, burns, and fractures of the hands.

Because the hand structures are delicate, deep lacerations should be immobilized to prevent possible disability. With a suspected finger or thumb dislocation, *do not* attempt to put the bones back into place.

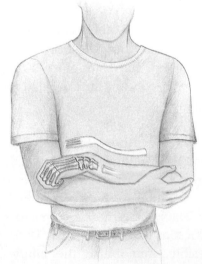

Figure 12-8 Fractures of both forearm bones often cause a characteristic s-shaped deformity.

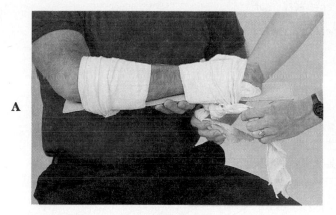
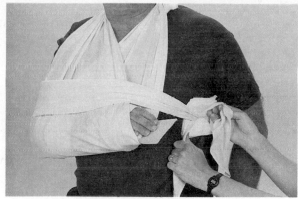

Figure 12-9 **A,** If the forearm is fractured, place a splint under the forearm and secure with two cravats. **B,** Put the arm in a sling and secure it to the chest with cravats.

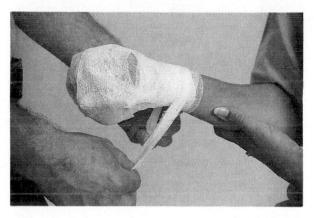

Figure 12-10 A bulky dressing is an effective splint for a hand or finger injury.

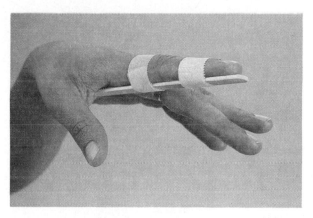

Figure 12-11 An ice cream stick can be used to splint a finger injury.

Q
1. Why should a lacerated hand be immobilized?

First aid for forearm, wrist, and hand injuries. First control any external bleeding with direct pressure. Then care for the injured forearm, wrist, or hand by immobilizing the injured part. Support the injured part by placing a splint underneath the forearm, extending it beyond both the hand and elbow. Place a roll of gauze or a similar object in the palm to keep the palm and fingers in a normal position. Then secure the splint with cravats or

roller gauze (Fig. 12-9, *A*). Put the arm in a sling and secure it to the chest with cravats (Fig. 12-9, *B*). For a hand or finger injury, a bulky dressing is effective (Fig. 12-10). For a possible fractured or dislocated finger, fasten a small splint, such as an ice cream stick, to the finger with tape (Fig. 12-11). Always apply ice and elevate injuries to the forearm, wrist, and hand.

◆ Lower Extremity Injuries

Injuries to the leg can involve both soft tissue and musculoskeletal damage. The major bones of the **thigh** and **lower leg** are large and

FRONT VIEW

BACK VIEW

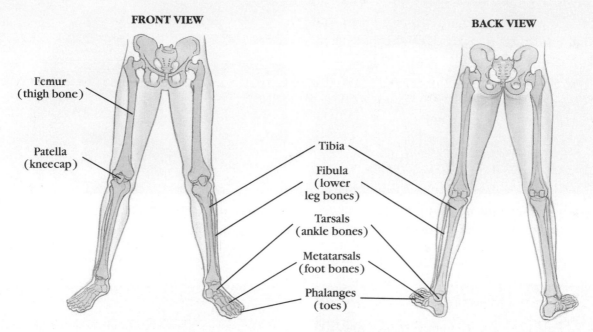

Femur
(thigh bone)

Patella
(kneecap)

Tibia

Fibula
(lower
leg bones)

Tarsals
(ankle bones)

Metatarsals
(foot bones)

Phalanges
(toes)

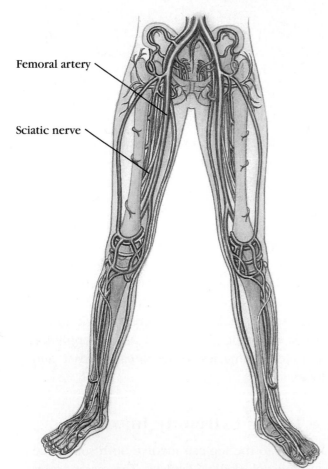

Femoral artery

Sciatic nerve

Figure 12-12   The lower extremities

strong in order to carry the body's weight. Bones of the leg include the thighbone (femur), the kneecap (patella), the two bones in the lower leg (tibia and fibula), and the bones of the foot (tarsals and metatarsals) and toes (phalanges). Because of the size and strength of the bones in the thigh and lower leg, a significant amount of force is required to cause a fracture.

The femoral artery is the major supplier of blood to the legs and feet. If it is damaged, which may happen with a fracture of the femur, the blood loss can be life-threatening.

Figure 12-12 shows the major structures of the lower extremities. When caring for lower extremity injuries, follow the same general principles of care described in Chapter 9. Serious injury to the lower extremities can result in an inability to bear weight. Since the victim will be unable to walk to a car, you should contact EMS personnel to transport him or her to a medical facility.

Specific Injuries to the Lower Extremities

Thigh and lower leg injuries

The femur is the largest bone in the body. Because it bears most of the weight of the body, it is most important in walking and running. Thigh injuries range from bruises and torn muscles to severe injuries such as fractures or dislocations. The upper end of the femur meets the pelvis at the hip joint (Fig. 12-13). Most femur fractures involve the upper end of the bone. Even though the hip joint itself is not involved, such injuries are often called hip fractures.

A fracture of the femur usually produces a characteristic deformity. When the fracture occurs, the thigh muscles contract. Because the thigh muscles are so strong, they pull the broken bone ends together, causing them to overlap. This may cause the injured leg to be noticeably shorter than the other leg. The injured leg may also be turned outward (Fig. 12-14). Other signals of a fractured femur include severe pain and inability to move the leg.

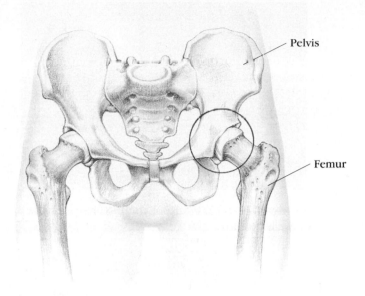

Figure 12-13 The upper end of the femur meets the pelvis at the hip joint.

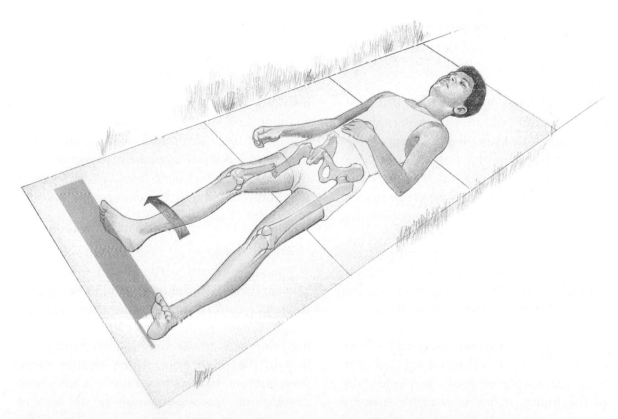

Figure 12-14 A fractured femur often produces a characteristic deformity. The injured leg is shorter than the uninjured leg and may be turned outward.

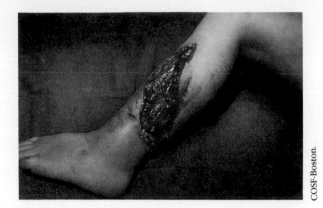

Figure 12-15 A fracture of the lower leg can be an open fracture.

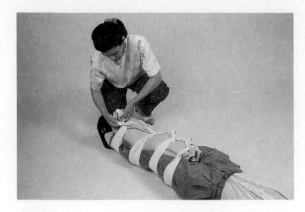

COSF-Boston.

Figure 12-16 To splint an injured leg, secure the injured leg to the uninjured leg with several wide cravats.

A fracture in the lower leg may involve one or both bones. Often both are fractured simultaneously. However, a blow to the outside of the lower leg can cause an isolated fracture of the smaller bone (fibula). Because these two bones lie just beneath the skin, open fractures are common (Fig. 12-15). Lower leg fractures may cause a severe deformity in which the lower leg is bent at an unusual angle (angulated), as well as pain and inability to move the leg.

First aid for thigh and lower leg injuries.
Initial care for the victim with a serious injury to the thigh or lower leg is to stop external bleeding and immobilize the injured area. Call EMS personnel immediately. They are much better prepared than a layperson to care for and transport a victim with a serious leg injury. While waiting for EMS personnel to arrive, immobilize the injured area and help the victim rest in the most comfortable position. What most people fail to consider is that the ground acts as an excellent splint. If the victim's leg is supported by the ground, do not move it. In other situations, you can secure the injured leg to the uninjured leg with several wide cravats placed above and below the site of the injury. If one is available, place a pillow or rolled blanket between the legs and bind the legs together above and below the

site of the injury (Fig. 12-16). Apply ice or a cold pack to reduce pain and swelling. Do not be alarmed if EMS personnel later undo the splint and apply a more rigid splint or a mechanical device called a traction splint. This device reduces the deformity of the leg by applying traction to overcome the pull of the thigh muscles that are causing the bone ends to overlap.

A fractured femur can injure the femoral artery, and serious bleeding can result. The likelihood of shock is great. Therefore, take steps to minimize shock. Keep the person lying down and try to keep him or her calm. Maintain normal body temperature, and make sure that EMS personnel have been called. Monitor the ABCs and watch for changes in the victim's level of consciousness.

Knee injuries

The knee joint is very vulnerable to injury. The knee involves the lower end of the femur, the upper ends of the tibia and fibula, and the patella (kneecap). The kneecap is a free-floating bone that moves on the lower front surface of the thigh bone. Knee injuries range from cuts and bruises to sprains, fractures, and dislocations. Deep lacerations in the area of the knee can cause severe joint infections. Sprains, fractures, and dislocations of the knee

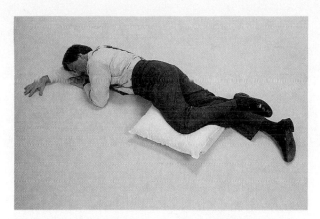

Figure 12-17 Support a knee injury in the bent position if the victim cannot straighten the knee.

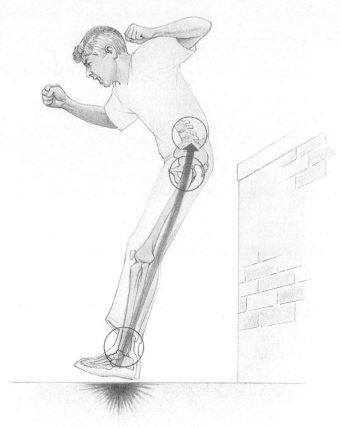

Figure 12-18 In a jump or fall from a height, the impact can be transmitted up the legs, causing injuries to the thighs, hips, or spine.

are common in athletic activities that involve quick movements or exert unusual force on the knee.

The kneecap is unprotected in that it lies directly beneath the skin. This part of the knee is very vulnerable to bruises and lacerations, as well as dislocations. Violent forces to the front of the knee, such as those caused by hitting the dashboard of a motor vehicle or by falling and landing on bent knees, can fracture the kneecap.

First aid for knee injuries. To care for an injured knee, first control any external bleeding. If the knee is bent and cannot be straightened without pain, support it in the bent position (Fig. 12-17). If the knee is straight or can be straightened without pain, secure it to the uninjured leg as you might do for an injury of the thigh or lower leg. Apply ice or a cold pack. Help the victim to rest in the most comfortable position. Call EMS personnel to have him or her transported to a medical facility for examination.

Ankle and foot injuries

Ankle and foot injuries are commonly caused by twisting forces. Injuries range from minor sprains with little swelling and pain that heal with a few days' rest, to fractures and dislocations. As with other joint injuries, you can-

not always distinguish between minor and severe injuries. You should initially care for all ankle and foot injuries as if they are serious. As with other lower extremity injuries, if the ankle or foot is painful to move, if it cannot bear weight, or if the foot or ankle is swollen, a physician should evaluate the injury. Foot injuries may also involve the toes. Although these injuries are painful, they are rarely serious.

Fractures of the feet and ankles can occur from forcefully landing on the heel. With any great force, such as falling from a height and landing on the feet, fractures are possible. The force of the impact may also be transmitted up the legs. This can result in an injury elsewhere in the body such as the thigh, pelvis, or spine (Fig. 12-18).

Quick Recovery

The train tracks that once criss-crossed the injured knees of Olympic skiers, professional football players, and arthritis sufferers have almost disappeared. Both the scars and the trauma of knee surgery have been diminished with the advent of a new medical technique, arthroscopy.

Arthroscopy has aided thousands of athletes cursed with bad knees. It put Chicago Bears defensive tackle Dan Hampton back on the football field countless times and saved the careers of gymnast Mary Lou Retton and marathon runner Joan Benoit just before the 1984 Olympics. Their recoveries were remarkable, considering that, 15 years ago, knee surgery meant a five-day hospital stay, a cast, and three- to four-months' rehabilitation. With arthroscopic surgery, many athletes leave the hospital the same day and begin rehabilitation within days of the procedure.

The most agile of joints, the knee is also the most vulnerable. It joins the two longest bones of the body. Four ligaments attach to the bones and hold the knee together. Two cartilage disks serve as shock absorbers on the ends of the bones. Repeated and excessive shocks to the knee will splinter the cartilage pads and stretch or fray ligaments.

The arthroscope, a thin, steel, 10-inch telescope for surgeons, allows physicians to perform delicate joint surgery without cutting muscles and ligaments and lifting the kneecap to get to the injured area. After injecting a saline solution to distend the knee joint, the surgeon inserts the arthroscope through small puncture wounds into the space of the knee joint. By projecting magnified images inside the knee onto a screen, the arthroscope allows orthopedic surgeons to use microsurgical instruments to smooth arthritic surfaces, remove chipped bones and cartilage, and sew up torn ligaments.

The procedure is not limited to rich and famous knees. More than a million people undergo arthroscopic surgery each year. Arthroscopes, some less than 1.7 millimeters in diameter, are being used to repair shoulders, ankles, wrists, and even jaws. Not all joint problems can be repaired with arthroscopy, but most surgeons would agree that advances in arthroscopy have had a profound impact on the lives of people who might otherwise be incapacitated.

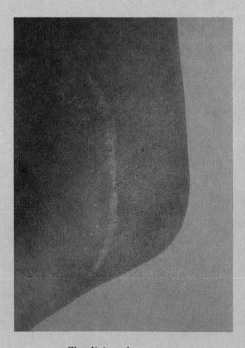

Traditional surgery

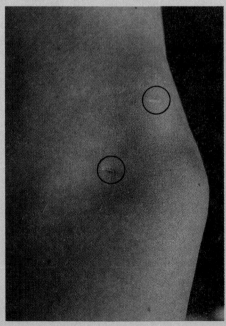

Arthroscopic surgery

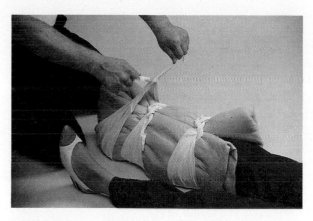

Figure 12-19 An injured ankle can be immobilized with a pillow or rolled blanket secured with two or three cravats.

First aid for ankle and foot injuries. Care for ankle and foot injuries by controlling external bleeding and immobilizing the ankle and foot. Immobilize by using a soft splint such as a pillow or rolled blanket. Wrap the injured area with the soft splint, and secure it with two or three cravats (Fig. 12-19). Then elevate the injured ankle or foot to help reduce the swelling. Apply ice or a cold pack. Suspect that any victim who has fallen or jumped from a height may also have injuries elsewhere. Call EMS personnel and keep the victim from moving until EMS personnel arrive and evaluate his or her condition.

2. How are soft splints, such as pillows and folded blankets, as effective as rigid splints in immobilizing body parts such as the foot or ankle?

◆ Summary

Injuries are a leading health problem in America. When the body experiences violent forces, many kinds of injuries can occur. As you have learned in Chapters 8 through 12, injuries may affect soft tissues, nerves, muscles, bones, ligaments, and tendons. These injuries can have permanent, disabling effects on the body and can even be life-threatening.

The musculoskeletal system and the soft tissues are complex groups of structures that provide protection, support, and movement for the body. You can care for musculoskeletal and soft tissue injuries to the extremities by providing care that focuses on minimizing pain, shock, and further damage to the injured area. You can do this by—

* Managing airway or breathing problems.
* Controlling external bleeding.
* Immobilizing the injured area of the body.
* Applying ice or a cold pack to the injured area.
* Limiting movement of the victim.
* Calming and reassuring the victim.
* Maintaining normal body temperature.
* Seeking advanced medical care.

Answers to Application Questions

1. Structures of the hands are delicate. Nerves, muscles, tendons, and blood vessels are easily damaged by lacerations. Because it is difficult to determine the extent of injury, a lacerated hand should be immobilized to prevent possible further damage to these underlying tissues.

2. Although a pillow or rolled blanket is soft, it secures a fractured limb in a stationary position because of the bulk. The more bulky the object, the better it prevents movement.

Study Questions

1. Match each term with the correct definition.

   a. Upper arm
   b. Forearm
   c. Thigh
   d. Lower leg
   e. Immobilization

   _____ The part of the leg above the knee.
   _____ The use of a splint or other method to keep an injured body part from moving.
   _____ The part of the arm between the elbow and the wrist.
   _____ The part of the leg between the knee and the ankle.
   _____ The part of the arm between the shoulder and the elbow.

2. Name the most frequent cause of upper extremity injuries.

3. List at least three signals that suggest a serious extremity injury.

4. List two specific signals of a fractured femur.

5. List three steps of general care for injuries to the extremities.

In questions 6 through 8, circle the letter of the correct answer.

6. A man who has fallen down a steep flight of stairs is clutching his right arm to his chest. He says his shoulder hurts and he cannot move his arm. To care for him, you—

   a. Allow him to continue supporting the arm.
   b. Splint the arm to the chest in this position.
   c. Have him move the arm into its normal position.
   d. a and b

7. A child has fallen from a bicycle onto the pavement and landed on her elbow. The elbow is bent and the girl says she cannot move it. What do you do?

   a. Straighten the arm and splint it.
   b. Call EMS personnel.
   c. Immobilize the elbow in the bent position.
   d. Ask her to continue to try to move the arm.
   e. b and c

8. A person with an open fracture of the femur is lying on the ground. You should—

   a. Call EMS personnel at once.
   b. Raise the injured leg in order to splint it.
   c. Use the ground as a splint and do not move the leg.
   d. Control external bleeding.
   e. a, c, and d

9. An elderly woman has tripped and fallen over some gardening tools. She is lying on the ground, conscious and breathing. Her lower leg is bleeding profusely from a gash and seems to be bent at an odd angle. List the steps of care you would provide.

Answers are in Appendix A.

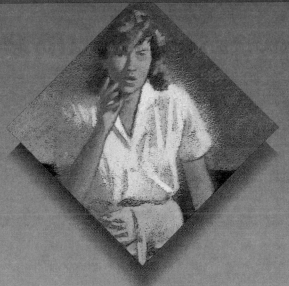

Medical Emergencies

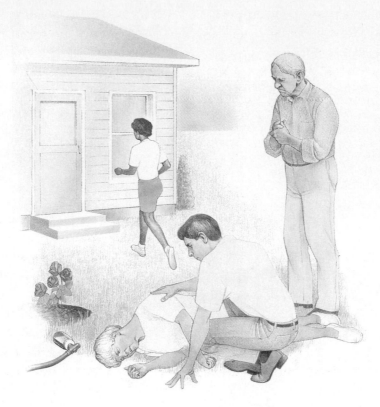

Figure V-1

♦ Introduction

As Steve is walking up to the front door of his friend Jackie's house, he hears a cry for help from the backyard next door. Just then Jackie opens the door and also hears the cry. They rush to the neighbor's backyard.

An elderly woman is lying on her side on the ground. An elderly man stands by helplessly. There is an insecticide spray bottle on the ground nearby. Steve notices that the woman's eyes are open and her body is limp. Saliva is dribbling from her mouth. Her face seems distorted, her mouth drooping to one side. She does not respond when he speaks to her and taps her on the shoulder. Steve bends over her and observes that she is breathing. Her skin is cool and she is sweating heavily.

Jackie asks the man what happened and how long his wife has been like this. He says he is not sure. He came outside and found her lying on the ground, twitching violently. Steve asks Jackie to call for an ambulance. Steve asks if the woman has any medical problems, is taking any medications, or is allergic to anything. The man looks confused and replies "no" to each question.

Thoughts race through Steve's mind. What could her problem be? Poisoning? An allergic reaction? A stroke? A diabetic problem? A head injury from a fall? What about the twitching the man described? Did the man understand the questions and answer them accurately?

Steve knows that the paramedics will arrive in about 10 minutes. He tries to remain calm. He asks the man for a blanket to help warm the woman's cool body. He decides not to move her but examines her carefully for any signals of what the problem could be. He wants to help the woman, but because he does not know what the problem is, he is unsure about how to proceed. He feels helpless. What should he do?

♦ The Dilemma of Medical Emergencies

Steve's dilemma in the preceding scenario is not rare. You too could someday face a situation involving an unknown medical emergency. Unlike easily identified problems such as external bleeding, medical emergencies are rarely as clear. Therefore, you may feel more uncertain about providing care.

When you face an emergency you do not understand, it is normal to feel helpless or indecisive. Yet everyone still wants to help to the best of his or her ability. Take comfort from the fact that giving initial care, even for unknown medical emergencies, does not require extensive knowledge. You do not have to "diagnose" or choose among possible problems in order to provide appropriate care. By following the emergency action principles and the guidelines for care in previous chapters, you will provide appropriate care until advanced medical help arrives. Knowing this, you can approach an unknown medical emergency with confidence.

Put yourself in Steve's place. Do you think he responded appropriately? The elderly woman was experiencing a diabetic emergency, but Steve could not have known this. Her husband was confused and did not give Steve correct information. Did it matter that Steve did not know that she was a diabetic? Not at all. Steve correctly focused on the following basics of care:

- Do no further harm—Steve was right not to try to move the woman from lying on her side. She was not conscious, and there was no immediate threat to her or anyone else requiring her to be moved.
- Monitor the ABCs—Keeping her positioned on her side kept her airway clear by letting fluid drain from her mouth so it would not obstruct her airway. Steve determined that she was breathing by watching and listening to her inhale and exhale. Since she was breathing, he knew she had a pulse. He did not see any severe external bleeding.
- Notify EMS personnel—Steve made sure EMS personnel were notified promptly, ensuring a rapid response. By sending a bystander to make the call, Steve was able to continue to provide care.

- Do a secondary survey to check for any additional injuries—Steve looked over the woman's body for any clues or additional problems but did not find any. Therefore no further care was needed.
- Minimize shock by maintaining normal body temperature—Steve recognized that the woman was cool. He asked for a blanket to help warm her.

Steve did all he should have done for the woman until EMS personnel arrived. What if Steve had other information such as seeing a medical alert bracelet indicating she was a diabetic? Would that have helped him care for this person? No. Even if Steve had known she was a diabetic, it would not have affected the care he gave. Since she was not conscious, Steve's care would have been the same. Almost all the care you will give a person having a medical emergency, whether the person is conscious or unconscious, is as simple as following these five basics of care.

◆ The Onset of Medical Emergencies

Medical emergencies can develop very rapidly (acute) or gradually over a period of time (chronic). They can result from illness or disease. They include chronic problems from degenerative diseases such as heart and lung disease. They can involve hormone imbalances such as diabetes. They can involve sudden unexplained conditions such as fainting. Medical emergencies can also involve illnesses, such as allergies or epilepsy, in which exposure to a certain substance causes a reaction or an occasional seizure occurs. Overexposure to heat and cold can also cause serious illness.

In the previous unit, you learned that injury is the leading cause of death and disability for people between the ages of 1 and 44. In this unit, you will learn about those medical conditions that can also cause death and disability in this age group and that are a major problem for those over age 45.

Sudden Illnesses

Objectives

After reading this chapter, you should be able to—

1. Identify at least four general signals of sudden illness.

2. Describe the care for a person who faints.

3. Describe the care for a person who you suspect is having a diabetic emergency.

4. Describe the care for a person having a seizure.

5. List at least three instances when you should call EMS personnel for a person having a seizure.

6. List at least two risk factors that can be controlled to help prevent stroke.

7. Describe the care for a person who you suspect has had a stroke.

8. Define the key terms for this chapter.

After reading this chapter and completing the class activities, you should be able to—

1. Make appropriate decisions regarding care when given an example of a situation in which someone has suddenly become ill.

◆ Introduction

Certain illnesses occur suddenly. Often there are no warning signals to alert you that something is happening. At other times, the victim may feel ill or state that he or she feels that something is wrong.

Sudden illnesses may be signaled in a variety of ways. They may cause changes in a person's level of consciousness. A person may complain of feeling light-headed, dizzy, or weak. He or she may feel nauseated or may vomit. Breathing, pulse, and skin color may change. The fact that a person looks and feels ill means there is a problem.

Many different conditions, such as diabetes, **stroke, epilepsy,** poisoning, and shock, can cause a change in consciousness. In an emergency, you may not know what caused the change, but the cause is not important. You do not need to know the exact cause to provide appropriate care for the victim. In this chapter, you will learn that knowing and following the emergency action principles and the basic principles of care are all you need to care for a victim of sudden illness.

Faced with an unknown illness, you may not be sure whether to call for emergency medical help. Sometimes, as with simple **fainting,** the illness quickly passes. In this case, EMS personnel may not be needed. However, if the problem is not resolved quickly and easily, or if you have any doubts about its severity, always call your local emergency number for help. It is better to err on the side of caution. Refer to Chapter 3 for conditions for which you should call EMS personnel.

This chapter provides information about some sudden illnesses you may encounter—fainting, **diabetic emergency, seizure,** and stroke. As you read, you will see that the care for these illnesses follows the same general guidelines:

* Do no further harm.
* Monitor the ABCs.
* Notify EMS personnel when necessary.

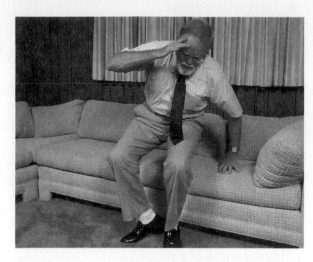

Figure 13-1 A sudden change in positions can sometimes trigger fainting.

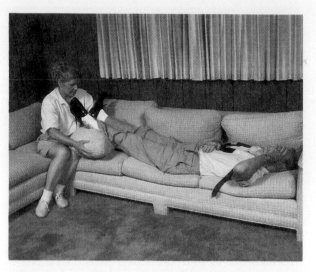

Figure 13-2 To care for fainting, place the victim on his back, elevate the feet, and loosen any restrictive clothing such as a belt, tie, or collar.

- Help the victim to rest comfortably.
- Minimize shock by maintaining normal body temperature.
- Provide reassurance.
- Provide any specific care needed.

♦ Specific Sudden Illness

Fainting

One of the most common sudden illnesses is fainting. Fainting is a partial or complete loss of consciousness. It is caused by a temporary reduction of blood flow to the brain, such as when blood pools in the legs and lower body, reducing blood flow to the head. When the brain is suddenly deprived of its normal blood flow, it momentarily shuts down and the person faints.

Fainting can be triggered by an emotional shock such as the sight of blood. It may be caused by pain, by specific medical conditions such as heart disease, by standing for long periods of time, or by overexertion. Some people, such as pregnant women or the elderly, are more likely to faint when suddenly changing positions, such as moving from sitting or lying to standing up (Fig. 13-1). Any time changes inside the body momentarily reduce the blood flow to the brain, fainting may occur.

Signals of fainting

Fainting may occur with or without warning. Often, the victim may initially feel light-headed or dizzy. Because fainting is one form of shock, he or she may show signals of shock, such as pale, cool, moist skin. The victim may feel nauseated and complain of numbness or tingling in the fingers and toes.

Q

1. How is fainting a form of shock?

Care for fainting

Usually, fainting resolves by itself. When the victim collapses, normal circulation to the brain resumes. The victim usually regains consciousness within a minute.

Fainting itself does not usually harm the victim, but injury may occur from falling. If you can reach the person starting to collapse, lower him or her to the ground or other flat surface and position on the back. If possible, elevate the victim's legs 8 to 12 inches.

Loosen any restrictive clothing such as a belt, tie, or collar (Fig. 13-2). Check the ABCs. Do not give the victim anything to eat or drink. Also, do not splash water on the victim's face. This does little to stimulate the victim, and the victim could aspirate the water.

Usually the victim of fainting recovers quickly with no lasting effects. However, since you will not be able to determine whether the fainting is linked to a more serious condition, EMS personnel should be summoned.

Q

2. Why do people who have fainted regain consciousness after collapsing to the ground?

Diabetic Emergencies

In order to function normally, body cells need sugar as a source of energy. Through the digestive process, the body breaks down food into sugars, which are absorbed into the bloodstream. However, sugar cannot pass freely from the blood into the body cells. Instead, it needs an escort. **Insulin**, a hormone produced in the pancreas, takes sugar into the cells. Without a proper balance of sugar and insulin, the cells will starve and the body will not function properly (Fig. 13-3).

The condition in which the body does not produce enough insulin is called diabetes mellitus, or more commonly, sugar diabetes. The person with this condition is a **diabetic**. There are between 11 and 12 million diabetics in the United States.

There are two major types of diabetes. Type I, insulin-dependent diabetes, occurs when the body produces little or no insulin. Since this type of diabetes tends to begin in childhood, it is often called juvenile diabetes. Most insulin-dependent diabetics have to inject insulin into their bodies daily.

Type II, noninsulin-dependent diabetes, occurs when the body produces insulin but not in sufficient quantity for the body's needs. This condition is called maturity-onset diabetes and usually occurs in older adults.

Anyone with diabetes must carefully monitor his or her diet and exercise. Insulin-depen-

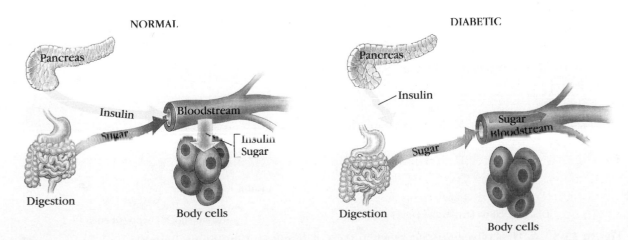

Figure 13-3 The hormone insulin is needed to take sugar from the blood into the body cells.

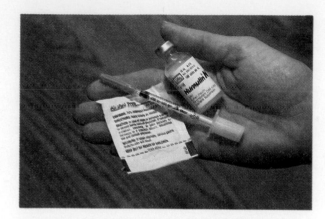

Figure 13-4 Insulin-dependent diabetics inject insulin to regulate the amount in the body.

dent diabetics must also regulate their use of insulin (Fig. 13-4). When a diabetic fails to control these factors, either of two problems can occur—too much or too little sugar in the body. This imbalance causes illness.

When the insulin level in the body is too low, the sugar level in the blood is high. This condition is called **hyperglycemia** (Fig. 13-5, *A)*. Sugar is present in the blood but cannot be transported from the blood into the cells without insulin. When this occurs, body cells become starved for sugar. The body attempts to meet its need for energy by using other stored food and energy sources such as fats. However, converting fat to energy produces waste products and increases the acidity level in the

blood, causing a condition called acidosis. As this occurs, the person becomes ill. If it continues, the hyperglycemic condition deteriorates into its most serious form, diabetic coma.

On the other hand, when the insulin level in the body is too high, the person has a low sugar level. This condition is known as **hypoglycemia** (Fig. 13-5, *B)*. The sugar level can become too low if the diabetic—

◆ Takes too much insulin.
◆ Fails to eat adequately.
◆ Overexercises and burns off sugar faster than normal.
◆ Experiences great emotional stress.

In this situation, the small amount of sugar is used up rapidly, and there is not enough for the brain to function properly. This results in an acute condition called insulin reaction.

Signals of diabetic emergencies

The signals of hyperglycemia and hypoglycemia differ somewhat, but the major signals are similar. These include—

◆ Changes in the level of consciousness, including dizziness, drowsiness, and confusion.
◆ Rapid breathing.
◆ Rapid pulse.
◆ Feeling and looking ill.

DIABETIC EMERGENCIES

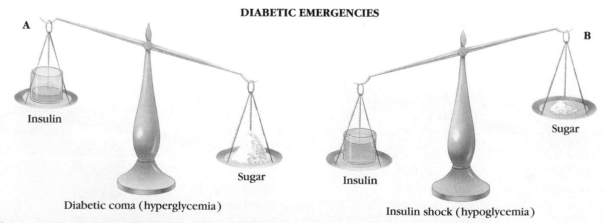

A
Insulin
Sugar
Diabetic coma (hyperglycemia)

B
Insulin
Sugar
Insulin shock (hypoglycemia)

Figure 13-5 A, Hyperglycemia occurs when there is insufficient insulin in the body, causing a high level of sugar in the blood. **B,** Hypoglycemia occurs when the insulin level in the body is high, causing a low level of sugar in the blood.

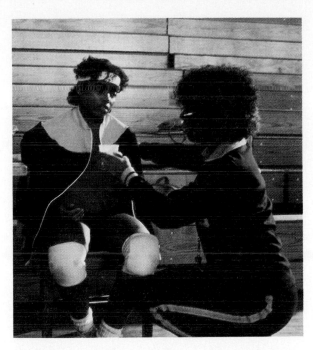

Figure 13-6 If the victim of a diabetic emergency is conscious, give him or her food or fluids containing sugar

It is not important for you to differentiate between insulin reaction and diabetic coma. The basic care for both conditions is the same.

Care for diabetic emergencies

First, do a primary survey and care for any life-threatening conditions. If the victim is conscious, do a secondary survey of the victim, looking for anything visibly wrong. Ask if he or she is a diabetic or look for a medical alert tag. If the person tells you that he or she is a diabetic and exhibits the signals, then suspect a diabetic emergency. If the conscious victim can take food or fluids, give him or her sugar (Fig. 13-6). Most candy, fruit juices, and nondiet soft drinks have enough sugar to be effective. Common table sugar, either dry or dissolved in a glass of water, also works well to restore the victim to normal. If the person's problem is low sugar (hypoglycemia), the sugar you give will help quickly. If the person already has too much sugar (hyperglycemia), the excess sugar will do no further harm. Often diabetics know what is wrong and will ask for something with sugar in it. They may carry a readily available source of sugar for such occasions.

If the person is unconscious, do not give anything by mouth. Instead, monitor the ABCs and maintain normal body temperature. If the victim is unconscious, or is conscious but does not feel better within approximately five minutes after taking sugar, EMS personnel should be called immediately.

Seizures

When the normal functions of the brain are disrupted by injury, disease, fever, or infection, the electrical activity of the brain becomes irregular. This irregularity can cause a loss of body control known as a seizure.

Seizures may be caused by an acute or chronic condition. The chronic condition is known as epilepsy. About 2 million Americans have epilepsy. Epilepsy is usually controlled with medication. Still, some people with epilepsy have seizures from time to time. Others who go a long time without a seizure may think the condition has gone away and stop taking their medication. These people may then have a seizure again.

Signals of seizure

Before a seizure occurs, the person may experience an aura. An aura is an unusual sensation or feeling such as a visual hallucination; a strange sound, taste, or smell; or an urgent need to get to safety. If the person recognizes the aura, he or she may have time to tell bystanders and sit down before the seizure occurs.

Seizures range from mild blackouts that others may mistake for daydreaming to sudden, uncontrolled muscular contractions (convulsions) lasting several minutes. Infants and young children are at risk for seizures brought on by high fever. These are called febrile (heat-induced) seizures.

Care for seizure

Although it may be frightening to see someone unexpectedly having a seizure, you can easily help care for the person. Remember that he or she cannot control the seizure and the violent muscular contractions that may occur. Do not try to stop the seizure. Do not hold or restrain the person. Holding the person can cause musculoskeletal injuries.

Your objectives for care are to protect the victim from injury and manage the airway. First, move away nearby objects, such as furniture, that might cause injury. Protect the person's head by placing a thin cushion, such as folded clothing, beneath it. If there is fluid, such as saliva, blood, or vomit, in the person's mouth, position him or her on one side so that the fluid drains from the mouth.

Do not try to place anything between the person's teeth. People having seizures rarely bite their tongues or cheeks with enough force to cause any significant bleeding. However, some blood may be present, so positioning the person on his or her side will help any blood drain out of the mouth.

When the seizure is over, the person will be drowsy and disoriented. Do a secondary survey, checking to see if he or she was injured during the seizure. Be reassuring and comforting. If the seizure occurred in public, the victim may be embarrassed and self-conscious. Ask bystanders not to crowd around the victim, who will be tired and want to rest. Stay with the victim until he or she is fully conscious and aware of the surroundings.

If the victim is known to have periodic seizures, you do not need to call EMS immediately. The victim will usually recover from a seizure in a few minutes. However, EMS personnel should be called if—

◆ The seizure lasts more than a few minutes.
◆ The victim has repeated seizures.
◆ The victim appears to be injured.
◆ You are uncertain about the cause of the seizure.
◆ The victim is pregnant.
◆ The victim is a known diabetic.
◆ The victim is an infant or child.

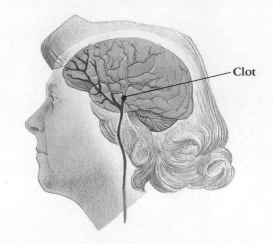

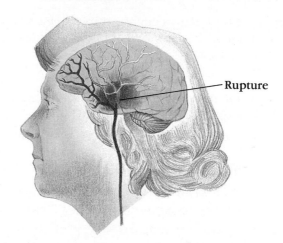

Figure 13-7 A stroke can be caused by a blood clot or bleeding from a ruptured artery in the brain.

◆ The seizure takes place in water.
◆ The victim fails to regain consciousness after the seizure.

Stroke

A stroke, also called a cerebrovascular accident (CVA), is a disruption of blood flow to a part of the brain that is serious enough to damage brain tissue (Fig. 13-7).

Most commonly, stroke is caused by a blood clot, called a thrombus or embolism, that forms or lodges in the arteries that supply blood to the brain. Another common cause is bleeding from a ruptured artery in the brain. A head injury, high blood pressure, a weak area in an artery wall (aneurysm), or fat deposits lining an artery (atherosclerosis) may cause stroke. Less commonly, a tumor or swelling from a head injury may compress an artery and cause a stroke.

A **transient ischemic attack (TIA)** is a temporary episode that is like a stroke. TIAs are sometimes called "mini-strokes." Like a stroke, a TIA is caused by reduced blood flow to part of the brain. Unlike a stroke, the signals of a TIA disappear within a few minutes or hours, although the person is not out of danger. Someone who experiences a TIA has a nearly 10 times greater chance of having a stroke in the future. Since you cannot tell a stroke from a TIA, you need only remember that any strokelike signals require an immediate call to EMS personnel for help.

3. Why does stroke result in damage to brain tissue?

Signals of stroke

As with other sudden illnesses, the primary signals of stroke or TIA are looking or feeling ill or abnormal behavior. Other signals of stroke include sudden weakness and numbness of the face, arm, or leg. Usually, this occurs only on one side of the body. The victim

---

The Brain Makes a Comeback

Neuroscientists have been mystified for years by the capricious effects of stroke. For many stroke survivors, talking becomes a tangle of words, a word like "piddlypop" spilling out in place of "hello." One man spoke normally unless he was asked to name fruits and vegetables. Each stroke survivor seemed to have a unique, perplexing set of problems, and doctors found recovery equally unpredictable.

But research into brain function after a stroke has shed new light on the way the brain works. Many strokes are caused when blood flow to the brain is cut off by a blood clot or hemorrhage. The oxygen-deprived brain cells rupture and die. Neuroscientists once believed that the cells died from lack of oxygen. However, their conclusion did not explain why stroke survivors sometimes got worse over a period of several hours.

The oxygen-deprived brain cells actually start an avalanche of death when they rupture. The ruptured cells release huge quantities of the amino acid glutamate that gushes into surviving brain cells and destroys them. Normally, small amounts of glutamate act as transmitters between the cells, but large amounts are extremely damaging. Researchers believe that, if they could inhibit the reaction of glutamate within the cell, they could stop the avalanche.

Researchers are developing several drugs to try to block the amino acid avalanche after a stroke. Oddly enough, they have found that drugs similar to phencyclidine, a potent animal tranquilizer and street drug known as PCP, have proven the most effective. Like PCP, the drugs cause temporary hallucinations. But doctors say the promising results outweigh the side effects.

Strokes still present many mysteries, but, with more than 2 million people surviving strokes in the United States, doctors are hopeful that the drugs will eventually eliminate the long-term effects.

REFERENCE
Blakeslee, S. "Pervasive Chemical Crucial to the Body Is Indicted as an Agent in Brain Damage," *The New York Times,* November 29, 1988.

may have difficulty talking or understanding speech. Vision may be blurred or dimmed; the pupils of the eyes may be of unequal size. The person may also experience a sudden, severe headache; dizziness, confusion, or changes in mood; or ringing in the ears. The victim may become unconscious or lose bowel or bladder control.

Care for stroke

If the victim is unconscious, make sure he or she has an open airway, and care for any life-threatening conditions that may occur. If there is fluid or vomitus in the victim's mouth, position him or her on one side to allow any fluids to drain out of the mouth. You may have to use a finger sweep to remove some of the material from the mouth. Call EMS personnel immediately; stay with the victim, and monitor his or her ABCs.

If the victim is conscious, do a secondary survey. If you see signals of a stroke, call EMS personnel. A stroke can make the victim fearful and anxious. Offer comfort and reassurance. Often he or she does not understand what has happened. Have the victim rest in a comfortable position. Do not give him or her anything to eat or drink. If the victim is drooling or having difficulty swallowing, place him or her on one side to help drain any fluids or vomitus from the mouth (Fig. 13-8).

Ten years ago, a stroke almost always caused irreversible brain damage. Today this is not necessarily true. New drugs and medical procedures can limit or, in some cases, reduce the damage caused by stroke. Therefore you should quickly activate the EMS system in order to get the best care for the victim as soon as possible.

Q
4. If you suspect that a conscious person has had a stroke, you should not give the person anything to eat or drink. Why?

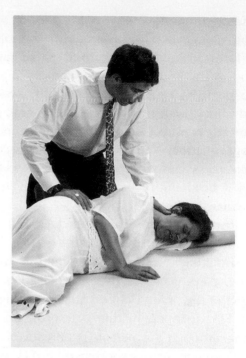

Figure 13-8 Position a victim on the side to help fluids or vomitus drain from the victim's mouth.

Preventing stroke

The risk factors for stroke and TIA are similar to those for heart disease. Some risk factors are beyond your control, such as age; gender; or family history of stroke, TIA, diabetes, or heart disease.

You can control other risk factors. One of the most important is hypertension, or high blood pressure. Hypertension increases your risk of stroke approximately seven times. High blood pressure puts pressure on arteries and makes them more likely to burst. Even mild hypertension can increase your risk of stroke. You can often control high blood pressure by losing weight, changing your diet, exercising routinely, and managing stress. If those measures are not sufficient, your physician may prescribe medication.

Cigarette smoking is another major risk factor for stroke. Smoking is linked to heart disease and cancer, as well. It increases blood pressure and makes blood more likely to clot. If you do not smoke, do not start. If you do smoke, seek help to try to stop. No matter how difficult or painful quitting may be, it's well worth it. The benefits of not smoking start as soon as you stop.

Diets that are high in saturated fats and cholesterol increase your chance of stroke by increasing the possibility of fatty materials building up on the walls of your blood vessels. Keep your intake of these foods at a moderate level.

Regular exercise reduces your chances of stroke by increasing blood circulation, which develops more channels for blood flow. These additional channels provide alternate routes for blood if the primary channels become blocked.

Q

5. Should a citizen responder try to diagnose the exact cause of a sudden illness? Why or why not?

◆ Summary

Sudden illness can strike anyone at any time. Usually you will not know the cause of the illness. Fortunately, you can provide proper care without knowing the cause. Following the emergency action principles and the basics of care for any emergency will help prevent the condition from becoming worse.

Diabetic emergencies, seizures, fainting, and stroke are all sudden illnesses, each with an individual, specific cause. Recognizing their *general* signals, such as changes in consciousness, sweating, confusion, weakness, and the appearance of illness, will indicate to you the necessary *general* care you should give the victim until EMS personnel arrive to take over.

Answers to Application Questions

1. Fainting is a form of shock because it involves the failure of the circulatory system to adequately circulate blood to all parts of the body.

2. When people collapse to the ground after fainting, the body does not have to work against gravity to pump blood to the brain. When the body is flat on the ground, blood that has pooled in the legs and trunk can now more readily return to the heart. Normal blood flow to the brain resumes, allowing consciousness to return.

3. Stroke causes damage to brain tissues by disrupting blood flow and, therefore, delivery of oxygen to the brain. Without oxygen, cells die—the brain is no exception.

4. You cannot tell the extent of damage suffered by the victim of a suspected stroke or TIA. Damage may have occurred that limits the victim's ability to eat and drink.

5. A citizen responder does not need to diagnose the *cause* of a sudden illness. The role of the citizen responder is to recognize that an emergency exists, get help by calling EMS personnel, and provide basic care for life-threatening conditions.

Study Questions

1. Match each term with the correct definition

   a. Diabetic

   b. Epilepsy

   c. Fainting

   d. Hyperglycemia

   e. Hypoglycemia

   f. Insulin

   g. Seizure

   h. Stroke

   _____ A hormone that enables the body to use sugar.

   _____ A temporary reduction of blood to the brain, resulting in loss of consciousness.

   _____ A disruption of blood flow to the brain that causes brain tissue damage.

   _____ An interruption of the brain's electrical activity, causing loss of consciousness and body control.

   _____ A condition in which too little sugar is in the bloodstream.

   _____ A person whose body cannot produce or use adequate insulin.

   _____ A condition in which too much sugar is in the bloodstream.

   _____ A chronic condition characterized by seizures and usually controlled by medication.

2. List at least four signals of a sudden illness.

3. List at least four basic principles of care that should be applied in any emergency.

4. List at least three instances in which you should call EMS personnel for a seizure victim.

5. List at least two risk factors that, when controlled, decrease the chances of stroke or TIA.

In questions 6 through 12, circle the letter of the correct answer.

6. If you were caring for someone who looked pale, was unconscious and was breathing irregularly, what would you do?

   a. Call EMS personnel.
   b. Maintain body temperature and monitor the ABCs.
   c. Give sugar to the victim.
   d. Tell the victim to call his or her physician.
   e. a and b

7. A friend who is a diabetic is drowsy and seems confused. He is not sure if he took his insulin that day. What should you do?

   a. Give him some sugar.
   b. Suggest he rest for an hour or so.
   c. Tell him to take his insulin.
   d. b and c
   e. a, b, and c

8. Your father is a diabetic. He also suffered a stroke a year ago. You find him lying on the floor unconscious. What should you do?

   a. Phone his doctor.
   b. Lift his head up and try to give him a sugary drink.
   c. Call the local emergency number and monitor his ABCs.
   d. Inject him with insulin yourself and then call EMS personnel.

9. In caring for the victim of a seizure, you should—

   a. Move any objects that might cause injury.
   b. Try to hold the person still.
   c. Place a spoon between the person's teeth.
   d. Douse the person with water.
   e. Try to keep the person upright.

10. To manage the airway of a seizure victim—

   a. Place an object between the victim's teeth.
   b. Position the victim on his or her side.
   c. Place a thick object, such as a rolled blanket, under the victim's head.
   d. Move the victim into a sitting position.
   e. a and b

11. Controlling high blood pressure reduces your risk of—

    a. Heart disease.
    b. Stroke or TIA.
    c. Diabetes.
    d. b and c
    e. a and b

12. At the office, your boss complains that he has had a severe headache for several hours. His speech suddenly becomes slurred. He loses his balance and falls to the floor. What would you do?

    a. Give him two aspirin.
    b. Help him find and take his high blood pressure medication.
    c. Suggest he go home.
    d. Call EMS professionals.
    e. Tell him to rest for a while.

13. Describe how to care for a seizure victim once the seizure is over.

Answers are in Appendix A.

Poisoning, Bites, and Stings

Objectives

After reading this chapter, you should be able to—

1. List the four ways poisons enter the body.

2. List at least six signals of poisoning.

3. Describe the role of a Poison Control Center (PCC).

4. Identify the general principles of care for any poisoning emergency.

5. Describe the specific care for a victim of ingested, inhaled, and absorbed poison.

6. Describe the specific care for an insect bite or sting, marine life sting, snakebite, tick bite, and animal bite.

7. List at least four ways to protect yourself from insect and tick bites.

8. Describe the signals of anaphylaxis.

9. List at least three ways to prevent poisoning.

10. Define the key terms for this chapter.

After reading this chapter and completing the class activities, you should be able to—

1. Make appropriate decisions regarding care when given an example of an emergency situation in which someone may be poisoned.

Key Terms

Absorbed poison: A poison that enters the body through the skin.

Anaphylaxis (an ah fi LAK sis): A severe allergic reaction; a form of shock.

Ingested poison: A poison that is swallowed.

Inhaled poison: A poison breathed into the lungs.

Injected poison: A poison that enters the body through a bite, sting, or hypodermic needle.

Lyme disease: An illness transmitted by a certain kind of infected tick.

Poison: Any substance that causes injury, illness, or death when introduced into the body.

Poison Control Center (PCC): A specialized kind of health center that provides information in cases of poisoning or suspected poisoning emergencies.

Rabies: A disease caused by a virus transmitted through the saliva of infected animals.

For Review

Before reading this chapter, you should review the information on breathing emergencies (Chapter 4) and sudden illnesses (Chapter 13).

◆ Introduction

Chapter 13 described sudden illnesses caused by conditions inside the body. Poisoning can also be a sudden illness, but unlike sudden illnesses, such as fainting, stroke, and others, poisoning results when external substances enter the body. The substance may be a chemical, or it may be a germ or virus that enters the body via a bite or sting. In this chapter, you will learn how to recognize and care for poisoning.

It is estimated that between one and two million poisonings occur each year in the United States. More than 90 percent of all poisonings take place in the home. Unintentional poisonings far outnumber intentional ones. Although most unintentional poisonings still occur to children under age 5, fewer than 5 percent of these children die. The death rate from poisoning in children under age 5 has dropped dramatically in the last 30 years. In the same period, however, poisoning fatalities among adults 18 and older has markedly increased.

This increase in fatalities among adults can be linked to two factors: (1) increases in intentional poisonings (suicides), and (2) increases in drug-related poisonings. Although illegal street drugs like cocaine attract more attention, the misuse and abuse of prescription medications is actually a bigger problem. About two thirds of all unintentional poisonings involve drugs and medications. Half of all drug overdoses are caused by misused or abused prescribed medication. Drug and other substance misuse or abuse is discussed in detail in Chapter 15.

◆ Poisoning

How Poisons Enter the Body

A **poison** is any substance that causes injury or illness when introduced into the body. Some poisons can cause death. Poisons include solids, liquids, and fumes (gases and vapors). A poison can enter the body in four ways: ingestion, inhalation, absorption, and injection (see Figure 14-1 on the next page.)

Ingestion means swallowing. **Ingested poisons** include foods, such as certain mushrooms and shellfish; substances, such as alcohol; medications, such as aspirin; and household and garden items, such as cleaning products, pesticides, and plants (see Figure 14-2 on the next page). Many substances not poison-

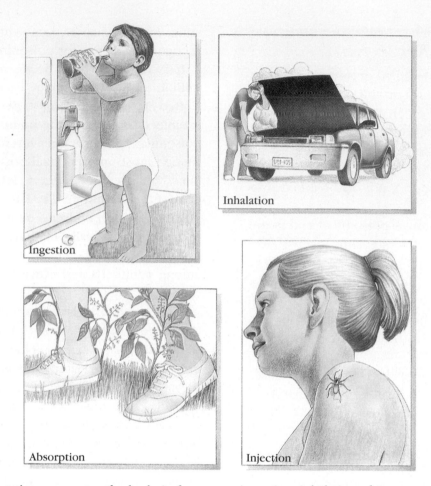

Figure 14-1 A poison can enter the body in four ways: ingestion, inhalation, absorption, and injection.

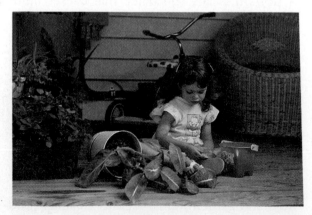

Figure 14-2 Many common household plants are poisonous.

ous in small amounts are poisonous in larger amounts.

Poisoning by inhalation occurs when a person breathes in toxic fumes. **Inhaled poisons** include—

◆ Gases, such as carbon monoxide, from an engine or other combustion.
◆ Gases, such as carbon dioxide, that can occur naturally from decomposition.
◆ Gases, such as nitrous oxide, used for medical reasons.
◆ Gases, such as chlorine, found in commercial swimming facilities.
◆ Fumes from household products, such as glues and paints.
◆ Fumes from drugs, such as crack cocaine.

An **absorbed poison** enters the body after

it comes in contact with the skin. Absorbed poisons come from plants such as poison ivy, poison oak, and poison sumac, as well as from fertilizers and pesticides used in lawn and plant care.

Injected poisons enter the body through bites or stings of insects, spiders, ticks, animals, and snakes, or as drugs or medications injected with a hypodermic needle.

Signals of Poisoning

The most important thing is to recognize *that a poisoning may have occurred.* As with other serious emergencies, such as a heart attack, shock, or a head and spine injury, evaluate the scene, the condition of the victim, and any information from the victim or bystanders. If you then have even a slight suspicion that the victim has been poisoned, seek medical assistance immediately.

As you approach the victim, survey the scene. Be aware of any unusual odors, flames, smoke, open or spilled containers, an open medicine cabinet, an overturned or damaged plant, or other signals of possible poisoning.

When you reach the victim, do a primary survey, then a secondary survey if the victim has no life-threatening conditions. The victim of poisoning generally looks ill and displays signals common to other sudden illnesses. The signals of poisoning include nausea, vomiting, diarrhea, chest or abdominal pain, breathing difficulty, sweating, loss of consciousness, and seizures.

Other signals of poisoning are burn injuries around the lips or tongue or on the skin. You may also suspect a poisoning based on any information you have from or about the victim. Look also for any drug paraphernalia or empty containers.

If you suspect a poisoning, try to get answers to the following questions:

- What type of poison was taken?
- How much was taken?
- When was it taken?

This information will help you provide the most appropriate care.

Poison Control Centers

A poisoning is sometimes a unique problem for the citizen responder as well as for responding EMS personnel. The severity of the poisoning depends on the type and amount of the substance, how it entered the body, and the victim's size, weight, and age. Some poisons act fast and have characteristic signals. Others act slowly and cannot be easily identified. Sometimes you will be able to identify the specific poison, sometimes not.

To help people deal with poisonings, a network of **Poison Control Centers (PCCs)** exists throughout the United States. Many centers are in the emergency departments of large hospitals. Medical professionals in these centers have access to information about virtually all poisonous substances. They will tell you how to counteract the poison. You should have your local PCC number posted by your phone (Fig. 14-3). You can obtain the phone number from your telephone directory, your doctor, a local hospital, or your local EMS system.

Poison Control Centers answer over a mil-

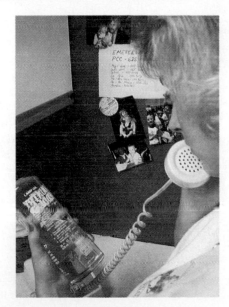

Figure 14-3 The local Poison Control Center phone number should be posted by your phone.

lion poisoning calls each year. Since many poisonings can be cared for without the help of EMS professionals, PCCs help prevent overburdening of the EMS system. If the victim is conscious, call your local or regional PCC first. The center will tell you what care to give and whether EMS personnel are needed.

If the victim is unconscious, or if you do not know your PCC number, call your local emergency number. Often the dispatcher will link you with the PCC. The dispatcher may also monitor your talk with the PCC and send an ambulance if needed (Fig. 14-4). This eliminates the need for a second call and saves time.

◆ First Aid for Poisoning

Follow these general principles for any poisoning emergency:

- Survey the scene to make sure it is safe to approach and to gather clues about what happened.
- Remove the victim from the source of the poison, if necessary.
- Do a primary survey to assess the victim's airway, breathing, and circulation.
- Care for any life-threatening conditions.
- If the victim is conscious, do a secondary survey to gather additional information.

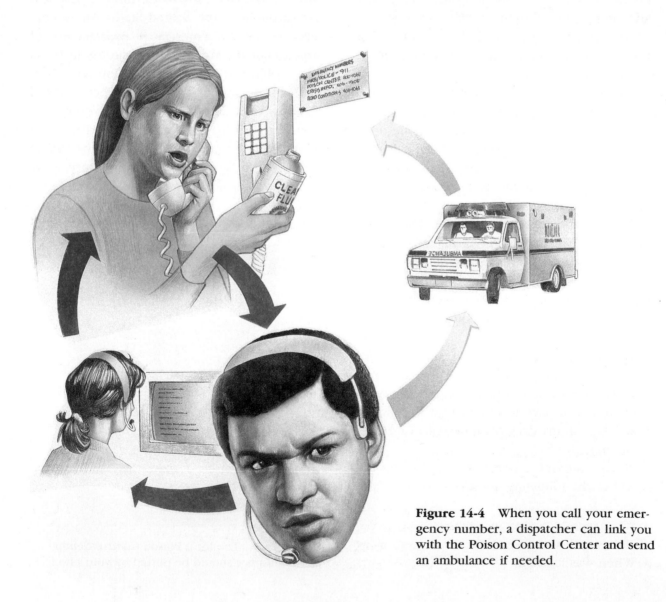

Figure 14-4 When you call your emergency number, a dispatcher can link you with the Poison Control Center and send an ambulance if needed.

- Look for any containers and take them to the telephone.
- Call your PCC or emergency number.
- Follow the directions of the PCC or the EMS dispatcher.

Do not give the victim anything to drink or eat unless advised by medical professionals. If the poison is unknown and the victim vomits, save some of the vomitus, which the hospital may analyze to identify the poison.

Ingested Poisons

Besides following these general principles for any poisoning, you may also need to provide additional care for specific types of poisons. Usually, if the person has ingested the poison in the last 30 minutes, the stomach should be emptied. The Poison Control Center may instruct you to induce vomiting.

To induce vomiting, give syrup of ipecac, which is available at your local pharmacy. It usually comes in a 30-ml bottle (about 2 tablespoons) (Fig. 14-5). Two tablespoons, followed by two glasses of water, is the normal dose for a person over 12 years of age. For children ages 1 to 12, the normal dose is 1 tablespoon followed by two glasses of water. Vomiting usually occurs within 20 minutes.

There are some instances when vomiting *should not* be induced. These include when the victim—

- Is unconscious.
- Is having a seizure.
- Is pregnant.
- Has ingested a corrosive substance (an acid or alkali) or a petroleum product (such as kerosene or gasoline).
- Is known to have heart disease.

Since vomiting removes only about half of the poison, you may need to counteract the remaining poison. Activated charcoal is used to absorb ingested poisons (Fig. 14-6). It is available in both liquid and powder forms. Before use, the powder should be mixed in water to form a solution with the consistency of a thin milk shake. For a person over 12 years of age, follow the directions on the bottle. For children ages 1 to 12, mix 4 tablespoons with water. Activated charcoal can also be purchased at your local pharmacy, but is not as readily available as syrup of ipecac. Syrup of ipecac and activated charcoal should be part of your home first aid supplies.

You can dilute some ingested poisons by giving the victim water to drink. Examples of such poisons are corrosive chemicals like ac-

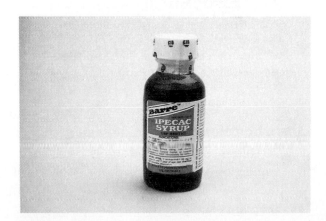

Figure 14-5 Syrup of ipecac is used to induce vomiting in victims who have swallowed certain kinds of poisons.

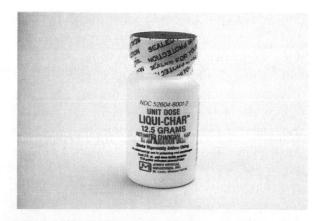

Figure 14-6 Activated charcoal is used to absorb swallowed poisons.

ids or alkalies that damage or destroy tissues. Vomiting these corrosives could burn the esophagus, throat, and mouth. Diluting the corrosive substance decreases the potential for damaging tissues.

Diluting poisons taken in tablet or capsule form is usually not a good idea. The increased fluid could dissolve them more rapidly in the stomach, speeding the body's absorption of the poison. As always, follow the advice of the PCC or other medical professionals.

Case Study

A hungry 22-year-old man hiking with his girlfriend ate a plant growing in water. Approximately one hour later, he experienced extreme stomach pains and difficulty breathing. These signals were soon followed by loss of consciousness and seizures. By the time paramedics arrived, the man was in cardiac arrest. He was transported by helicopter to the nearest hospital where he was pronounced dead less than three hours after eating the plant. An autopsy revealed that he had ingested the poisonous western water hemlock plant.

Inhaled Poisons

Toxic fumes come from a variety of sources. They may have an odor or be odor free. Carbon dioxide, for example, is an inhaled poison that comes from decomposing organic matter, wells, and sewers. It is also in fumes from certain industrial and home spray chemicals.

A more common inhaled poison is carbon monoxide (CO). It is present in car exhaust and can be produced by defective cooking equipment, fires, and charcoal grills. A pale or bluish skin color that indicates a lack of oxygen may signal carbon monoxide poisoning. For years, people were taught that carbon monoxide poisoning was indicated by a cherry-red color of the skin and lips. This, however, is a poor *initial indicator* of carbon

monoxide poisoning. The red color occurs later, usually after death.

All victims of inhaled poison need oxygen as soon as possible. First and foremost, however, remember the emergency action principles. Survey the scene to determine if it is safe for you to help. If you can remove the person from the source of the poison without endangering your own life, then do so. You can help a conscious victim by just getting him or her to fresh air and then calling EMS personnel. Remove an unconscious victim from the environment, maintain an open airway, and call EMS personnel. If the person is not breathing, give rescue breathing and call EMS personnel.

Case Study

An eight-year-old girl traveling in a 1974 automobile was found unconscious and not breathing on the back seat. Her 18-year-old sister, seated in the front passenger's seat, had checked on her about 15 minutes earlier and believed she was only sleeping. Rescue breathing was done while the driver sped to a hospital miles away. By the time she arrived at the hospital, the girl was in cardiac arrest. Advanced cardiac life support measures were successfully used to resuscitate her. However, she had repeated cardiac arrests while being transported to a hyperbaric chamber for treatment. Eleven hours after the incident occurred, she was pronounced dead. The autopsy confirmed that the cause of death was poisoning by carbon monoxide from engine fumes and improper ventilation.

Absorbed Poisons

People often contact poisonous substances that can be absorbed into the body. Millions of people each year suffer from contact with poisonous plants such as poison ivy, poison oak, and poison sumac (Fig. 14-7). Other poisons absorbed through the skin include dry and wet chemicals, such as those used in yard and

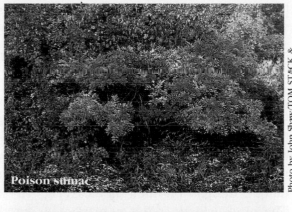

Poison sumac

Photo by John Shaw/TOM STACK & ASSOCIATES.

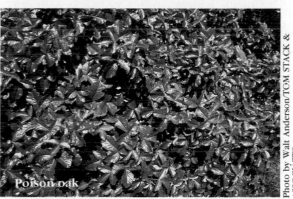

Poison oak

Photo by Walt Anderson/TOM STACK & ASSOCIATES.

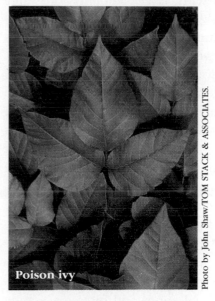

Poison ivy

Photo by John Shaw/TOM STACK & ASSOCIATES.

Figure 14-7 Annually, millions of people suffer from contact with poisonous plants whose poisons are absorbed into the body.

garden maintenance, which may also burn the surface of the skin.

To care for poison plant contact, immediately wash the affected area thoroughly with soap and water (Fig. 14-8, *A*). If a rash or weeping lesion has begun to develop, apply a paste of baking soda and water to the area several times a day to alleviate some of the discomfort.

Lotions such as Calamine^R or Caladryl^R may help soothe the area. Antihistamines such as Benadryl^R may also help dry up the lesions. If the condition worsens and large areas of the body or the face are affected, the person should see a doctor, who may administer antiinflammatory drugs, such as corticosteroids, or other medications to relieve discomfort.

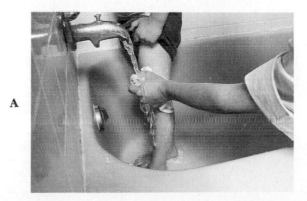

A

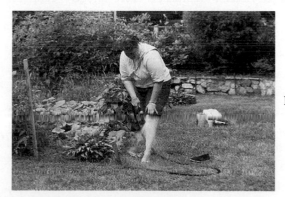

B

Figure 14-8 A, To care for skin contact with a poisonous plant, immediately wash the affected area with soap and water. **B,** Whenever chemical poisons come in contact with the skin or eyes, flush the affected area continuously with large amounts of water.

If other poisons, such as dry or wet chemicals, contact the skin, flush the affected area continuously with large amounts of water (Fig. 14-8, *B*). Activate the EMS system immediately. Continue to flush the area until EMS personnel arrive.

If running water is not available, dry chemicals, such as lime, should be brushed off. Take care not to get any in your eyes or the eyes of the victim or any bystanders. Dry chemicals are activated by contact with water. But if continuous running water is available, it will flush the chemical from the skin before activating it. Running water reduces the threat to you and quickly and easily removes the substance from the victim.

Injected Poisons

Insect and animal stings and bites are among the most common sources of injected poisons. This text cannot consider all possible types of stings and bites that could result in poisoning. The following sections describe the care for common stings and bites of insects, spiders, ticks, marine life, snakes, and animals.

Insects

Although insect stings are painful, they are rarely fatal. Fewer than 100 reported deaths occur each year. Some people, however, have a severe allergic reaction to an insect sting that results in the life-threatening condition, **anaphylaxis,** discussed later in this chapter. See also Chapter 4.

To give care for an insect sting, first examine the sting site to see if the stinger is in the skin. If it is, remove it to prevent any further poisoning. Scrape the stinger away from the skin with your fingernail or a plastic card such as a credit card. Often the venom sac will still be attached to the stinger. Do not remove the stinger with tweezers, since putting pressure on the venom sac can cause further poisoning.

Next, wash the site with soap and water. Cover it to keep it clean. Apply a cold pack to the area to reduce the pain and swelling. Observe the victim periodically for signals of an allergic reaction.

Spiders and scorpions

Few spiders in the United States have venom that causes death. But the bites of the black widow and brown recluse spiders can be fatal. These spiders live in most parts of the United States. You can identify them by the unique designs on their bodies (Fig. 14-9). The black widow spider is black with a reddish hourglass shape on its underbody. The brown recluse spider is light brown with a darker brown, violin-shaped marking on the top of its body.

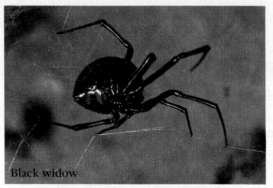

Black widow

Photo by Rod Planck/TOM STACK & ASSOCIATES.

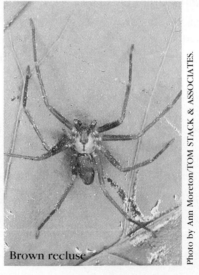

Brown recluse

Photo by Ann Moreton/TOM STACK & ASSOCIATES.

Figure 14-9 The black widow spider and brown recluse spider have characteristic markings.

Both spiders prefer dark, out-of-the-way places where they are seldom disturbed. Bites usually occur on the hands and arms of people reaching into places such as wood, rock, and brush piles or rummaging in dark garages and attics. Often, the victim will not know that he or she has been bitten until signals develop.

The bite of the black widow spider is the more painful and often the more deadly of the two. In fact, its venom is even deadlier than that of a rattlesnake, although the smaller amount of venom injected usually produces less of a reaction than a snakebite.

If the victim recognizes the spider as either a black widow or brown recluse, he or she should seek professional help at a medical facility as soon as possible. Professionals will clean the wound and give medication to reduce the pain and inflammation. An antivenin is available for black widow bites.

Scorpions live in dry regions of the southwestern United States and Mexico (Fig. 14-10). Like spiders, only a few species of scorpions are fatally poisonous. They live under rocks and logs and under the bark of certain trees and are most active at night.

Signals of spider bites and scorpion stings include—

* Nausea and vomiting.
* Difficulty breathing or swallowing.
* Sweating and salivating profusely.

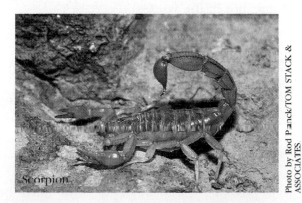

Photo by Rod Panck/TOM STACK & ASSOCIATES

Figure 14-10 Only a few species of scorpions found in the United States are fatally poisonous.

* Irregular heart rhythms that can lead to cardiac arrest.
* Severe pain in the sting or bite area.
* Swelling of the site.
* A mark indicating a possible bite or sting.

In the event of a scorpion sting, call EMS personnel. The victim may need to go to a medical facility where he or she can receive antivenin. While waiting for EMS personnel, wash the wound and apply a cold pack to the site.

Marine life

The stings of some forms of marine life are not only painful but can also make you sick (see Figure 14-11 on next page). The side affects include allergic reactions that can cause breathing and heart problems and paralysis. Always remove the person from the water as soon as possible. Call 9-1-1 if the victim doesn't know what stung him or her, has a history of allergic reactions to marine life stings, is stung on the face or neck, or starts to have difficulty breathing.

If you know the sting is from a jellyfish, sea anemone, or Portugese man-of-war, soak the injured part in vinegar as soon as possible. Vinegar often works best to offset the toxin. Rubbing alcohol or baking soda may also be used. Do not rub the wound or apply fresh water or ammonia as this will increase pain. Meat tenderizer is no longer recommended.

If you know the sting is from a sting ray, sea urchin, or spiny fish, flush the wound with tap water. Ocean water may also be used. Immobilize the injured part, usually the foot, and soak the affected area in nonscalding hot water (as hot as the person can stand) for about 30 minutes or until the pain goes away. If hot water is not available, packing the area in hot sand may have a similar effect if the sand is hot enough. Then carefully clean the wound and apply a bandage. Watch for signs of infection and check with a health care provider to determine if a tetanus shot is needed.

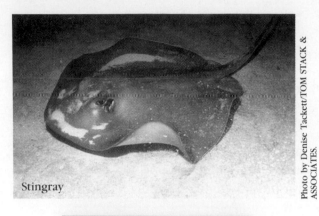

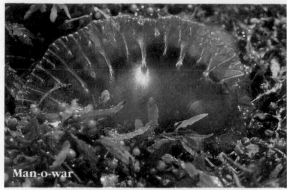

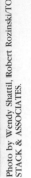

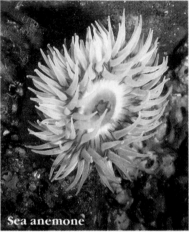

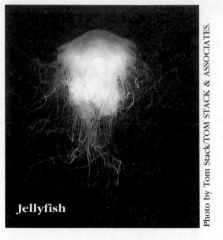

Figure 14-11 The painful sting of some marine animals can cause serious problems.

Snakes

Few areas of medicine have provoked more controversy about care for an injury that claims so few lives. Snakebite care issues, such as whether to use a tourniquet, cut the wound, apply ice, apply suction, use electric shocks, and capture the snake, have been discussed at length over the years. All this controversy is rather amazing since, of the 8,000 people bitten annually in the United States, fewer than 12 die. Rattlesnakes account for most snakebites and nearly all deaths from snakebites. Figure 14-12 shows the four kinds of poisonous snakes found in the United States. Most deaths occur because the victim has an allergic reaction or weakened body system, or because much time passes before the victim receives medical care.

Advice to citizen responders has varied greatly over the years. Elaborate care is usually unnecessary because in most cases the victim can reach professional medical care within 30 minutes. Often care can be reached much faster, since most bites occur near the home, not in the wild.

Follow these guidelines to care for someone bitten by a snake:

◆ Wash the wound, if possible.
◆ Immobilize the affected part. Apply a sling to an injured arm.
◆ Keep the affected area lower than the heart if possible.
◆ Call EMS professionals.
◆ If possible, carry a victim who must be transported, or have him or her walk slowly.
◆ If you know the victim cannot get profes-

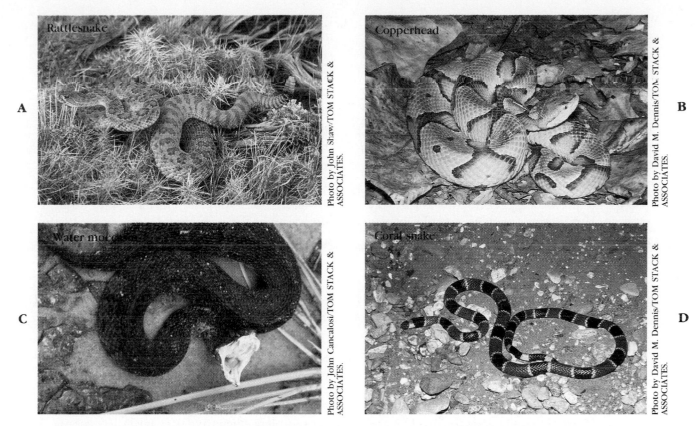

Figure 14-12 There are four kinds of poisonous snakes found in the United States: **A**, Rattlesnake. **B**, Copperhead. **C**, Water moccasin. **D**, Coral snake.

sional medical care within 30 minutes, consider suctioning the wound using a snakebite kit. People at risk of snakebites in the wild (away from medical care) should carry a snakebite kit and know how to use its contents.

Regardless of what you may have otherwise heard or read—

- *Do not* apply ice. Recent studies show that cooling the bite can cause as much harm as good.
- *Do not* cut the wound. Cutting the wound can further injure the victim and has not been shown to remove any significant amount of venom.
- *Do not* apply a tourniquet. A tourniquet severely restricts blood flow to the limb, which could result in the loss of the limb.
- *Do not* use electric shock. This technique

has not been conclusively shown to affect the poison and can be dangerous. It is inappropriate in the majority of snakebite cases in the United States, since professional help is readily attainable.

Q

1. Why should you keep a snakebite wound lower than the level of the heart?

Animals

The bite of a domestic or wild animal carries the risk of infection as well as soft tissue injury. The most serious possible result is **rabies**. Rabies is transmitted through the saliva of diseased animals such as skunks, bats, raccoons, cats, dogs, cattle, and foxes.

Animals with rabies may act in unusual

ways. For example, nocturnal animals, such as raccoons, may be active in the daytime. A wild animal that usually tries to avoid humans may not run away when you approach. Rabid animals may salivate, appear partially paralyzed, or act irritable, aggressive, or strangely quiet. Do not pet or feed wild animals, and do not touch the body of a dead wild animal.

If not treated, rabies is fatal. Anyone bitten by an animal suspected to be rabid must get medical attention. To prevent rabies from developing, the victim receives a series of vaccine injections to build up immunity. In the past, caring for rabies meant a lengthy series of painful injections that had many unpleasant side effects. The vaccines used now require fewer injections and have less severe side effects.

If someone is bitten by an animal, try to get him or her away from the animal without endangering yourself. Do not try to restrain or capture it. If the wound is minor, wash it with soap and water. Then control any bleeding and apply an antibiotic ointment and a dressing. Watch for signals of infection. If the wound is bleeding seriously, control the

Spiders and Snakes

Some scientists believe the venoms of these feared creatures may unlock the mysteries of some neurological disorders and cancers. Researchers have been studying the venom of different spiders and snakes to isolate the powerful chemicals that allow the animals to kill and eat their prey.

In Cambridge, Massachusetts, scientists are focusing on the protein chemicals the spider uses to paralyze its prey.[1] They believe that certain compounds in the venom may offer help for strokes and other neurological disorders.

The compound glutamate is vital to communication between nerve cells in both humans and insects. It serves as a transmitter between cells. With too little glutamate, the cells cannot transmit information through the nerve network, causing paralysis. Too much glutamate damages the cells.

Brain damage from cerebral palsy, epilepsy, and stroke is caused in part by excess glutamate. Damaged cells release excess quantities of glutamate when they rupture, causing the undamaged cells to rupture in a chain reaction that is very dangerous. Researchers say the spider venom contains glutamate blockers that may prevent this chain reaction. Researchers are currently studying the reactions in test tubes and hope to begin testing on rodents in the years to come.

In Seattle, Washington, doctors are studying the actions of chemicals found in snake venom.[2]

They isolated proteins from the venoms of different snake varieties and incubated them with human cancer cells to see if the proteins could destroy the tumors. After experimenting with the venoms of many different kinds of snakes and scorpions, they have narrowed their experiments to the Western Diamondback rattlesnake.

The cancer cells are killed by a small protein that comes from the snake's digestive juices, researchers say. Unfortunately, the protein kills normal cells as well. To combat this problem, researchers are linking the protein with an antibody that attaches only to certain cancer cells. They hope that the antibody, with its bound toxin, can attach itself to the outside of the cancer cell, inject the poison and destroy it. This would spare the normal cells.

After studying the reactions in test tubes, doctors have begun injecting the venom/antibody in mice that have tumors. If they are successful in this first stage of testing, they will begin tests on monkeys.

REFERENCES
1. Goldin, Stan. Director of Biochemistry, Cambridge NeuroScience Research Inc., 1 Kendell Square, Cambridge, Massachusetts 02139. Interview, April 1990.
2. Twardzik, Daniel, Ph.D. Affiliate Professor of Medicine, University of Washington School of Medicine. Research Fellow, Oncogen/Bristol Myers/Squibb in Seattle, Washington. Interview, April 1990.

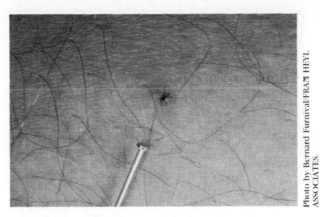

Figure by Bernard Furnival/FRAN HEYL ASSOCIATES.

Figure 14-13 A deer tick can be as small as the head of a pin.

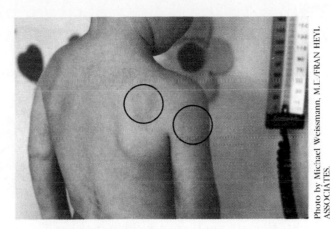

Photo by Michael Weissmann, M.L./FRAN HEYL ASSOCIATES.

Figure 14-14 A person with Lyme disease may develop a rash.

bleeding first. Do not clean the wound. The wound will be properly cleaned at a medical facility. Seek medical attention.

If possible, try to remember what the animal looked liked and the area in which it was last seen. Call your local emergency number. The dispatcher will get the proper authorities, such as animal control, to the scene.

Ticks

Ticks can contract disease, carry disease, and transmit it to humans. In the past, Rocky Mountain Spotted Fever was widely publicized as a tick disease. It is still occurring today, but more recently, attention has been focused on a new disease transmitted by ticks known as **Lyme disease.**

Lyme disease, or Lyme borreliosis, is an illness that people get from the bite of an infected tick. Lyme disease is affecting a growing number of people in the United States. The areas most affected are New York, New Jersey, Rhode Island, and Connecticut in the East; Wisconsin and Minnesota in the Midwest; and California and Oregon in the West. Lyme disease has occurred in more than 40 states, however, and everyone should take appropriate precautions to protect against it.

Not all ticks carry Lyme disease. Lyme disease is spread primarily by a type of tick that commonly attaches itself to field mice and

deer. It is sometimes called a deer tick. This tick is found around beaches and in wooded and grassy areas. Like all ticks, it attaches itself to *any* warm-blooded animal that brushes by it, including humans.

Deer ticks are very tiny and difficult to see. They are much smaller than the common dog tick or wood tick. They can be as small as a poppy seed or the head of a pin (Fig. 14-13). Even in the adult stage, they are only as large as a grape seed. A deer tick can attach to you without your knowing it is there. Many people who develop Lyme disease cannot recall having been bitten.

You can get Lyme disease from the bite of an infected tick at any time of the year. However, in northern states, the risk is greatest between May and late August, when ticks are most active and people spend more time outdoors.

The first signal of infection may appear a few days or a few weeks after a tick bite. Typically, a rash starts as a small red area at the site of the bite. It may spread up to five to seven inches across (Fig. 14-14). In fair-skinned people, the center is lighter in color, and the outer edges red and raised, sometimes giving the rash a bull's-eye appearance. In dark-skinned people, the area may look black and blue, like a bruise.

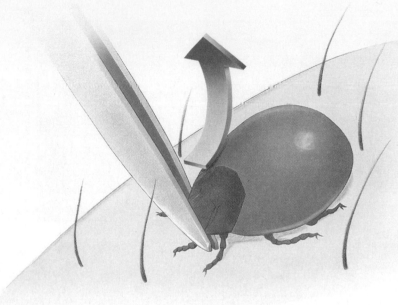

Figure 14-15 Remove a tick by pulling steadily and firmly with fine-tipped tweezers.

Other signals of Lyme disease include fever, headache, weakness, and joint and muscle pain similar to the pain of "flu." These signals may develop slowly and may not occur at the same time as a rash. In fact, you can have Lyme disease without developing a rash.

Lyme disease can get worse if not treated. In its advanced stages it may cause arthritis, numbness, memory loss, problems in seeing or hearing, high fever, and stiff neck. Some of these signals could indicate brain or nervous system problems. An irregular or rapid heartbeat could indicate heart problems.

If you find a tick, remove it by pulling steadily and firmly. Grasp the tick with fine-tipped tweezers, as close to the skin as possible, and pull *slowly* (Fig. 14-15). If you do not have tweezers, use a glove, plastic wrap, a piece of paper, or a leaf to protect your fingers. If you use your bare fingers, wash your hands immediately. Do not try to burn a tick off with a hot match or a burning cigarette. Do not use other home remedies, like coating the tick with Vaseline or nail polish or pricking it with a pin.

If you cannot remove the tick, or if its mouthparts stay in your skin, obtain medical care. Once the tick is removed, wash the area immediately with soap and water. If an antiseptic or antibiotic ointment is available, apply it to prevent wound infection. Observe the site periodically thereafter. If a rash or flu-like symptoms develop, seek medical help.

A physician will usually use antibiotics to treat Lyme disease. Antibiotics work best and most quickly when taken *early*. If you suspect Lyme disease, do not delay seeking treatment. Treatment is slower and less effective in advanced stages.

Additional information on Lyme disease may be available from your local or state health department.

◆ Anaphylaxis

Severe allergic reactions to poisons are rare. But when one occurs, it is truly a life-threatening medical emergency. This reaction is called anaphylaxis and was discussed in Chapter 4. Anaphylaxis is a form of shock. It can be caused by an insect bite or sting or by contact with drugs, medications, foods, and chemicals. Anaphylaxis can result from any of the kinds of poisoning described in this chapter.

Signals of Anaphylaxis

Anaphylaxis usually occurs suddenly, within seconds or minutes after contact with the substance. The skin or area of the body that came in contact with the substance usually swells and turns red (Fig. 14-16). Other signals include hives, itching, rash, weakness, nausea, vomiting, dizziness, and breathing difficulty that includes coughing and wheezing. This breathing difficulty can progress to an obstructed airway as the tongue and throat swell. Death from anaphylaxis usually occurs because the victim's breathing is severely impaired.

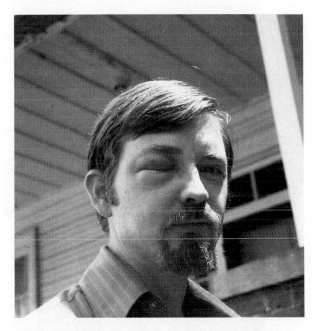

Figure 14-16 In anaphylaxis, the skin usually swells and turns red.

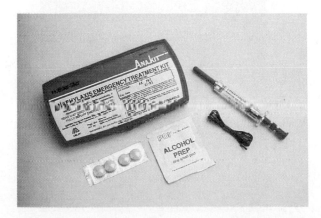

Figure 14-17 The contents of an anaphylaxis kit.

Case Study

A 20-year-old woman who boasted to friends, "I'm not allergic to anything," while on an outdoor wilderness trip would have changed her statement if she had lived long enough. The woman was stung five times in the face and arm after accidentally reaching into a hornet's nest. With more than a two-hour hike to get out of the remote area, a group of three young adults did what they could for her, while two others went for help. However, severe swelling of her throat and tongue blocked her airway. The woman lost consciousness less than a half hour after she was stung. Soon after, her heart stopped. Members of the group attempted CPR for nearly 30 minutes, but gave up because they could not get any air into her lungs. Flight paramedics made no attempts to resuscitate her when they arrived 2½ hours after the incident occurred.

Care for Anaphylaxis

If an unusual inflammation or rash is noticeable immediately after contact with a possible source, it could be an allergic reaction. Observe the person carefully because any allergic reaction can develop into anaphylaxis. Assess the person's airway and breathing. If the person has any breathing difficulty or complains that his or her throat is closing, call EMS personnel immediately. Help him or her into the most comfortable position for breathing. Monitor the ABCs and offer reassurance.

People who know they are extremely allergic to certain substances usually try to avoid them, although this is sometimes impossible. These people may carry an anaphylaxis kit in case they have a severe allergic reaction. Such kits are available by prescription only (Fig. 14-17). The kit contains a single dose of the drug epinephrine that can be injected into the body to counteract the anaphylactic reaction. If you are allergic to a substance, contact your doctor to discuss whether you need such a kit.

◆ Poisoning Prevention

The best approach to poisoning emergencies is to prevent them from occurring in the first place. This is a simple principle, but often people do not take enough precautions. Of all the child poisoning cases reported, the vast majority occurred when the child was under the direct supervision of a parent or guardian. It takes only a brief lapse of supervision for a child to get into trouble. Children are curious and can get into things in ways you might not consider possible.

Many substances commonly found in or around the house are poisonous. Children are especially vulnerable to these because of their tendency to put everything in their mouths.

When giving medication to a child, do so carefully. Medicine is not candy and should never be called candy to entice a child to take it. Cough syrup looks like a soft drink to children, and many coated medicine tablets look like candy. Some children's medicine has a pleasant candy flavor so that children will take it more easily. When giving any of these substances, make it clear to the child that this is medicine. Take care also to keep the medication out of reach.

By following these general guidelines, you will be able to prevent most poisoning emergencies:

• Keep all medications and household products well out of the reach of children. Special clamps are available to keep children from opening cabinets. Use these or other methods to keep children from reaching any substances that can poison them. Consider all household or drugstore products to be potentially harmful.
• Use childproof safety caps on containers of medication and other potentially dangerous products.
• Keep products in their original containers with the labels in place.
• Use poison symbols to identify dangerous substances and teach children what the symbols mean.

• Dispose of outdated products.
• Use potentially dangerous chemicals only in well-ventilated areas.
• Wear proper clothing for work or recreation that may put you in contact with a poisonous substance (Fig. 14-18).

Preventing bites and stings from insects, spiders, ticks, or snakes is the best protection

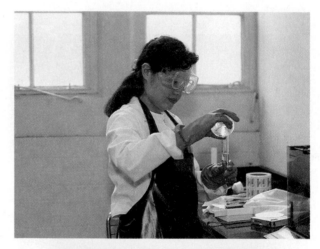

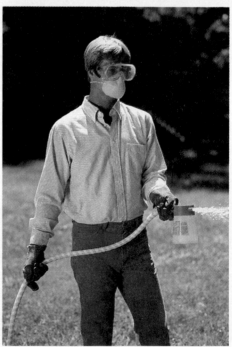

Figure 14-18 Wear proper clothing for any activity that may put you in contact with a poisonous substance.

against the transmission of injected poisons. When in wooded or grassy areas, follow these general guidelines to prevent bites and stings:

- Wear long-sleeved shirts and long pants.
- Tuck your pant legs into your socks or boots. Tuck your shirt into your pants.
- Wear light-colored clothing to make it easier to see tiny insects or ticks.
- Use a rubber band or tape the area where pants and socks meet so that nothing can get under clothing.
- When hiking in woods and fields, stay in the middle of trails. Avoid underbrush and tall grass.
- Wear sturdy hiking boots.
- Avoid walking in areas known to be populated with snakes.
- If you encounter a snake, look around, there may be others. Turn around and walk away on the same path you came on.
- Inspect yourself carefully for insects or ticks after being outdoors or have someone else do it. If you are outdoors for a long period of time, check yourself several times during the day. Check especially in hairy areas of the body (back of the neck and the scalp line).
- If you have pets that go outdoors, spray them with repellent made for your type of pet. Apply the repellent according to the label, and check your pet for ticks often.

If you will be in a grassy or wooded area for a length of time, or if you know the area is highly infested with insects or ticks, you may want to use a repellent. Diethyltolusmide (DEET) is an active ingredient in many skin-applied repellents that are effective against ticks and other insects. Repellents containing DEET can be applied on exposed areas of skin and clothing. However, repellents containing permethrin, another common repellent, should be used *only* on clothing.

If you use a repellent, follow these general rules:

- Keep all repellents out of the reach of children.

Table 14-1 Some Poisonous Substances	
Household products and medications	**Plants**
Acetaminophen	Azalea
Acids	Carolina jessamine
Ammonia	Castor bean
Aspirin	Dieffenbachia
Bleach	Elderberry
Cosmetics	Foxglove
Drain cleaner	Holly berries
Heating fuel	Lantana
Iodine	Lily of the valley
Kerosene	Mountain laurel
Lye	Mistletoe berries
Lighter fluid	Mushrooms and
Paint	toadstools
Strong detergents	Oleander
Rat poison	Nightshade
Rust remover	Poinsettia
Toilet bowl cleaner	Potato vines
Turpentine	Rhododendron
Weed killer	Rhubarb leaves
	Water hemlock
	Yellow jessamine

- To apply repellent to the face, first spray it on your hands, and then apply it from your hands to your face. Avoid sensitive areas such as the lips and the eyes.
- Never spray repellents containing permethrin on your skin or a child's skin.
- Never use repellents on a wound or irritated skin.
- Never put repellents on children's hands. They may put them in their eyes or mouth.
- Use repellents sparingly. One application will last four to eight hours. Heavier or more frequent applications will not increase effectiveness.
- Wash treated skin with soap and water and remove treated clothing after you come indoors.
- If you suspect you are having a reaction to a repellent, wash the treated skin immediately and call your physician.

◆ Summary

Poisonings can occur in one of four ways: ingestion, inhalation, absorption, and injection. For suspected poisonings, call your local or regional Poison Control Center (PCC) and/or your local emergency number. Beyond giving the general steps for caring for a suspected poisoning, medical professionals may advise you to provide some specific care such as inducing vomiting. The best way to avoid poisoning is to take steps to prevent it. In the next chapter, you will learn how misuse and abuse of substances such as drugs and medications can poison the body.

Answer to Application Question

1. Keeping a snakebite wound lower than the level of the heart slows the progress of the venom from the site of the wound to the heart. This ultimately slows the progress of the venom throughout the body.

Study Questions

1. Match each term with the correct definition.

   a. Absorbed poison
   b. Anaphylaxis
   c. Ingested poison
   d. Inhaled poison
   e. Injected poison
   f. Lyme disease
   g. Poison Control Center (PCC)
   h. Rabies

   _____ An illness people get from the bite of a specific type of infected tick.
   _____ A poison introduced into the body through bites, stings, or a hypodermic needle.
   _____ A life-threatening allergic reaction.
   _____ A center staffed by professionals who can tell you how to provide care in a poisoning emergency.
   _____ A poison that is swallowed.
   _____ A poison that enters the body through contact with the skin.
   _____ A disease caused by a virus transmitted through the saliva of infected animals.
   _____ A poison that enters the body through breathing.

2. List at least six common signals of poisoning.

3. List at least four factors that determine the severity of a poisoning.

4. List the steps of care for a tick bite.

5. Describe at least four ways to prevent bites and stings.

6. List at least four rules for using any repellent.

7. List the steps of care for a snakebite.

8. Describe how to care for a person who has spilled a poisonous substance on his or her skin, or has touched a poisonous plant such as poison ivy.

9. List at least six steps you can take to prevent poisoning emergencies in your home.

In questions 10 through 16, circle the letter of the correct answer.

10. You suspect a man has swallowed poison. You should—

    a. Give him something to drink.
    b. Induce vomiting.
    c. Call your local Poison Control Center.
    d. Have him lie down.

11. You suspect an unconscious child has swallowed poison. You should—

    a. Dilute the poison by giving something to drink.
    b. Give rescue breathing.
    c. Call the PCC or local emergency number.
    d. Do a finger sweep.
    e. a and d

12. In caring for the victim of an inhaled poison, you should—

    a. Be sure the scene is safe for you to enter.
    b. Remove the victim from the source of the poison.
    c. Monitor the ABCs.
    d. Call the Poison Control Center or EMS personnel.
    e. All of the above

13. In caring for an insect sting, you should—

    a. Remove the remaining stinger by scraping it from the skin.

    b. Remove a remaining stinger using tweezers.

    c. Wash the sting site, then cover it.

    d. a and c

14. When spending time outdoors in woods or tall grass, to prevent bites and stings you should—

    a. Wear dark-colored clothing.

    b. Wear loose-fitting clothing.

    c. Tuck pant legs into boots or socks.

    d. All of the above

15. Signals of Lyme disease may include—

    a. A rash with red, raised outer edges.

    b. Headache, fever, weakness, joint and muscle pain.

    c. Hysteria.

    d. a and b

    e. a, b, and c

16. In caring for a tick bite, you should—

    a. Remove the tick by pulling it slowly from the skin.

    b. Burn the tick off.

    c. Use nail polish to suffocate the tick.

    d. All of the above

17. You and a friend are hiking in the woods and your friend is stung by a wasp. You provide first aid. Your friend appears fine. You ask how she feels. She responds, "Fine, I'm just a little worried. My father is allergic to wasp stings. I don't know if I am or not." List at least four signals that would tell you if your friend needs further care.

Answers are in Appendix A.

Substance Misuse and Abuse

Objectives

After reading this chapter, you should be able to—

1. Identify the three main categories of commonly abused or misused substances.

2. Identify four signals that may indicate substance abuse or misuse.

3. Describe the general care for someone suspected of misusing or abusing a substance.

4. Explain how you can help prevent unintentional drug misuse.

5. Define the key terms for this chapter.

After reading this chapter and completing the class activities, you should be able to—

1. Make appropriate decisions regarding care if you suspect drug abuse or misuse.

Key Terms

Addiction: The compulsive need to use a substance. Stopping use would cause the user to suffer mental, physical, and emotional distress.

Dependency: The desire to continually use a substance.

Depressants: Substances that affect the central nervous system to slow down physical and mental activity.

Drug: Any substance other than food intended to affect the functions of the body.

Hallucinogens: Substances that affect mood, sensation, thought, emotion, and self-awareness; alter perceptions of time and space; and produce delusions.

Inhalants: Substances inhaled to produce an effect.

Medication: A drug given to prevent or correct the effects of a disease or condition or otherwise enhance mental or physical welfare.

Overdose: A situation in which a person takes enough of a substance that it has toxic (poisonous) or fatal effects.

Stimulants: Substances that affect the central nervous system to speed up physical and mental activity.

Substance abuse: The deliberate, persistent, excessive use of a substance without regard to health concerns or accepted medical practices.

Substance misuse: The use of a substance for unintended purposes or for intended purposes but in improper amounts or doses.

Tolerance: A condition that occurs when a user of a substance has to increase the dose and frequency of use to obtain the desired effect.

Withdrawal: The condition produced when a person stops using or abusing a substance to which he or she is addicted.

For Review

Before reading this chapter, you should have a basic understanding of the functions of the central nervous system (Chapter 2) and the basic signals of and care for sudden illness (Chapter 13). You should also be familiar with how poisons enter the body and the basic care for poisoning (Chapter 14).

◆ Introduction

When you hear the term **substance abuse**, what thoughts flash through your mind? Narcotics? Cocaine? Marijuana? Because of the publicity they receive, we tend to think of illegal **drugs** when we hear of substance abuse. But, in the United States today, alcohol and over-the-counter **medications** such as aspirin, sleeping pills, and certain **stimulants** are among the most often misused or abused substances.

The term substance abuse refers to a broad range of improperly used medical and nonmedical substances. Substance abuse costs the United States billions of dollars each year in medical care, insurance, and loss of productivity. Even more important, however, are the lives lost or permanently impaired each year from injuries or medical emergencies related to substance abuse or misuse.

This chapter will teach you about common forms of **substance misuse** and abuse, how to recognize these problems, and how to care for the victims. In an emergency caused by substance abuse or misuse, the care you give can save a life.

◆ Effects of Misuse and Abuse on Health

Substance abuse and misuse pose a very serious threat to the health of millions of Americans. According to the Drug Abuse Warning Network (DAWN), drug-related emergency department admissions are at an all-time high.

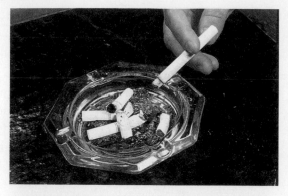

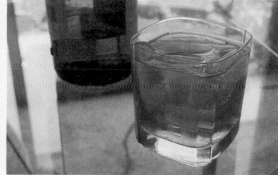

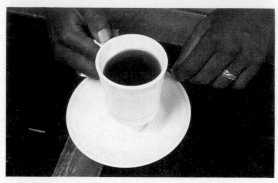

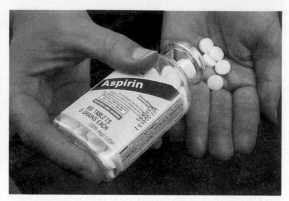

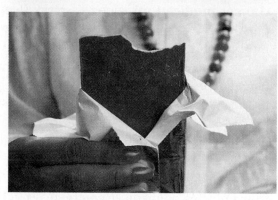

Figure 15-1 Substance abuse and misuse involve a broad range of improperly used medical and nonmedical substances.

The number of emergency department patients saying they have used illegal substances has risen dramatically. The greatest increase is in the number that admit to using cocaine. In addition, the human immunodeficiency virus (HIV) that causes AIDS is now transmitted more commonly through intravenous drug use than ever before.

◆ Forms of Substance Misuse and Abuse

Substance misuse is the use of a substance for unintended purposes, or for appropriate purposes but in improper amounts or doses. Sub-

stance abuse is the deliberate, persistent, and excessive use of a substance without regard to health concerns or accepted medical practices. Many substances that are abused or misused are not illegal. Other substances are legal when prescribed by a physician. Some are illegal only for those under age. Figure 15-1 shows some misused and abused substances.

A drug is any substance other than food taken to affect body functions. A drug used to prevent or treat a disease or otherwise enhance mental or physical welfare is a medication. Any drug can cause **dependency**, the desire to continually use the substance. The victim feels that he or she needs the drug to function normally. Those with a compulsive need for a substance and who would suffer mental, physical, and emotional distress if they stopped taking it are said to have an **addiction** to that substance.

When one continually uses a substance, its

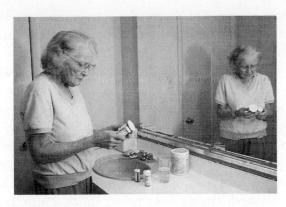

Figure 15-2 Misuse of a medication can occur unintentionally for an elderly person or a person with failing eyesight.

effects on the body decrease—a condition called **tolerance**. The user then has to increase the dose and frequency of substance use to obtain the desired effect.

An **overdose** occurs if someone takes enough of a substance that it has toxic (poisonous) or fatal effects. An overdose may occur if the person takes more than is needed for medical purposes. It may occur unintentionally when a person takes too much medication at one time. An elderly person, for example, may not remember if he or she took the medication and then takes another dose (Fig. 15-2). Or a person with failing eyesight may mistake one medication for another.

An overdose may also be intentional, such

as in suicide attempts. Sometimes the suicide victim takes a sufficiently high dose of a substance to be certain to cause death. Other times, to gain attention or help, the victim takes enough to need medical attention but not enough to cause death.

The term **withdrawal** describes the condition produced when a person stops using or abusing a drug to which he or she is addicted. This may occur as a deliberate decision or because the person is unable to obtain the specific drug. Withdrawal from certain substances, such as alcohol, can cause severe mental and physical discomfort and become a serious medical condition.

◆ Commonly Misused and Abused Substances

Substances are categorized according to their effects on the body. The basic categories are stimulants, **depressants**, and **hallucinogens**. The category to which a substance belongs depends mostly on the effects it has on the central nervous system. Some substances depress the nervous system, whereas others speed up its activity. Some are not easily categorized because they have various effects. Figure 15-3 shows a variety of misused and abused substances.

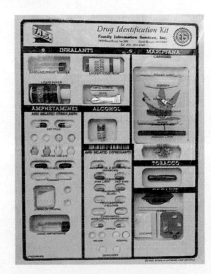
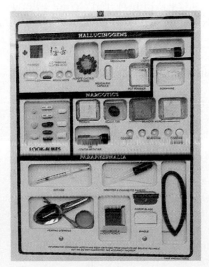

Figure 15-3 Misused and abused substances

Stimulants

Stimulants affect the central nervous system to speed up physical and mental activity. They have limited medical value. They produce temporary feelings of alertness, improve task performance, and prevent sleepiness. They are sometimes used for weight reduction because they suppress appetite.

Many stimulants are ingested as pills, but some can be absorbed or inhaled. Amphetamine, dextroamphetamine, and methamphetamine are stimulants. Their street (slang) names include uppers, bennies, black beauties, speed, crystal, meth, and crank. One of the most recent and dangerous new stimulants is called ice. This is a smokable form of methamphetamine that is extremely addictive.

Cocaine is one of the most publicized and powerful stimulants. Cocaine can be taken into the body in different ways. The most common is sniffing it in powder form, known as "snorting." In this method, the drug is absorbed into the blood through capillaries in the nose. A purer and more potent form of cocaine is crack. Crack is smoked. The vapors that are inhaled into the lungs reach the brain within 10 seconds, causing immediate effects. Crack poses a serious threat because it is highly addictive.

"Getting Fried!"

"This is your brain. This is your brain on drugs. Any questions?" These words from this advertisement from the Partnership for a Drug-Free America, depicting the brain on drugs, is well-known to most of us, but what does it really mean?

Your nervous system, directed by the brain, continually monitors and responds appropriately to the environment. It receives messages, interprets them, and responds by transforming them into mental or physical activity. Drugs alter the quality of messages received and transmitted by the brain. They interfere with the nervous system's ability to transmit messages. Transmission may be delayed, extended, distorted, interrupted, or obliterated. Your brain may never receive vital messages from body parts, and vice versa. For example, some drugs can impair and distort messages from the brain to the heart, causing the heart to beat abnormally fast, slow, or irregularly. Others alter perceptions, sometimes creating frightful images and thoughts of death. Most drugs affect the part of the brain that controls behavior, causing users to be overly aggressive, passive, or unable to judge the consequences of certain actions. Some drugs damage the brain's respiratory center, impairing its ability to control and regulate breathing. No matter how you look at it, drugs affect the brain. The misuse or abuse of drugs can have devastating consequences. So, how do you want your brain?

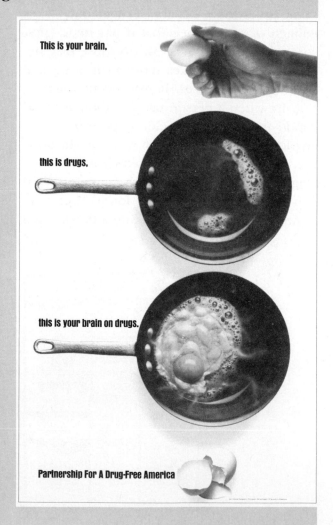

This is your brain,

this is drugs,

this is your brain on drugs.

Partnership For A Drug-Free America

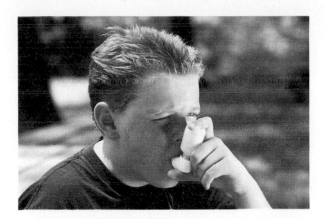

Figure 15-4 Medication used to treat asthma is a common legal stimulant.

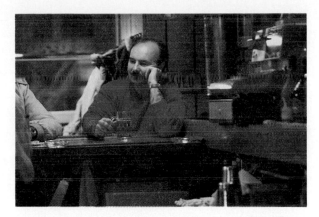

Figure 15-5 Alcohol is one of the most widely used and abused substances in the United States.

The most common stimulants in America are legal. Leading the list is caffeine, present in coffee, tea, many kinds of sodas, chocolate, diet pills, and pills used to combat fatigue. Next is nicotine, found in tobacco products. Other stimulants used for medical purposes are inhaled to treat asthma (Fig. 15-4).

Hallucinogens

Hallucinogens have no present medical uses. They cause changes in mood, sensation, thought, emotion, and self-awareness. They alter one's perception of time and space and produce delusions.

Among the most widely abused are lysergic acid diethylamide (LSD), commonly called acid; psilocybin, called mushrooms; phencyclidine (PCP), also known as angel dust; and mescaline, otherwise referred to as peyote, buttons, or mesc. These substances are usually ingested, but PCP is also often inhaled.

Hallucinogens often have physical effects similar to stimulants but are classified differently because of the other effects they produce. Hallucinogens sometimes cause what is called a "bad trip." A bad trip can involve intense fear, panic, paranoid delusions, vivid hallucinations, profound depression, tension, and anxiety. The victim may be irrational and feel threatened by any attempt others make to help.

Depressants

Depressants affect the central nervous system to slow down physical and mental activity. Unlike stimulants and hallucinogens, which have little or no medical value, depressants are commonly used for medical purposes. Common depressants are barbiturates, benzodiazepines, narcotics, alcohol, and **inhalants**. Most depressants are ingested or injected. Their street names include downers, rainbows, barbs, goofballs, yellow jackets, purple hearts, nemmies, tooies, or reds.

All depressants alter consciousness to some degree. They relieve anxiety, promote sleep, depress respiration, relieve pain, relax muscles, and impair coordination and judgment. Like other substances, the larger the dose or the stronger the substance, the greater its effects.

Narcotics have effects similar to those of other depressants. They are powerful and are used to relieve anxiety and pain. All narcotics are illegal without a prescription, and some are not prescribed at all. The most common natural narcotics are morphine and codeine. Most other narcotics, including heroin, are synthetic.

Alcohol is the most widely used and abused depressant substance in the United States (Fig. 15-5). In small amounts, its effects are fairly mild. In higher doses, its effects can be toxic.

Alcohol is like other depressants in its effects and the risks for overdose. Frequent drinkers may become dependent on the effects of alcohol and increasingly tolerant of them.

Alcohol taken in large or frequent amounts has many unhealthy consequences. The digestive system may be irritated. Alcohol can cause the esophagus to rupture or can injure the stomach lining, causing the victim to vomit blood. Chronic drinking can affect the brain and cause a lack of coordination, memory loss, and apathy. Other problems include liver disease such as cirrhosis (Fig. 15-6). In addition, many psychological, family, social, and work problems are related to chronic drinking.

Substances inhaled to produce an intoxicating effect are called inhalants. Inhalants also have a depressing effect on the central nervous system. In addition, inhalant use can damage the heart, lungs, brain, and liver. Solvents such as acetone, toluene, and butane, found in glues, gasoline, kerosene, lighter fluid, paints, nail polish and remover, and aerosol sprays, all have been inhaled for their effects. The effects are similar to those of alcohol. The user at first appears to be drunk.

An Incalculable Cost

The hospital morgue is full. There is a teenager who drowned while boating, an elderly man who died of a chronic liver disease, and a third victim who was shot by her boyfriend. The group seems to share no connection other than they are lying in the same morgue.

But there is a connection—alcohol.

Public health officials are seeing a growing number of injuries, illnesses, and other social problems in which alcohol plays a role. More than 100,000 people die each year from alcohol-related causes.[1] From the child abused by her alcoholic parent to the driver who drinks and causes a six-car pileup, our country feels the influence of alcohol abuse.

Because alcohol impairs judgment and coordination, even a first-time drinker who overindulges can become a death statistic. Nearly half of all deaths from motor vehicle crashes, one third of all drownings, and about half of all deaths caused by fire involve alcohol.[2] Researchers say strength, judgment, stamina, motor skills, speed, and intellect are all factors in injury prevention. Alcohol impairs many of these abilities. Subsequently, alcohol is a major risk factor for nearly every type of injury.

Tragically, it is a risk often taken by young people. Bruce Kimball was a 25-year-old Olympic diving champion when he drove into a group of teenagers at the end of a country road, killing two people and injuring four others. His blood alcohol concentration was 0.20 percent, twice the legal limit. In one night, both his life and the lives of many others were destroyed.[3]

Reckless and violent behavior has been linked to alcohol use in study after study. Nearly half of all homicides, a third of all suicides, and two thirds of all assaults involve alcohol.[4] One of the best predictors of violence is alcohol abuse, a study of violent men showed. In one 1986 survey of state prison populations, 18.5 percent of inmates reported that they were under the influence of alcohol at the time of the crime. Another 18 percent reported that they were under the influence of both alcohol and drugs. Other crimes and social problems are linked to alcohol. Social workers find alcohol use a factor in nearly 50 percent of their child abuse cases. Prevalence of alcohol abuse among the homeless ranges from 20 to 45 percent.

These personal and social consequences create a tremendous economic burden. A report to the U.S. Congress by the Secretary of Health and Human Services estimates that, by 1995, the cost of alcohol abuse will reach $150 billion annually. The bulk of the cost comes in lost employment and reduced productivity.

Health care costs account for $15 to $20 billion of alcohol costs, and research documenting the detrimental health effects of alcohol is growing. Doctors now say that moderate drinking increases risks of high blood pressure, cirrhosis of the liver, and decreased motor development for children whose mothers drink while pregnant.

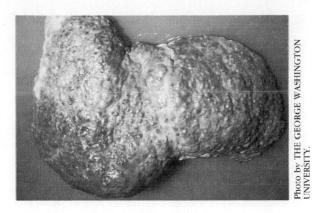

Figure 15-6 Chronic drinking can result in cirrhosis, a disease of the liver.

Heavy drinking—more than four drinks a day—causes more serious long-term effects on your health, including risk of heart attack, many cancers, stroke, kidney failure, and problems of the nervous system like shaking and dementia.

Our morgues are filling up with people ravaged by a drug they could or did not control. In terms of economic cost, lives, and productivity, alcohol abuse outdistances cocaine, heroin, and all other drugs. Avoid alcohol or drink moderately so you won't end up an unfortunate statistic.

REFERENCES

1. Centers for Disease Control. "Alcohol-Related Mortality and Years of Potential Life Lost—United States, 1987." *Morbidity and Mortality Weekly Report,* 39(11) (1990):173.

2. Ibid.

3. Associated Press. *The New York Times,* January 31, 1989, p. 87.

4. National Clearinghouse for Alcohol and Drug Information. *The Fact Is. . ., "OSAP Responds to National Crisis."* Rockville, MD, Summer 1990, p. 2.

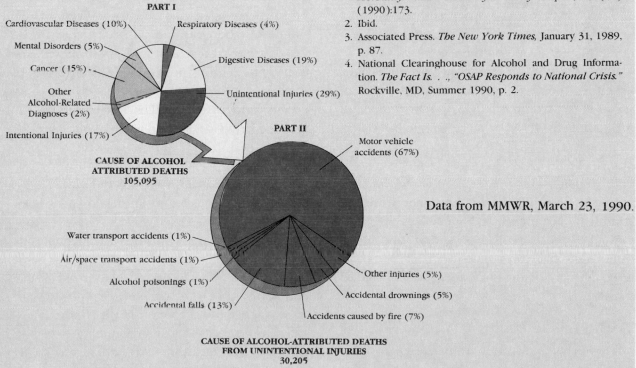

PART I

Cardiovascular Diseases (10%)

Respiratory Diseases (4%)

Mental Disorders (5%)

Digestive Diseases (19%)

Cancer (15%)

Other Alcohol-Related Diagnoses (2%)

Unintentional Injuries (29%)

Intentional Injuries (17%)

CAUSE OF ALCOHOL ATTRIBUTED DEATHS
105,095

PART II

Motor vehicle accidents (67%)

Data from MMWR, March 23, 1990.

Water transport accidents (1%)

Air/space transport accidents (1%)

Alcohol poisonings (1%)

Other injuries (5%)

Accidental drownings (5%)

Accidents caused by fire (7%)

Accidental falls (13%)

CAUSE OF ALCOHOL-ATTRIBUTED DEATHS
FROM UNINTENTIONAL INJURIES
30,205

Photo by THE GEORGE WASHINGTON UNIVERSITY.

Other Substances

Some other substances do not fit neatly into these categories. These include designer drugs, marijuana, steroids, and also over-the-counter substances that can be purchased without a prescription.

Designer drugs

In the early 1980s, the spread of designer drugs was a frightening possibility. Today, it is a reality. Like designer clothes, designer drugs are produced to appeal to a wide audience.

Designer drugs are variations of medically prescribed substances such as narcotics and amphetamines. Through simple and inexpensive methods, the molecular structure of substances produced for medicinal purposes can be modified by street chemists into extremely potent and dangerous street drugs; hence the name "designer drug." One designer drug, a form of the commonly used surgical anesthetic "Fentanyl," can be made 2,000 to 6,000 times stronger than its original form.

When the chemical makeup of a drug is altered, such as with designer drugs, the user can experience a variety of unpredictable and dangerous effects. In many cases, the chemist has no knowledge of what the effects of the new designer drug could be.

One of the more commonly used designer drugs is "Ecstasy" (MDMA). Although "Ecstasy" is structurally related to stimulants and hallucinogens, its effects are somewhat different from either. "Ecstasy" can evoke a euphoric high that makes it popular among young adults.

The signals of "Ecstasy" use range from the stimulant-like effects of high blood pressure, rapid heartbeat, profuse sweating, and agitation, to the hallucinogenic-like effects of paranoia, visual distortion, and erratic mood swings.

Marijuana

Marijuana is derived from the plant *cannabis sativa.* It is typically smoked in cigarette form or in a pipe. The effects include

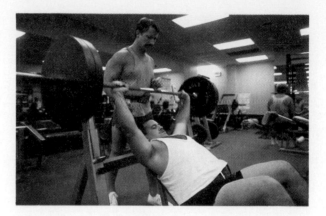

Figure 15-7   Steroids are drugs sometimes abused by athletes to enhance performance and increase muscle mass.

feelings of elation, distorted perceptions of time and space, and impaired judgment. Marijuana irritates the throat, reddens the eyes, and causes a rapid pulse, dizziness, and often an increased appetite.

Anabolic steroids

Anabolic steroids are drugs sometimes used by athletes to enhance performance and increase muscle mass (Fig. 15-7). Their medical uses include bringing about weight gain for persons unable to gain weight naturally. They should not be confused with corticosteroids, which are used to counteract the toxic effects of poisons such as poison ivy. Chronic use of anabolic steroids can lead to sterility, liver cancer, and personality changes such as aggressive behavior. Steroid use by younger people may also disrupt normal growth.

Over-the-counter substances

Aspirin, laxatives, and antihistamine sprays are commonly misused or abused over-the-counter substances. Aspirin is an effective minor pain reliever found in a variety of medicines. People use aspirin for many reasons and conditions. As useful as aspirin is, misuse can have a poisonous effect on the body. Typically, aspirin can cause inflammation of the stomach and small intestine that results in bleeding ulcers. Aspirin can also impair normal blood clotting.

Steroids: Body Meltdown

You've seen Arnold Schwarzenegger and you want to look just like him. If you think steroids are the answer, think again. These drugs may build up bodies on the outside, but they can cause a body meltdown on the inside.

Anabolic steroids are synthetic chemicals that mimic the hormone testosterone. Testosterone gives the male his masculine characteristics—his deeper voice, his beard and mustache, and other sex characteristics. Steroids also help create proteins and other substances used to build muscle tissue, which is why they are popular with athletes.

The problem is that some young athletes and bodybuilders are listening to their gym buddies rather than their doctors. Steroids are being used in greater doses than ever before and at earlier ages. Doctors just don't know what these dosages will do to the body.

Most doctors don't prescribe anabolic steroids because the Food and Drug Administration limits usage to certain medical problems. Before you listen to some gym guru's opinion of steroids, consider these effects:

Stunted growth. In children, steroids cause the growth plates in the bones to close prematurely. As a teenager, you may have been destined to be six-foot-four, but by taking steroids, you can permanently stunt your growth.

Heart disease and stroke. Steroids cause dangerous changes in cholesterol levels. One study found dramatic drops in the amount of good cholesterol, which helps remove the fatty deposits on the artery walls, in steroid users. The research also found dramatic increases in bad cholesterol, which clogs the arteries and causes heart problems.[1] Your steroid-doped body may look fine on the outside, but inside, your body may look like the body of a man in his 50s whose arteries are so clogged that he needs heart surgery.

Aggressive personality and psychological disorders. Some men who take anabolic steroids become unnaturally aggressive. A few have developed documentable mental disorders. In a *Sports Illustrated* article, a South Carolina football player on steroids described his nightmare with steroids.[2] He described pulling a gun on a pizza delivery boy in his dorm and how his family intervened when he began threatening suicide. Many doctors feel the psychiatric effects of steroids may be the most threatening side effect.

Lowered white blood cell count. Taking steroids also affects the number of white blood cells in your body. With fewer white blood cells, your body has fewer antibodies to fight off infections, including cancers and other diseases.

Sexual dysfunction and disorders. Synthetic steroids cause your body to cut off its own natural production of steroids. This can result in shrinking testicles and shrinking sexual interest. If you are a woman, you may grow facial hair, your breast size may decrease, and your voice may get permanently deeper.

Disabled liver. Steroids seriously affect the liver's ability to function. They act as an irritant to the liver, causing tissue damage and an inability to clear bile. Doctors also have found blood-filled benign tumors in the liver.

There are dangers beyond the physiological side effects. Because steroids are often sold on the black market, they are increasingly sold by drug traffickers who obtain their wares from unsanitary laboratories. Pills that cost $5 to make cost $18 to the dealer and $50 for consumers.

Doctors are also concerned that sharing needles to inject steroids increases the danger of transmission of diseases such as hepatitis, and HIV, which causes AIDS. Doctors and other public health officials are particularly concerned about the long-term effects of high doses.

Arnold Schwarzenegger, director of the President's Council on Physical Fitness and Sports, maintains his massive biceps and quadriceps naturally.

In his early bodybuilding days, he used steroids, but that was before doctors knew the risks. "It was an experimental thing in the 60s and 70s," Schwarzenegger says. "Then we didn't have the knowledge that we have now. Now we know that it is harmful."

With steroids, it's not "bodybuilding," he adds. It's "body destroying."

REFERENCES
1. Altman, L. "New 'Breakfast of Champions': A Recipe for Victory or Disaster?", *The New York Times*, November 20, 1988.
2. Chaikin, T., and Telander, R. "The Nightmare of Steroids," *Sports Illustrated*, 69(1988):18.

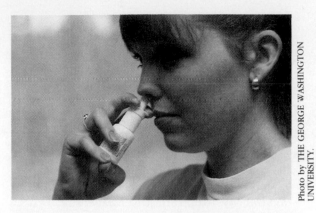

Photo by THE GEORGE WASHINGTON UNIVERSITY.

Figure 15-8 Antihistamines, such as nasal sprays, are used to relieve the congestion of colds and allergies but, if misused, can cause a dependency.

Laxatives, another over-the-counter substance, are used to relieve constipation. They come in mild and strong forms. If used improperly, laxatives can cause uncontrolled diarrhea that can result in dehydration. The very young and the elderly are particularly susceptible to dehydration.

Antihistamines, such as nasal sprays, can help relieve the congestion of colds or hay fever (Fig. 15-8). If misused, they can cause physical dependency. Using the spray over a long period can cause nosebleeds and changes to the lining of the nose that make it difficult to breathe without the spray.

◆ Signals of Substance Misuse or Abuse

Many of the signals of substance misuse and abuse are similar to the signals of other medical emergencies. You should not necessarily assume, for example, that someone who is stumbling, is disoriented, or has a fruity, alcohol-like odor on the breath, is intoxicated by alcohol, since he or she may be a victim of a medical emergency.

The misuse or abuse of stimulants can have many unhealthy effects on the body. A stimulant overdose can cause moist or flushed skin, sweating, chills, nausea, vomiting, fever, headache, dizziness, rapid pulse, rapid breathing, high blood pressure, and chest pain. In some

instances, it can cause respiratory distress, disrupt normal heart rhythms, or cause death. The victim may appear very excited, restless, talkative, or irritable or suddenly lose consciousness. Stimulant use can lead to dependency and can cause heart attack or stroke.

Specific signals of hallucinogen abuse may include sudden mood changes and a flushed face. The victim may claim to see or hear something not present. He or she may be anxious and frightened.

Specific signals of depressant abuse may include drowsiness, confusion, slurred speech, slow heart and breathing rates, and poor coordination. An alcohol abuser may smell of alcohol.

Specific signals of alcohol withdrawal, a potentially dangerous condition, include confusion and restlessness, trembling, and hallucinations. Always call EMS personnel if you suspect a person is suffering from alcohol withdrawal or from any form of substance abuse.

Remember that, as in other medical emergencies, you do not have to diagnose substance misuse or abuse to provide care. However, you may be able to find clues that suggest the nature of the problem. Often these clues will come from the victim, bystanders, or the scene itself. Look for containers, drug paraphernalia, and signals of other medical problems. Try to get information from the victim or from any bystanders or family members. Since many of these physical signals of substance abuse mimic other conditions, you may not be able to determine that a person has overdosed on a substance. To provide care for the victim, you need only recognize abnormalities in breathing; pulse; skin color, temperature, and moisture; and behavior that may indicate a condition requiring professional help.

◆ First Aid for Substance Misuse or Abuse

Since substance abuse or misuse is a form of poisoning, care follows the same general principles. Your initial care for substance misuse or abuse does not require that you know the specific substance taken. Follow these general principles as you would for any poisoning:

* Survey the scene to be sure it is safe to help the person.
* Do a primary survey and care for any life-threatening conditions.
* Call the local Poison Control Center or your local emergency telephone number, and follow their directions.
* Question the victim or bystanders during your secondary survey to try to find out what substance was taken, how much was taken, and when it was taken.
* Calm and reassure the victim.
* Help maintain normal body temperature.
* Withdraw from the area if the victim becomes violent or threatening.
* If you suspect that someone has used a designer drug, tell EMS personnel. This is important because a person who has overdosed on a designer drug frequently may not respond to usual medical treatment.

◆ Preventing Substance Abuse

Preventing substance abuse is a complex process, not yet well-understood or successfully carried out. Various approaches, including educating people about substances and their effects on health and attempting to instill fear of penalties, have not by themselves proved particularly successful. It is becoming clearer that, to be effective, prevention efforts must involve a better understanding of the individual and his or her environment and society.

Understanding the many factors that can lead a person to substance misuse and abuse is an important step toward prevention. These factors include—

* Lack of parental supervision.
* The breakdown of traditional family structures.
* A wish to escape unpleasant surroundings and stressful situations.
* Widespread availability of substances.

* Peer pressure.
* Low self-esteem.
* Media glamorization, especially of alcohol and tobacco.

Perhaps one of the most compelling factors is the belief that using substances can cause you to feel good and have fun.

Each point below has a bearing on an individual's behavior regarding substance use.

* Substance abuse is frequently linked to your past and present home and community environments.
* Self-destructive behavior such as substance abuse is linked to how you feel about yourself. If you have positive feelings of self-worth, you are less likely to become a substance abuser.
* It is important that you choose friends and activities that promote positive attitudes.
* Young people model the behavior of peers and older adults. Before you "light up" or have a drink, or misuse or abuse a substance, think of those around you and how your actions may influence others. If you choose to use substances, do so responsibly, and recognize the rights of others not to do so.
* The more you know about substances, their effects, and the penalties for their use, the better you are able to make educated choices about your behavior regarding them.

A person's best defense against substance misuse or abuse, however, is his or her own values and beliefs. This fact cannot be overemphasized. Your values and beliefs result from upbringing, and from your life experiences and choices. Preventing substance misuse and abuse in your life begins by examining your knowledge, values, attitudes, and beliefs. Furthermore, discussing your values with others can help to strengthen convictions and lower chances of becoming a victim of substance misuse or abuse. Completing the statements in Table 15-1 may help you clarify your feelings about substance misuse and abuse.

Table 15-1 Expressing Yourself: A Values Clarification Exercise

Complete each statement according to your feelings:

* I view substance abuse as . . .
* The thought of using an illegal substance . . .
* Substance abuse begins . . .
* The thought that alcohol, tobacco, and food are drugs . . .
* Substance abusers should . . .
* If I found out that a close friend was abusing an illegal substance, I would . . .
* If I found out that a close friend was abusing a legal substance, I would . . .
* Substance Abuse Treatment Programs are . . .

* Those abusing substances while pregnant should . . .
* If I were faced with a situation of providing emergency care to a known intravenous substance abuser, I would feel . . .
* Raising the drinking age to 21 has . . .
* If I could change something about myself, . . .
* How do I feel about myself? I feel . . .
* The greatest fear I would have about seeking help for a substance abuse problem is . . .

Table 15-2 Sources of Help for Victims of Substance Abuse

Al-Anon Family Group Headquarters
1372 Broadway
7th Floor
New York, NY 10018
(800) 356-9996

Alcohol Hotline
(800) ALCOHOL

Alcoholics Anonymous
P.O. Box 459
Grand Central Station
New York, NY 10163
Treatment Hotline (212) 686-1100

Alcoholism & Drug Addiction Treatment Center (McDonald Center)
9904 Genesse Ave.
La Jolla, CA 92037
(800) 382-4357
(619) 458-4300

Mothers Against Drunk Driving (MADD)
(214) 744-6233
(800) 438-6233   (victims only)

National Cocaine Hotline Treatment Center
(800) COCAINE

National Council on Alcoholism
(800) 622-2255

National Institute on Drug Abuse
Drug Information/ Treatment Hotline
12280 Wilkins Ave.
1st Floor
Rockville, MD 20852
(800) 662-HELP

Remove Intoxicated Drivers (RID)
(518) 372-0034

Students Against Driving Drunk (SADD)
(508) 481-3568

Many resources offer help to victims of substance abuse. Community-based programs offered through schools and churches often provide help and access to hotlines and local groups that give help and support for substance abuse problems. Look in the advertising pages of the phone book under Counseling, Drug Abuse and Addiction Information, Social Service Organizations, Clinics, and Health Services for services in your area.

Many of the agencies listed in Table 15-2 may have groups in your area.

◆ Preventing Substance Misuse

As you have read, not all substance misuse is intentional. By being careful, you can prevent unintentional misuse or overdoses. Use common sense with all medications. Read the product information and use only as directed. Ask your doctor or pharmacist about the effects, side effects, and possible interaction effects if you are taking other medications. Never use another person's prescribed medications; what is right for one person is seldom right for another. Always keep medications in their appropriate, marked containers. Since time can alter the chemical composition of medications, causing them to be less effective and possibly even toxic, you should destroy all out-of-date medications.

Q
1. Describe three situations that represent substance misuse.

◆ Summary

Substance abuse and misuse can produce a variety of signals, some of which are common to other medical emergencies. However, you do not need to be able to determine the cause of the emergency in order to provide care. If you see any of the signals of a medical emergency, follow the emergency action principles.

When you survey the scene, look for clues that may indicate the nature of the problem. Try to get information from the victim, from any bystanders, or from family members. If you suspect that the victim's condition is caused by substance misuse or abuse, provide care for a poisoning emergency. Call your Poison Control Center or local emergency number and follow their directions. Call EMS personnel, if necessary. If the victim becomes violent or threatening, retreat to safety, and wait for EMS personnel to arrive.

Answer to Application Question

1. Examples of substance misuse include—

* Taking somebody else's medication prescribed for similar symptoms.
* Taking medication prescribed for you at an earlier time.
* Unintentionally mistaking one medication for another.
* Putting more than one medication in the same container.

* Ignoring directions concerning when and how to take medication.
* Ignoring directions concerning alcohol use when taking a medication.
* Inappropriate use of laxatives, for example, to avoid weight gain.
* Ignoring directions concerning driving or operating machinery when taking medication.

Study Questions

1. Match each term with its definition.

a. Addiction

b. Dependency

c. Medication

d. Drug

e. Overdose

f. Substance Abuse

g. Tolerance

h. Withdrawal

_____ Deliberate, persistent, excessive use of a substance.

_____ A drug given to prevent or correct a disease or otherwise enhance mental or physical welfare.

_____ Any substance other than food intended to affect the functions of the body.

_____ Taking enough of a substance to produce a toxic or fatal effect in the body.

_____ The compulsive need to use a substance.

_____ The condition produced when a person stops using or abusing a substance to which he or she is addicted.

_____ A desire to continually use a substance, feeling that it is needed to function normally.

_____ A condition that occurs when a substance user has to increase the dose and frequency of use of a substance to obtain the desired effect.

2. List four signals that might indicate substance abuse or misuse.

3. List four commonly misused or abused legal substances.

4. List four things you can do to prevent unintentional substance misuse.

5. Describe the care for a victim of suspected substance misuse or abuse.

6. Match each type of substance with the effects it has on the body.

a. Depressants   c. Inhalants
b. Hallucinogens   d. Stimulants

_____ Produce psychological changes in mood, sensation, thought, emotion, and self-awareness, alter perception of time and space, and produce delusions.

_____ Produce intoxicating effects similar to those of alcohol.

_____ Alter consciousness to some degree, causing relaxation, anxiety and pain relief, impaired judgment and coordination.

_____ Speed up the physical and mental activity of the brain, producing temporary feelings of alertness and improved task performance.

In questions 7 and 8, circle the letter of the correct answer.

7. Which of the following is true of substance abuse?

a. It occurs only among the elderly who are forgetful and may have poor eyesight.
b. It is the use of a substance for intended purposes but in improper amounts or doses.
c. It is the use of a substance without regard to health concerns or accepted medical practices.
d. Its effects are minor and rarely result in medical complications.

8. The effects of designer drugs are—

a. Well-known.
b. Unpredictable.
c. Sometimes dangerous.
d. Easily controlled.
e. b and c

---

9. List two clues at the scene of an emergency that might indicate substance abuse or misuse.

Answers are in Appendix A.

Heat and Cold Exposure

Objectives

After reading this chapter, you should be able to—

1. Identify three conditions that can result from overexposure to heat.

2. List at least four signals that would lead you to suspect a heat-related illness.

3. Identify two signals of heat-related illness that indicate EMS personnel should be called.

4. Describe how to care for a person you suspect is suffering from heat-related illness.

5. List at least two signals of frostbite.

6. List at least three signals that would lead you to suspect hypothermia.

7. Describe how to care for frostbite.

8. Describe how to care for a person you suspect is suffering from hypothermia.

9. Describe at least three precautions you can take to prevent heat- and cold-related illnesses.

10. Define the key terms for this chapter.

After reading this chapter and completing the class activities, you should be able to—

1. Make appropriate decisions for care when given an example of a situation in which someone has become ill because of overexposure to heat or cold.

Key Terms

Frostbite: A serious condition in which body tissues freeze, more commonly in the fingers, toes, ears, and nose.

Heat cramps: Painful spasms of skeletal muscles following exercise or work in warm or moderate temperatures; usually involve the calf and abdominal muscles.

Heat exhaustion: A form of shock, often resulting from strenuous work or exercise in a hot environment.

Heat stroke: A life-threatening condition that develops when the body's cooling mechanisms are overwhelmed and body systems begin to fail.

Hypothermia: A life-threatening condition in which the body's warming mechanisms fail to maintain normal body temperature and the entire body cools.

For Review

Before reading this chapter, you should have a basic understanding of the functions of the circulatory and integumentary systems (Chapter 2). You should also know the signals of and care for shock (Chapter 7) and sudden illness (Chapter 13).

◆ Introduction

Only one more mile to go in the race. You have trained hard all year and you're one of the leaders. After the first two legs of the triathlon, you have your best time yet. You are close to exhaustion but imagine the people cheering as you cross the finish line with the top runners. You summon up your last energies to push ahead, but instead, your legs begin to falter. You are suddenly aware that you feel a chill, even though it is a hot day. You feel weak, dizzy, and nauseated.

You have been struggling to keep up with the leaders for the last several miles. Now you are wondering if you should have trained harder. Could you have better paced yourself? The race officials warned you to drink the water at the aid stations along the course, but you did not want to disrupt your pace. Now you look on helplessly, as if in slow motion, as others are passing you by. Your head seems to spin. You do not realize that you have slowed to a walk and are staggering. Suddenly things go black.

You do not remember falling. You barely remember voices shouting for help and indistinguishable people moving your limp body to a tub of cool water nearby. Things are now coming into focus. The sounds around you are becoming clearer, but your vision is still blurry. You hear a siren very near. You think that someone must need help. You hear voices close by—calling your name. You feel your body being moved. You are suddenly overwhelmed by the realization that you are the one in trouble. You realize that you are on your way to the hospital in an ambulance. Your moment of glory ended just yards from the finish line. You have fallen victim to the heat—victim of a condition to which not even champions are immune.

The human body is equipped to withstand extremes of temperature. Usually, its mechanisms for regulating body temperature work very well. However, when the body is overwhelmed by extremes of heat and cold, illness occurs.

Extreme temperatures can occur anywhere, both indoors and outdoors, but a person can develop a heat- or cold-related illness even if temperatures are not extreme. The effects of humidity, wind, clothing, living and working environment, physical activity, age, and an individual's health are all factors in heat- and cold-related illnesses.

Illnesses caused by exposure to temperature extremes are progressive and can become life-threatening. Once the signals of a heat- or cold-related illness begin to appear, a victim's condition can rapidly deteriorate and lead to death. If the victim exhibits any of the signals of sudden illness, the environmental conditions should alert you to look for the presence of a heat- or cold-related illness and give the appropriate care. Immediate care can prevent the illness from becoming life-threatening. In this chapter, you will learn how extremes of heat and cold affect the body, how to recognize temperature-related emergencies, and how to provide care.

◆ How Body Temperature Is Controlled

Body temperature must remain constant for the body to work efficiently. Normal body temperature is 98.6° F. Body heat is generated primarily through the conversion of food to energy. Heat is also produced by muscle contractions, as in exercise or shivering.

Heat always moves from warm areas to cooler ones. Since the body is usually warmer than the surrounding air, it tends to lose heat to the air. The body maintains its temperature by constantly balancing heat loss with heat production (Fig. 16-1). The heat produced in routine activities is usually enough to balance normal heat loss.

When body heat increases, the body removes heat through the skin. Blood vessels near the skin dilate, or widen, to bring more

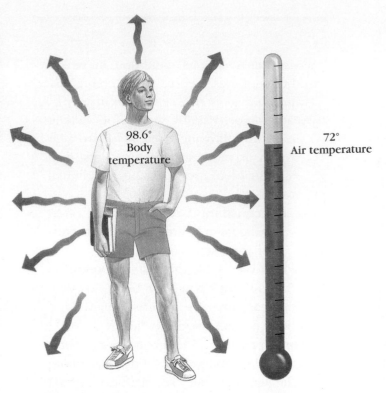

Figure 16-1   Since the body is usually warmer than the surrounding air, it tends to lose heat to the air.

warm blood to the surface. Heat then escapes and the body cools (Fig. 16-2, *A).*

The body is also cooled by the evaporation of sweat. When the air temperature is very warm, dilation of blood vessels is a less effective means of removing heat. Therefore, sweating increases. But when the humidity is high, sweat does not evaporate as quickly. It stays longer on the skin and has little or no cooling effect.

When the body reacts to cold, blood vessels near the skin constrict and move warm blood to the center of the body. Thus less heat escapes through the skin, and the body stays warm (Fig. 16-2, *B).* When constriction of blood vessels fails to keep the body warm, shivering results. Shivering produces heat through muscle action.

Three main factors can affect how well the body maintains its temperature: air temperature, humidity, and wind. Humidity and wind

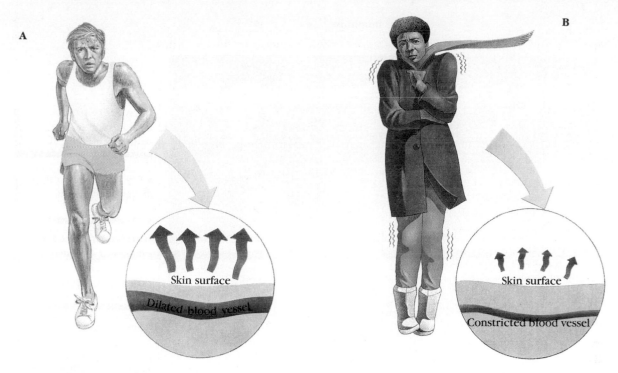

Figure 16-2 **A,** Your body removes heat by dilating the blood vessels near the skin's surface. **B,** The body conserves heat by constricting the blood vessels near the skin.

multiply the effects of heat or cold. Extreme heat or cold accompanied by high humidity hampers the body's ability to effectively maintain temperature (see Figure 16-3 on the next page). A cold temperature combined with a strong wind rapidly cools exposed body parts. The combination of temperature and wind speed form what is called the "wind chill factor."

Other factors, such as the clothing you wear, how often you take breaks from exposure to extreme temperature, how much and how often you drink water, and how intense your activity is, also affect how well your body manages extremes of temperature. These are all factors you can control to prevent illnesses related to heat or cold.

People at Risk for Heat- or Cold-Related Illnesses

People at risk for heat or cold illnesses include—

- Those who work or exercise strenuously outdoors.
- Elderly people.
- Young children.
- Those with health problems.
- Those who have had a heat- or cold-related illness in the past.
- Those who have cardiovascular disease or other conditions that cause poor circulation.
- Those who take medications to eliminate water from the body (diuretics).

Usually people seek relief from an extreme temperature before they begin to feel ill. However, some people do not or cannot easily escape these extremes (see Figure 16-4 on page 337). Athletes and those who work outdoors often keep working even after they develop the first signals of illness. Many times, they may not even recognize the signals.

Heat- and cold-related illnesses occur more

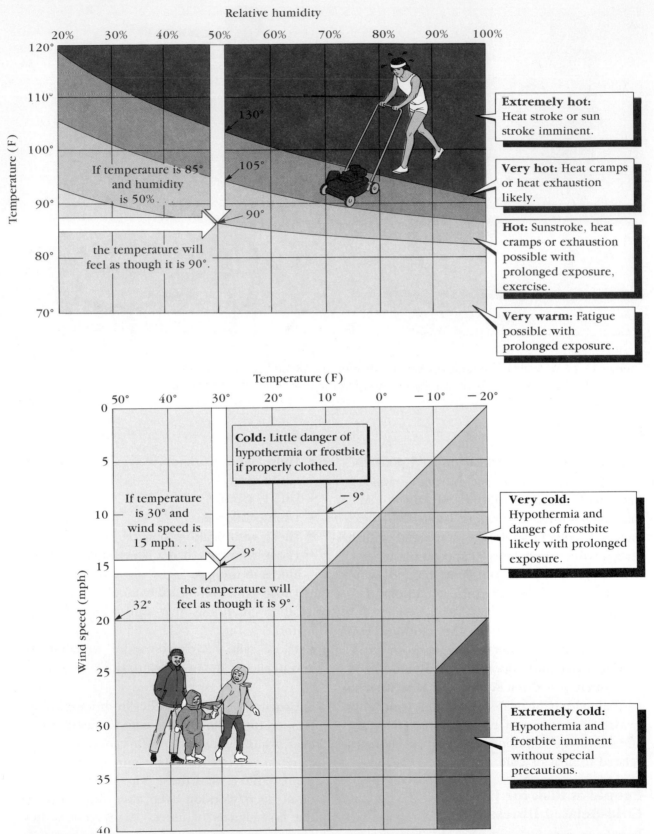

Figure 16-3 Temperature, humidity, and wind are the three main factors affecting body temperature.

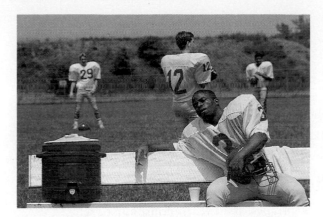

Figure 16-4 In certain situations, it is difficult to escape temperature extremes.

frequently with the elderly, especially those living in poorly ventilated or poorly insulated buildings or those with poor heating or cooling systems. Young children and people with health problems are also at risk because their bodies do not respond as effectively to temperature extremes.

◆ Heat Emergencies

Heat cramps, heat exhaustion, and **heat stroke** are conditions caused by overexposure to heat. Heat cramps are the least severe but, if not cared for, may lead to heat exhaustion and heat stroke. Heat exhaustion and heat stroke are heat-related illnesses.

Heat Cramps

Heat cramps are painful spasms of skeletal muscles. The exact cause is not known, although it is believed to be a combination of fluid and salt loss due to heavy sweating. Heat cramps develop fairly rapidly and usually occur after heavy exercise or work outdoors in warm or even moderate temperatures. Heat cramps are characterized by severe muscle contractions, usually in the legs and the abdomen, but can occur in any voluntary muscle. Body temperature is usually normal, and the skin is moist. However, heat cramps may also indicate that a person is in the early stages of a more severe heat-related emergency.

To care for heat cramps, have the victim rest comfortably in a cool place. Provide cool water or a commercial sports drink. Usually, rest and fluids are all the body needs to recover. Lightly stretch the muscle and gently massage the area (Fig. 16-5). The victim should not take salt tablets or salt water. Ingesting high concentrations of salt, whether in tablet or liquid form, can hasten the onset of heat-related illness.

When the cramps stop, if there are no other signals of illness, the person can usually resume activity again but should be watched carefully for signals of developing heat-related illness. He or she should continue to drink plenty of fluids during and after activity.

Heat-Related Illnesses

Heat exhaustion

Heat exhaustion is the early stage and the most common form of heat-related illness. It typically occurs after long periods of strenuous exercise or work in a hot environment. Although heat exhaustion is commonly associated with athletes, it also affects firefighters, construction workers, factory workers, and others who wear heavy clothing in a hot, humid environment. Heat exhaustion is an early

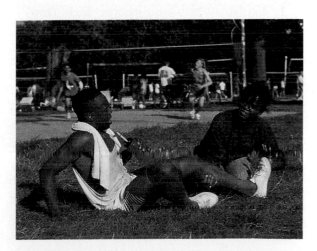

Figure 16-5 Resting, lightly stretching the affected muscle, and replenishing fluids is usually enough for the body to recover from heat cramps.

indication that the body's temperature-regulating mechanism is becoming overwhelmed. It is not always preceded by heat cramps. Over time, the victim loses fluid through sweating, which decreases the blood volume. Blood flow to the skin increases, reducing blood flow to the vital organs. Because the circulatory system is affected, the person goes into mild shock.

The signals of heat exhaustion include—

* Normal or below normal body temperature.
* Cool, moist, pale, or red skin.
* Headache.
* Nausea.
* Dizziness and weakness.
* Exhaustion.

Heat exhaustion in its early stage can usually be reversed with prompt care. Often the victim soon feels better when he or she rests in a cool place and drinks cool water. If heat exhaustion progresses, however, the victim's condition worsens. Body temperature continues to climb. A victim may vomit and begin to show changes in his or her level of consciousness. Without prompt care, heat exhaustion can quickly advance to a more serious stage of heat-related illness—heat stroke.

Q

1. Explain why some people feel "faint" in hot weather.

Heat stroke

Heat stroke is the least common and most severe heat emergency. It most often occurs when people ignore the signals of heat exhaustion. Heat stroke develops when the body systems are overwhelmed by heat and begin to stop functioning. Sweating stops because body fluid levels are low. When sweating stops, the body cannot cool itself effectively, and body temperature rapidly rises. It soon reaches a level at which the brain and other vital organs, such as the heart and kidneys, begin to fail. If the body is not cooled, convulsions, coma, and death will result. Heat stroke is a *serious* medical emergency. You must recognize the signals of this later stage of heat-related illness and provide care immediately.

The signals of heat stroke include—

* High body temperature (often as high as 106° F).
* Red, hot, dry skin.
* Progressive loss of consciousness.
* Rapid, weak pulse.
* Rapid, shallow breathing.

Someone in heat stroke may at first have a strong, rapid pulse, as the heart works hard to rid the body of heat by dilating blood vessels and sending more blood to the skin. As consciousness deteriorates, the circulatory system begins to fail, and the pulse becomes weak and irregular. Without prompt care, the victim will die.

Caring for Heat-Related Illness

When any signals of sudden illness develop and you suspect the illness is caused by overexposure to heat, follow these general care steps immediately:

* Cool the body.
* Give fluids.
* Minimize shock.

When you recognize heat-related illness in its early stages, you can usually reverse it. Remove the victim from the hot environment and give him or her cool water to drink. Moving the victim out of the sun or away from the heat allows the body's own temperature-regulating mechanism to recover, cooling the body more quickly.

Loosen any tight clothing and remove clothing soaked with perspiration. Apply cool, wet cloths, such as towels or sheets, to the skin and fan the victim to increase evaporation.

If the victim is conscious, drinking cool wa-

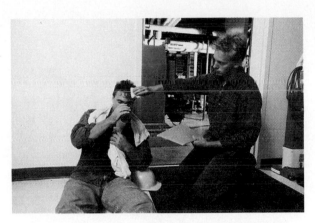

Figure 16-6 For the early stages of heat-related illness, apply cool, wet cloths and fan the victim to increase evaporation. Give cool water to drink.

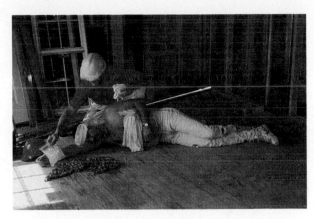

Figure 16-7 To cool the body of a victim of heat-related illness, cover with cool, wet towels and apply ice packs.

ter slowly will help replenish the vital fluids lost through sweating (Fig. 16-6). The victim is likely to be nauseated, and water is less likely than other fluids to cause vomiting and is more quickly absorbed into the body from the stomach. Do not let the victim drink too quickly. Give one half glass (4 ounces) about every 15 minutes. Let the victim rest in a comfortable position, and watch carefully for changes in his or her condition. A victim of heat-related illness should not resume normal activities the same day.

When to call EMS personnel

Refusing water, vomiting, and changes in the victim's level of consciousness are signals that the victim's condition is worsening. Call EMS personnel immediately if you have not already done so. If the person vomits, stop giving fluids and position the victim on the side. Make sure the airway is clear. Monitor the ABCs and check vital signs. Keep the victim lying down and continue to cool the body.

A change in the victim's level of consciousness is the first reliable signal that a victim's condition is deteriorating. If you observe changes in the victim's level of consciousness, cool the body by any means available. Soak towels or sheets and apply them to the victim's body. If you have ice packs or cold packs, place them on

each of the victim's wrists and ankles, on the groin, in each armpit, and on the neck to cool the large blood vessels (Fig. 16-7). *Do not* apply rubbing (isopropyl) alcohol. Alcohol closes the skin's pores and prevents heat loss. Maintain an open airway and monitor the ABCs. Immersing the victim in a tub of cool water is not always a good idea because doing so may make it difficult to maintain an open airway. A person in heat stroke may experience respiratory or cardiac arrest. Be prepared to do rescue breathing or CPR.

◆ Cold Emergencies

Frostbite and **hypothermia** are two types of cold emergencies. Frostbite occurs in body parts exposed to the cold. Hypothermia is a general body cooling that develops when the body can no longer generate sufficient heat to maintain normal body temperature.

Frostbite

Frostbite is the freezing of body tissues. It usually occurs in exposed areas of the body, depending on the air temperature, length of exposure, and the wind. Frostbite can affect superficial or deep tissues. In superficial frostbite, the skin is frozen, but the tissues below are not. In deep frostbite, also called freezing,

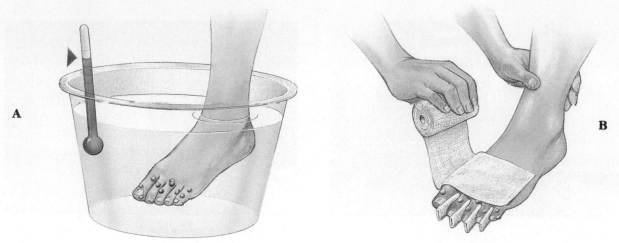

Figure 16-8 A, Warm the frostbitten area gently by soaking it in water. Do not allow the frostbitten area to touch the container. **B,** After rewarming, bandage the area with a dry, sterile dressing. If fingers or toes are frostbitten, place gauze between them.

both the skin and underlying tissues are frozen. Both types of frostbite are serious. The water in and between the body's cells freezes and swells. The ice crystals and swelling damage or destroy the cells. Frostbite can cause the loss of fingers, hands, arms, toes, feet, and legs.

The signals of frostbite include—

- Lack of feeling in the affected area.
- Skin that appears waxy.
- Skin that is cold to the touch.
- Skin that is discolored (flushed, white, yellow, blue).

Care for frostbite

When caring for frostbite, handle the affected area gently. Never rub an affected area. Rubbing causes further damage because of the sharp ice crystals in the skin. Warm the area gently by soaking the affected part in water no warmer than 100° F to 105° F. Use a thermometer to check the water, if possible. If not, test the water temperature yourself. If the temperature is uncomfortable to your touch, the water is too warm. Do not let the affected part touch the bottom or sides of the container (Fig. 16-8, *A).* Keep the frostbitten part in the water until it appears red and feels warm. Bandage the area with a dry, sterile dressing. If fingers or toes are frostbitten, place cotton or gauze between them (Fig. 16-8, *B).* Avoid breaking any blisters. Seek professional medical attention as soon as possible.

Hypothermia

In hypothermia, the entire body cools when its warming mechanisms fail. The victim will die if not given care. In hypothermia, body temperature drops below 95° F. Most thermometers do not measure below 94° F. As the body temperature cools, the heart begins to beat erratically (ventricular fibrillation) and eventually stops. Death then occurs.

The signals of hypothermia include—

- Shivering (may be absent in later stages).
- Slow, irregular pulse.
- Numbness.
- Glassy stare.
- Apathy and decreasing levels of consciousness.

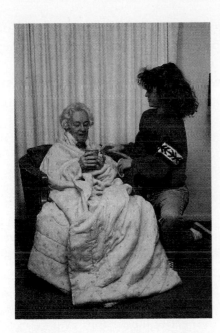

Figure 16-9 For a hypothermia victim, rewarm the body gradually.

The air temperature does not have to be below freezing for people to develop hypothermia. Elderly people in poorly heated homes, particularly people with poor nutrition and who get little exercise, can develop hypothermia at higher temperatures. The homeless and the ill are also at risk. Certain substances, such as alcohol and barbiturates, can also interfere with the body's normal response to cold, causing hypothermia to occur more easily. Medical conditions such as infection, insulin reaction, stroke, and brain tumor also make a person more susceptible. Anyone remaining in cold water or wet clothing for a prolonged time may also easily develop hypothermia.

Care for hypothermia

Hypothermia is a medical emergency. Do a primary survey and care for any life-threatening problems. Call EMS personnel. Remove any wet clothing and dry the victim.

Warm the body gradually by wrapping the victim in blankets or putting on dry clothing and moving him or her to a warm environment. If they are available, apply hot water bottles, heating pads (if the victim is dry), and/or other heat sources to the body. Keep a barrier, such as a blanket, towel, or clothing, between the heat source and the victim to avoid burning him or her. If the victim is alert, give warm liquids to drink (Fig. 16-9). *Do not warm the victim too quickly such as by immersing the victim in warm water. Rapid rewarming can cause dangerous heart rhythms.* Be extremely gentle in handling the victim.

In cases of severe hypothermia, the victim may be unconscious. Breathing may have slowed or stopped. The pulse may be slow and irregular. The body may feel stiff as the muscles become rigid. Monitor the ABCs, give rescue breathing if necessary, and continue to warm the victim until EMS personnel arrive. Be prepared to start CPR.

Q

2. Consuming alcohol usually makes a person feel warmer. Would you recommend that people drink alcohol in moderation on a cold day to keep warm? Why or why not?

◆ Preventing Heat or Cold Emergencies

Generally, illnesses caused by overexposure to extreme temperatures are preventable. To prevent heat or cold emergencies from happening to you or anyone you know, follow these guidelines:

* Avoid being outdoors in the hottest or coldest part of the day.
* Change your activity level according to the temperature.
* Take frequent breaks.
* Dress appropriately for the environment.
* Drink large amounts of fluids.

The easiest way to prevent illness caused by temperature extremes is to avoid being outside during the part of the day when temperatures are most intense. For instance, if you plan to work out-of-doors in hot weather, plan your activity for the early morning and evening hours when the sun is not as strong.

Likewise, if you must be out-of-doors on cold days, plan your activities for the warmest part of the day.

However, not everyone can avoid extremes of temperature. Often work or other situations

Shelter From a Storm

Robert Falcon Scott was one of the most famous people to freeze to death. The explorer perished while leading an expedition to the South Pole. Weakened by lack of food and slowed by blizzards, Scott and four of his men died in the frozen Antarctic wasteland in 1912.

Tales of freezing to death are usually associated with being trapped outdoors in a blizzard, but many cold exposure deaths today occur in drab little rooms where there is no heat and hardly even a blanket to keep warm. It may shock you to learn that the number of deaths by exposure to cold has doubled in the United States, according to the Centers for Disease Control. Between 1976 and 1986, the numbers rose from about 500 to nearly 1,000 deaths annually.

The numbers come as no surprise to Cynthia Jacobs, who runs an energy assistance program for the homebound in Washington, D.C. The Washington, D.C. Energy Office spends more than $3 million annually to supply heat to residents who cannot afford to pay their heating bills.

In her visits to people who need energy assistance, Jacobs often finds people in desperate situations. She found one elderly woman, huddled under six or seven blankets, sitting in a room where all the windows were broken. Another, a man, who was wheelchair-bound, told her he had been without heat for six or seven days.

"They're alone and nobody's there to help and it's cold," says Jacobs, who delivers about 500 blankets in addition to covering heating bills. "I feel so sad for them."

Very few of the elderly know about the risk of hypothermia, which is particularly dangerous for their age group. The body's natural defense system against the cold weakens with age. The elderly have decreased muscle tone and body fat. Their heart rate is slower, and their blood vessels have less capacity to constrict. Medicines commonly used by older people, such as antidepressants, tranquilizers, and those that affect the cardiovascular system, decrease sensitivity to cold. Alcohol also blunts the body's ability to regulate temperature.

With limited incomes, many elderly attempt to economize by keeping their heat down. Their landlords may fail to turn the heat up as the temperature drops. This puts them in serious danger, because temperatures do not have to become extremely cold for the elderly to be at risk.

Programs like Jacobs' are available throughout the country, but tragedies still happen. Homer Goodwin's body was frozen by the time a building superintendent and a gas-meter reader found him in the basement of an apartment house in the Bronx. The 47-year-old man, who worked odd jobs, lived in an empty room except for a couch and a bare light bulb dangling overhead. The heat in the building had failed several times during the bitter New York City winter.

Ron Barrington never came in from the cold. He died on a sleeping grate where he had curled up with other homeless men. They took him to the hospital when they realized he had stopped breathing.

If you know someone who has no heat during winter's arctic blasts, urge him or her to call the community or state energy office. The federal government provides funding to states and local communities to offer energy assistance for people who cannot afford to pay their heating bills. Homeless shelters operated by governments, churches, and other organizations provide an alternative to the streets.

Table 16-1   First Aid for Heat and Cold Emergencies

Cold emergencies

Frostbite

Cover affected area

Handle gently, never rub

Soak affected part in water 100° F to 105° F

Do not let affected part touch bottom or sides of container

Keep in water until red and warm

Bandage with dry, sterile dressing

Hypothermia

Call EMS personnel

Warm body gradually by wrapping in blankets or putting on dry clothing

Apply heat sources (hot water bottle, heating pad if victim is dry), if available

Give warm liquids to an alert victim

Do not rewarm too quickly

Handle gently

Heat emergencies

Heat cramps

Have victim rest in cool place

Give cool water or sports drink

Stretch muscle and massage area

Heat-related illness

Have victim rest in cool place

Give cool water

Monitor victim's condition for signals of worsening

Loosen tight clothing

Remove perspiration-soaked clothing

Apply cool, wet cloths to skin and fan victim

Monitor condition carefully

Call EMS immediately

Cool the body by any means available

- ◆ Wet towels or sheets
- ◆ Ice packs
- ◆ Immerse in tub of cool water (if can maintain airway)

Monitor ABCs

Be prepared to do rescue breathing or CPR

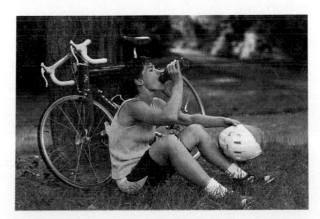

Figure 16-10 Taking frequent breaks when exercising in extreme temperatures allows your body to readjust to normal body temperature.

require exposure to extreme conditions. But you can take additional precautions such as changing your activity level and taking frequent breaks. For instance, in very hot conditions, exercise only for brief periods, then rest in a cool, shaded area. Frequent breaks allow your body to readjust to normal body temperature, enabling it to better withstand brief periods of exposure to temperature extremes (Fig. 16-10). Avoid heavy exercise during the hottest or coldest part of the day. Extremes of temperature promote fatigue, which hampers the body's ability to adjust to them.

Always wear clothing appropriate to the environmental conditions and your activity level. When possible, wear light-colored cotton clothing in the heat. Cotton absorbs perspiration and lets air circulate through the material. This lets heat escape and perspiration evaporate, cooling the body. Light-colored clothing reflects the sun's rays.

When you are in the cold, wear layers of clothing made of tightly woven fibers, such as wool, that trap warm air against your body. Wear a head covering in both heat and cold. A hat protects the head from the sun's rays in the summer and prevents heat from escaping in the winter. Also protect other areas of the body, such as the fingers, toes, ears, and nose, from cold exposure by wearing protective coverings.

Whether in heat or cold, always drink enough fluids. Drinking plenty of fluids is the most important thing you can do to prevent heat- or cold-related illnesses. Plan for fluids when you break. Just as you would drink cool fluids in the summer, drink warm fluids in the winter. Cool and warm fluids help the body maintain a normal temperature. If cold or hot drinks are not available, drink plenty of plain water. Do not drink beverages containing caffeine or alcohol. Caffeine and alcohol hinder the body's temperature-regulating mechanism.

◆ Summary

Overexposure to extreme heat and cold may cause a person to become ill. The likelihood of illness also depends on factors such as physical activity, clothing, wind, humidity, working and living conditions, and a person's age and physical condition.

Heat cramps are an early indication that the body's normal temperature-regulating mechanism is not working efficiently. They may signal that the person is in the early stage of a heat-related illness. For heat-related illnesses, it is important to stop physical activity, cool the victim, and call EMS personnel.

Frostbite and hypothermia are both serious cold-related conditions, and the victim of either needs professional medical care. Hypothermia can be life-threatening. For both hypothermia and frostbite, it is important to warm the victim.

Answers to Application Questions

1. In an effort to cool the body, blood flow to the skin is increased, bringing warm blood to the surface and allowing heat to escape. As more blood flows to the skin, blood flow to vital organs, such as the brain, is reduced. This reduction of blood flow causes a lack of oxygen-rich blood in the brain, creating a temporary decline in the level of consciousness and making the person feel weak and dizzy, or faint. A person who feels faint should rest in a cool place and sip cool water.

2. Although consuming alcohol makes you feel warm, it actually decreases body temperature. When you drink alcohol, blood vessels dilate and blood flow to the skin increases, causing the loss of body heat through the skin. Therefore, alcohol should not be consumed on a cold day to keep warm.

Study Questions

1. Match each term with the correct definition

   a. Frostbite
   b. Heat cramps
   c. Heat exhaustion
   d. Heat stroke
   e. Hypothermia

   _____ A form of shock caused by strenuous work or exercise in a hot environ-ment. Signals include cool, moist, pale, or red skin; headache; nausea; and dizziness.

   _____ A life-threatening body cooling that develops when the body's warming mechanisms fail to maintain normal body temperature.

   _____ A life-threatening condition that develops when the body's cooling mecha-nism fails.

   _____ The freezing of body tissues caused by overexposure to the cold.

   _____ Painful spasms of skeletal muscles that develop following heavy exercise or work outdoors in warm or moderate temperatures.

2. List at least four factors that affect body temperature.

3. List three conditions that can result from overexposure to heat.

4. List at least four signals of a heat-related illness.

5. List two signals of a heat-related illness for which EMS personnel should be called.

6. List two ways to cool a victim of a suspected heat-related illness.

7. List two conditions that result from overexposure to the cold.

8. List at least four ways to prevent heat and cold emergencies.

In questions 9 and 10, circle the letter of the correct answer.

9. To care for heat cramps—

    a. Have the victim rest comfortably.

    b. Give cool water.

    c. Give salt tablets.

    d. a and b

    e. a, b, and c

10. If the victim of a suspected heat-related illness begins to lose consciousness, you should—

    a. Cool the body using wet sheets, towels, or cold packs.

    b. Cool the body by applying rubbing alcohol.

    c. Give cool water.

    d. Call EMS personnel.

    e. a and d

Use the following scenario to answer questions 11 through 13.

You and your mom decide to work in the yard. It is a sunny, humid day. Your mom is wearing her usual gardening outfit, which includes a floppy hat and a white cotton shirt. You are wearing a navy blue tank top and a pair of jeans.

You have been working for nearly two hours when you feel a sudden chill. You shake it off and continue working. While your mom has gone inside, you take a drink of her water. Although she has had several glasses, you have not really felt thirsty and have not had anything to drink.

When your mother returns, she notices you look pale and are sweating heavily. She asks how you feel. You reply that you feel weak. In fact, you also feel a little nauseated and dizzy.

Your mother insists that you quit working and go inside or at least sit in the shade a while. As you stand up to move to the shade, you feel dizzy and weak.

11. List the signals of heat exhaustion you find in the scenario.

12. List the actions you could have taken to prevent heat exhaustion.

13. Now that you are out of the sun, what care should your mother give?

Use the following scenario to answer questions 14 and 15.

You and a friend have been skiing all morning. The snow is great, but it is really cold. Your buddy has complained for the last half hour or so that his hands and feet are freezing. Now he says he can't feel his fingers and toes. You decide to return to the ski lodge. Once inside, your friend has trouble removing his mittens and ski boots. You help him take them off and notice that his fingers look waxy and white and feel cold. Your friend says he still can't feel them.

14. List the signals of frostbite you find in the scenario.

15. How would you care for your friend's hands and feet?

Use the following scenario to answer questions 16 and 17.

You are working on a community service project delivering meals to elderly, home-bound individuals. It is a blustery winter day that has you running from the van to each front door. As you enter the last home, you notice that it is not much warmer inside the house than it is outside. An elderly woman, bundled in blankets, is sitting as close as possible to a small space heater. You speak to her, introducing yourself and asking how things are, but you get no response. The woman's eyes are glassy as she makes an effort to look at you. She seems weak and exhausted, barely able to keep her head up. You touch her arm but she does not seem to feel it.

16. List the signals in the scenario that would lead you to suspect a cold-related illness.

17. Describe the actions you would take to care for the woman.

Answers are in Appendix A.

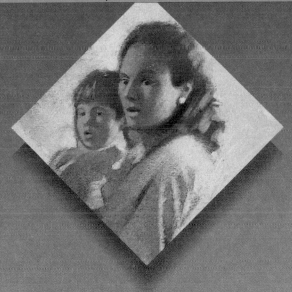

PART VI

Rescue

Reaching and Moving Victims

17

Reaching and Moving Victims

Objectives

After reading this chapter, you should be able to—

1. List at least four situations in which an emergency move of a victim is necessary.

2. List at least four limitations you should be aware of before you attempt to move someone.

3. Describe at least four guidelines you should follow when moving someone.

4. Describe how to perform at least four emergency moves.

5. Identify the most appropriate emergency move for a victim with a suspected head or spine injury.

6. Describe the three safest methods of rescuing a near-drowning victim.

7. Describe at least one method of self-rescue in water.

8. List at least three precautions to take around water.

9. Define the key terms for this chapter.

After reading this chapter and completing the class activities, you should be able to—

1. Make appropriate decisions when given an example of an emergency situation in which someone may need to be moved.

Key Terms

Drowning: Death by suffocation when submerged in water.

Near-drowning: A situation in which a person who has been submerged in water survives.

Personal flotation device (PFD): A buoyant device, such as a cushion or lifejacket, designed to be held or worn to keep a person afloat.

Survival floating: A facedown floating technique that enables a victim in warm water to conserve energy while waiting for rescue.

For Review

Before reading this chapter, you should have a basic understanding of how to recognize an emergency situation (Chapter 1) and how to ensure your own safety in an emergency situation (Chapter 3).

◆ Introduction

You awake in the middle of the night smelling smoke through the open bedroom window. Something is burning outside the house, but you cannot tell where. You quickly put on clothes and run from the bedroom toward the front door. There is a sudden crackling sound outside, followed by screams. Through the windows you see flames.

You rush outside and see the neighbor's house ablaze. A man carrying a young child staggers through the door. He collapses to the ground in the doorway. Smoke is blowing over him and the child. You can see flames inside the house. You hear the sound of sirens, but they are still far off in the distance.

You make a split-second decision to help, and run to the collapsed victims. Both the man and the child are unconscious. You rec-ognize the immediate danger and the need to get them to a safer place. You pick up the child and run toward your house. Other neighbors begin to gather. You hand the child to one of them and run back to help the man. With a neighbor's help, you drag him away from the fire.

The house is nearly fully ablaze when the firefighters arrive. Through the smoke and flames, you see that the place where the man and child lay is now covered with burning debris from a collapsed wall. You made a fast decision to rescue two people. You did it quickly and probably saved two lives.

In earlier chapters, you learned how to care for victims of injury and illness when it is safe to do so. Sometimes, however, the victim is in a dangerous situation and must be rescued before you can give care. In this chapter, you will learn how to safely move victims on land and rescue victims from water without endangering or injuring yourself.

◆ Moving Victims

Usually, when you give first aid, you will not face hazards that require moving the victim immediately. In most cases, you can follow the emergency action principles (EAPs) and give care where you find the victim. Moving a victim needlessly can lead to further injury. For example, if the victim has a closed fracture of the leg, movement could result in the end of the bone tearing the skin. Soft tissue damage, damage to nerves, blood loss, and infection all could result unnecessarily.

You should move a victim *only if there is immediate danger* such as fire, lack of oxygen, risk of drowning, risk of explosion, a collapsing structure, or uncontrollable traffic hazards (see Figure 17-1 on the next page).

Before you act, consider the following limitations in order to ensure moving one or more victims quickly and safely:

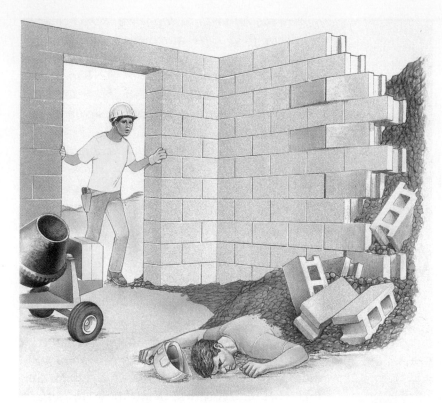

Figure 17-1 You should move a victim only if the victim is in immediate danger, such as from a collapsing structure.

- Dangerous conditions at the scene
- The size of the victim
- Your own physical ability
- Whether others can help you
- The victim's condition

Considering these limitations will help you decide how to proceed. For example, if you are injured, you may be unable to move the person and will only risk making the situation worse. If you become part of the problem, EMS personnel will now have one more person to rescue.

To protect yourself and the victim, follow these guidelines when moving a victim:

- Only attempt to move a person you are sure you can comfortably handle.
- Bend your body at the knees and hips.
- Lift with your legs, not your back.
- Walk carefully using short steps.
- When possible, move forward rather than backward.
- Always look where you are going.
- Support the victim's head and spine.
- Avoid bending or twisting a victim with possible head or spine injury.

Emergency Moves

There are many different ways to move a person to safety. But there is *no one best way.* As long as you can move a person to safety without injuring yourself or causing further injury to the victim, the move is successful. Four common types of emergency moves are the—

- Walking assist.
- Fireman's carry.
- Two-person seat carry.
- Clothes drag.

All of these emergency moves can be done by one or two people and without any equipment. This is important because, with most rescues, limited resources are available.

Walking assist

The most basic emergency move is the walking assist. Either one or two rescuers can use this method with a conscious victim. To do a walking assist, place the victim's arm across your shoulders and hold it in place with one hand. Support the victim with your other hand around the victim's waist (Fig.

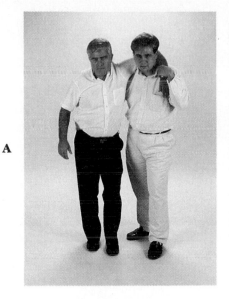

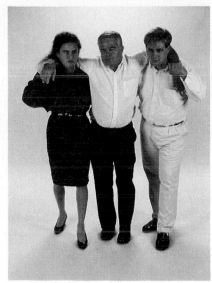

A

B

Figure 17-2   **A,** The most basic emergency move is the walking assist. **B,** A second rescuer can support the victim from the other side.

17-2, *A).* In this way, your body acts as a "crutch," supporting the victim's weight while you both walk. A second rescuer, if present, can support the victim in the same way from the other side (Fig. 17-2, *B).*

Fireman's carry

The fireman's carry is useful for quickly moving a person from a dangerous situation such as a fire. The advantage of this carry is that it leaves one of your hands free while you move the victim. This method can be used with both conscious and unconscious victims. The disadvantages are that you may need help to position the victim across your shoulders, and that the technique is not appropriate for victims of major trauma. It should not be used for a victim with suspected head, spine, or abdominal injury, since the victim's body is twisted, the head is not supported, and the victim's abdomen bears the weight.

To perform a fireman's carry, kneel down and bring the victim to a seated position facing you. Hoist the victim across your shoulders lengthwise, feet on one side, head on the other. Put your arm around the victim's legs. Grasp one of the victim's arms and stand up (Fig. 17-3).

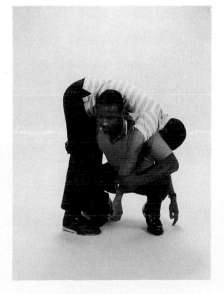

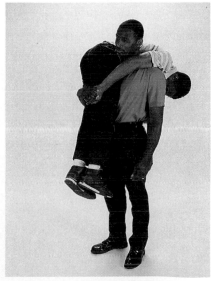

Figure 17-3   The fireman's carry is useful for quickly moving a victim from a dangerous situation.

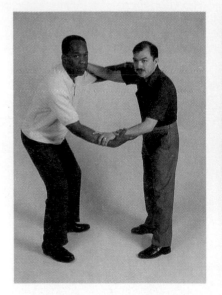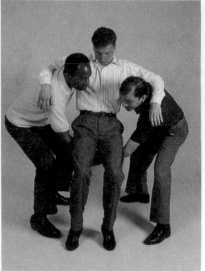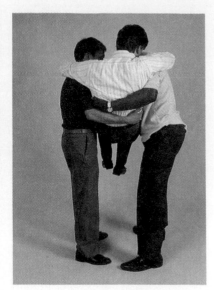

Figure 17-4 The two-person seat carry

Two-person seat carry

The two-person seat carry requires a second rescuer. Put one arm under the victim's thighs and the other across the victim's back. Interlock your arms with those of a second rescuer under the victim's legs and across the victim's back. Lift the victim in the "seat" formed by the rescuers' arms (Fig. 17-4).

Clothes drag

The clothes drag is most appropriate for moving a person suspected of having a head or spine injury. This move helps keep the head and neck stabilized. Gather the victim's clothing until tight from behind the victim's neck. Using the clothing, pull the victim to safety. During the move, the victim's head is cradled by both the clothing and the rescuer's hands (Fig. 17-5). This emergency move is exhausting and may cause back strain for the rescuer, even when done properly.

◆ Water Rescue

Drowning

Drowning is death by suffocation when sub-merged in water. Most people who are **near-drowning** cannot or do not call for help. Their energy is spent just trying to keep their head above water. In near-drowning the victim survives submersion, sometimes only temporarily. Drowning begins whenever small amounts of water are inhaled into the lungs by a person gasping for air while struggling to stay afloat. Stimulation by the water causes spasms of the muscles of the larynx (voice box), which close the airway to prevent more water from entering the lungs. As a result, the lungs of most drowning or near-drowning vic-

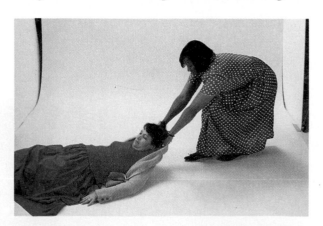

Figure 17-5 Use the clothes drag to move a person suspected of having a head or spine injury.

tims are relatively dry, unless the victims are submerged for a long time. However, the spasms that prevent water from entering the airway also prevent air from entering. The victim suffocates and soon becomes unconscious. At some point after unconsciousness, the muscles relax, the victim spontaneously breathes, and, if the victim is submerged, more water can enter the lungs.

Get to the victim as soon as possible without risking personal safety. If possible, use something that floats, such as a life jacket, ring buoy, rescue tube, boat, raft, surfboard, and so on, to aid in the rescue. Remove the victim from the water as quickly as possible. If you suspect the victim may have a head or spine injury, you must support the victim's neck and keep it aligned with the body. If it is necessary to turn the victim on his or her back, the victim's head, neck, chest, and the rest of the body must be aligned, supported, and turned as a unit.

Once the victim is out of the water, open the airway and check for breathing. Give rescue breaths if the victim is not breathing. If you cannot get air into the victim, the airway is probably obstructed. Give abdominal thrusts. Before giving thrusts, turn the victim's head to one side, unless you suspect head or spine injury. This will allow water or vomit to drain from the mouth. Once you are able to get air in, check circulation.

The pulse may be difficult to detect in a near-drowning victim. Check it for up to 1 minute. If you cannot feel a pulse, start CPR. The body needs to be on a hard, firm, horizontal surface for compressions to be effective.

Continue rescue breathing or CPR until medical help arrives. **Every near-drowning victim should be taken to a medical facility immediately for follow-up care.**

Assisting a Near-drowning Victim

You can assist a near-drowning victim in several ways. The safest methods are reaching, throwing, and wading assists. If possible, have someone call EMS personnel while you try to rescue the victim.

Do not endanger yourself. Rescues that require swimming out to a victim require special training. If you swim to a victim without this training, you put yourself in danger also and thus risk two lives. Likewise, leaping into water to help someone nearby may seem courageous. But choosing a different method is safer and usually more effective. You can help a victim only if you remain safe and in control of the situation.

Reaching assists

With a reaching assist, reach out to the victim while remaining in a safe position. First, firmly brace yourself. Extend your reach with any object that will reach the victim, such as a pole, oar or paddle, a tree branch, a shirt, a belt, or a towel (Fig. 17-6).

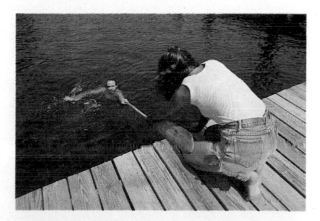

Figure 17-6 With a reaching assist, you remain safe while reaching out to the victim.

An Icy Rescue

Rescuers who pulled Michelle Funk from an icy creek near her home thought she was gone. The child's eyes stared dully ahead, her body was chilled and blue, and her heart had stopped beating. The 2½-year-old had been under the icy water for more than an hour. By all basic measurements of life, she was dead.

Years ago, Michelle's family would have prepared for her funeral. Instead, paramedics performed CPR on Michelle's still body as they rushed her to a children's medical center, where Dr. Robert G. Bolte took over care. Bolte had been reading about a rewarming technique used on adult hypothermia victims, and he thought it would work on Michelle. Surgeons sometimes intentionally cool a patient when preparing for surgery and use heart-lung machines to rewarm the patient's blood after surgery. This cooling helps keep oxygen in the blood longer. Bolte ordered Michelle to the heart-lung machine, which provided oxygen and removed carbon dioxide, in addition to warming the blood. When Michelle's temperature reached 77° F, the comatose child gasped. Soon her heart was pumping on its own.

Doctors once believed the brain could not survive more than five to seven minutes without oxygen, but miraculous survivals like Michelle's have changed opinions. Ironically, researchers have determined that freezing water actually helps to protect the body from drowning.

In icy water, a person's body temperature begins to drop almost as soon as the body hits the water. The body loses heat in water 32 times faster than it does in the air. Swallowing water accelerates this cooling. As the body's core temperature drops, the metabolic rate drops. Activity in the cells comes to almost a standstill, and they require very little oxygen. Any oxygen left in the blood is diverted from other parts of the body to the brain and heart.

This state of suspended animation allows humans to survive underwater four to five times as long as doctors once believed was possible. Nearly 20 cases of miraculous survivals have been documented in medical journals, although unsuccessful cases are rarely described. Most cases involve children who were 15 minutes or longer in water temperatures of 41° F or less.

Children survive better because their bodies cool faster than adult bodies.

Researchers once theorized that the physiological responses were caused by a "mammalian dive reflex" similar to a response found in whales and seals. They believed the same dive mechanism that allowed whales and seals to stay underwater for long periods of time was triggered in drowning humans. But experiments have failed to support the idea. Many researchers now say the best explanation for the slowdown is simply the body's response to extreme cold.

After being attached to the heart-lung machine for nearly an hour, Michelle was moved into an intensive care unit. She stayed in a coma for more than a week. She was blind for a short period, and doctors weren't sure she would recover. But slowly she began to respond. First she smiled when her parents came into the room, and soon she was talking like a 2½-year-old again. After she left the hospital, she suffered a tremor from nerve damage. But Michelle was one of the lucky ones—eventually she regained her sight, full balance, and coordination.

Although breakthroughs have saved many lives, parents still must be vigilant around their children and others near water. Most near-drowning victims are not as lucky as Michelle. One out of every three survivors suffers neurological damage. There is no replacement for close supervision.

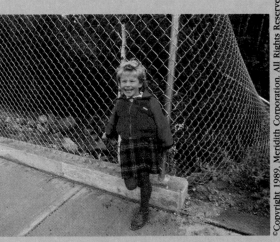

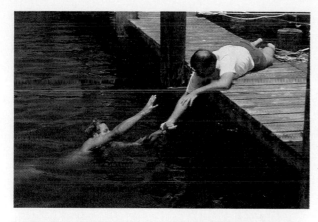

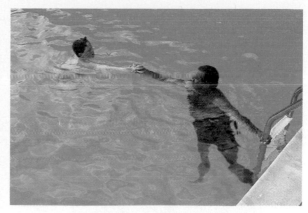

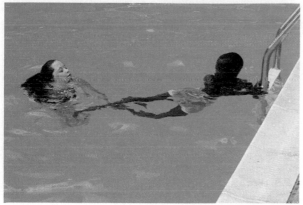

Figure 17-7 When no object is available to extend to the victim, try to extend your arm to the victim or extend your foot.

If you have no objects to extend your reach, try to extend your arm and grasp the victim, or extend your foot to the victim. To avoid going into the water, lie flat on a pool deck or pier and reach with your arm. If you are in the water, use one hand to get a firm grasp on a pool ladder, overflow trough, piling, or other secure object, and extend your free hand or one of your legs to the victim (Fig. 17-7).

Throwing assists

With a throwing assist, you throw a heaving line, ring buoy, throw bag, rescue tube, or any other device that the victim can grab to help stay afloat (Fig. 17-8). If a line is attached, you can pull the person to safety.

When throwing a device, follow these general principles:

1. Get into a safe position where you can keep your balance.
2. Step on or otherwise secure the nonthrowing end of the line (see Figure 17-9, *A*, on the next page).

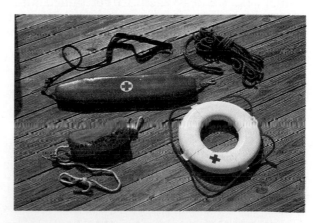

Figure 17-8 Throw any device the victim can grab to help stay afloat.

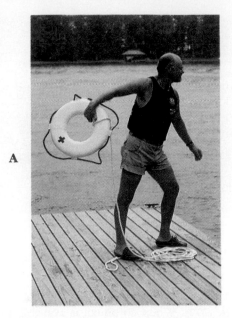

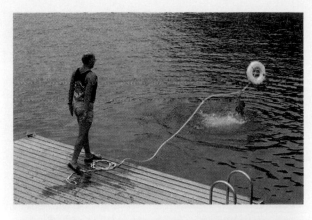

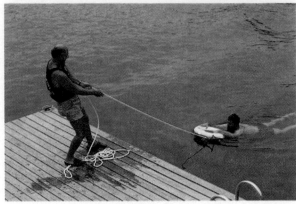

Figure 17-9 **A,** Step on or otherwise secure the nonthrowing end of the line before throwing. **B,** Try to throw the device beyond the victim. **C,** Lean your body away from the victim as you slowly pull the victim in.

3. Try to throw the device beyond the victim (Fig. 17-9, *B*).
4. Throw the device so that the wind or current will bring it back within the victim's reach.
5. Once the victim has grasped the device, slowly pull him or her to safety. Lean your body away from the victim as you pull, so that you are less likely to get pulled into the water (Fig. 17-9, *C*).
6. If there is no line on the device, tell the victim to hold on and kick to safety.

Wading assists

If you can enter the water without danger from currents, objects on the bottom, or an unexpected dropoff, wade in and reach to the victim. If possible, extend your reach using a floatable item such as a rescue tube, a ring buoy, a buoyant cushion, a raft, a kickboard, or a **personal flotation device (PFD)** such as a lifejacket. If you do not have a buoyant object,

reach out with a tree branch, a pole, or another object (Fig. 17-10).

Whatever object you have, use it for support in the water. Let the victim grasp the other side of it. You can then pull the victim to safety, or you can let go of an object that floats and tell the victim to kick with it toward safety. When you keep the safety device between you and the victim, even a panicky victim cannot grab you and pull you under.

Self-Rescue

Besides knowing the skills needed to rescue someone in trouble in the water, you should know what to do to help yourself if you suddenly get into trouble in the water.

If you unexpectedly fall into the water, you may need to remove clothing in order to swim or float. But some clothing, such as a long-sleeved shirt that buttons, will actually help you float and also help protect you from cold. If your shoes are light enough for you to

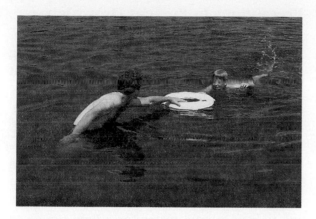 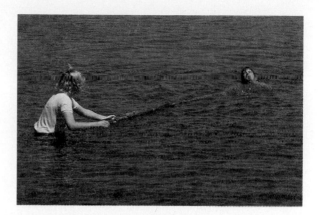

Figure 17-10 If you can enter the water without endangering yourself, wade in and reach to the victim. If possible, extend your reach with an object.

swim comfortably, leave them on. If they are too heavy, remove them.

Tread water to stay in an upright position while you signal for help or wait for rescue. You may need to tread water while you arrange your clothing for flotation. To tread water, stay vertical and submerged to your chin. Move your hands back and forth and use a kick that you can do effectively and comfortably, using the least amount of energy (Fig. 17-12).

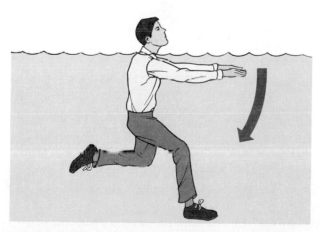

Figure 17-11 You can tread water by moving your hands back and forth and using a kick that requires little energy.

Survival swimming

There may be times when you find yourself in the water fully clothed. If this is the case, you may be able to use your clothes to your advantage. If you can trap air in the shoulders of your shirt, it may be easier to get to safety. If you need one hand to hold your shirt closed, swim with the other. To get air into your shirt, tuck your shirt in or tie the shirttail ends together. Fasten the top buttons of the shirt up to the neck. Unbutton one of the middle buttons. Take a deep breath, bend your head forward to the water, pull the shirt up to your face, and blow into the opening in the shirt. The front of the shirt must be under water. The air will rise and form a bubble in the shoulders of the shirt, which will help you float (see Figure 17-12 on the next page).

Many people can float on their backs fairly easily. To help stay afloat, gently spread your hands and arms away from your body. Then extend your fingers and hands outward, and push your hands in toward your feet. Repeat the movement. Kick only if needed.

If you find yourself in warm water, you can also use the facedown floating technique called **survival floating**. When you are facedown in the water, the lower part of your body tends to sink. Survival floating is based on this. It helps victims in warm water con-

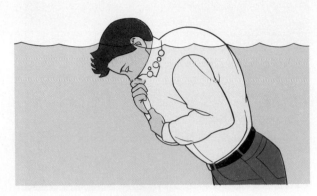

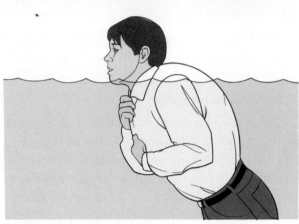

Figure 17-12 Trapping air in your shirt may make it easier for you to swim to safety.

serve their energy while they wait to be rescued. Each move you make should be slow and easy.

With your mouth above the surface of the water, breathe in, hold your breath, put your face in the water, and let your arms and legs dangle. Rest in this position for several seconds (Fig. 17-13, *A*). Then tilt your head back to raise your face above the surface but only high enough for your mouth to clear the water. As you raise your face, exhale. As your mouth clears the water, gently press down with your arms and bring your legs together (Fig. 17-13, *B*). This will help keep your mouth above the water. Take another breath and then return to the resting position. Repeat this cycle, conserving energy by repeated resting.

Precautions to Prevent Drowning

Most drowning victims never intended to enter the water. People fishing or hunting around ponds or streams, industrial workers at sites near water, or people on a boat ride may find themselves suddenly in the water (Fig. 17-14). Even shallow water can be a danger. Children have drowned around or in homes, even in the bathtub. People have drowned in wells, cisterns, and even standing rainwater.

Falling into cold water, and especially having to stay in cold water for a long time, can be particularly dangerous. Many hunters and fishermen who at first seemed to have drowned actually died from exposure to cold water.

The most important safety precaution is to

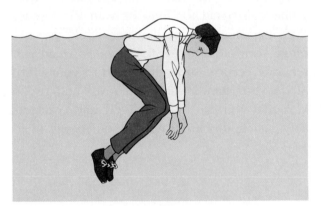

A

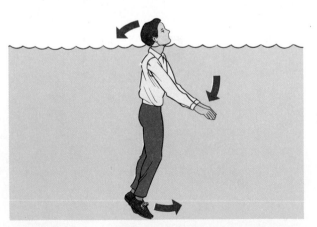

B

Figure 17-13 **A,** To do a survival float, rest in a facedown position for several seconds. **B,** To prepare to inhale, tilt your head back, press down with your arms, and bring your legs together.

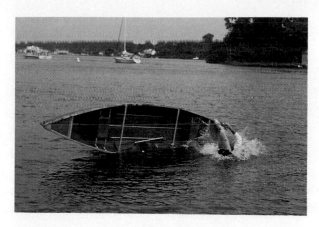

Figure 17-14 Most drowning victims never intended to enter the water.

respect the water—*always*. Water is dangerous even if you do not intend to go into it.

When you are around water, take the following precautions:

- Be aware of possible dangers. Urge companions to be careful, and set a good example yourself.
- Watch children at all times.
- Wear a Coast Guard-approved personal flotation device (PFD), or at least keep PFDs within reach to throw to someone who falls into the water.
- Stay with at least one other person whenever you are around water, and *never* swim alone, no matter how good a swimmer you are.

- Wear nonslip rubber shoes or boots on a boat or when around slippery rocks.
- When around water, do not use alcohol or other substances that impair judgment or physical ability.

◆ Summary

One of the more common mistakes citizen responders make is to move an ill or injured person unnecessarily. Remember to take the time to survey the scene for life-threatening or potentially life-threatening situations. If it is necessary to move a victim, remember the variety of emergency moves you can use. Use the safest and easiest method to rapidly move the victim without injury to either you or the victim.

In water emergencies, use the basic methods of reach, throw, or wade in order to rescue someone without endangering yourself. Only enter the water to make a rescue if you have been trained to do so. Many drownings could be prevented by following simple precautions when around water.

In the next chapter, you will learn how, by developing and maintaining a healthy lifestyle, you can do much to prevent or decrease your risks for many common illnesses and injuries that lead to death or disability.

Study Questions

1. List at least four situations in which it may be necessary to move a victim.

2. List four limitations you should consider before attempting to move a victim.

3. List four guidelines to follow when moving a victim.

4. Name four common types of emergency moves.

5. List the three safest methods of rescuing a conscious, near-drowning victim.

6. List three precautions to take around the water.

In questions 7 through 11, circle the letter of the correct answer.

7. To move the victim of a suspected head or spine injury, you would use the—

    a. Fireman's carry.
    b. Walking assist.
    c. Clothes drag.
    d. Two-person seat carry.

8. Which condition(s) is/are appropriate for a wading assist?

    a. You can reach the victim by extending a branch from the shore.
    b. You suspect or see strong currents.
    c. The bottom is clearly visible and free of objects.
    d. The ground under the water slopes gradually downward.
    e. c and d

9. You see a man struggling in the rushing waters of a flooded creek. What is the safest way for you to try to rescue him?

    a. Plunge into the water and grab him.
    b. Wade in and reach out to him with an object.
    c. From the bank, extend an object for him to reach.
    d. Yell to him to kick forcefully.

10. To safely rescue a near-drowning victim, you may—

    a. Extend an object for the victim to grab.
    b. Go immediately into the water and grab the victim.
    c. Throw a device that the victim can grab.
    d. Wade in and reach out to the victim with a floatable object.
    e. a, c, and d

11. Survival floating is appropriate to use when—

    a. You are in very cold water.
    b. You are in warm water.
    c. You can swim to safety.
    d. You are floating on your back.

12. As you come upon the scene of a car crash, you notice a downed electrical wire hanging across the damaged car. The driver is slumped over the steering wheel and appears unconscious. Several people gathered at the scene are discussing what to do and if the driver should be moved. Describe the actions you would take.

Answers are in Appendix A.

PART VII

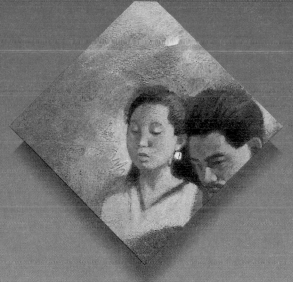

Healthy Lifestyles

18
Your Guide to a Healthier Life

Your Guide to a Healthier Life

Objectives

After reading this chapter, you should be able to—

1. Describe at least two ways you can improve your diet.

2. List at least three ways in which cardiovascular fitness helps make you healthier.

3. Identify two health hazards associated with smoking.

4. List at least three ways to help control alcohol consumption.

5. List at least four elements of a home safety plan.

6. List at least three elements of a fire escape plan.

7. List at least three things you can do to improve your safety at work.

8. Identify the best way to avoid injury in a motor vehicle crash.

9. List at least four ways you can avoid injury in sports or recreational activities.

◆ Introduction

What is a healthy lifestyle? A healthy lifestyle combines beliefs and practices to form good habits in many areas of your life, including nutrition, exercise, and safety.

By now you have learned first aid basics. You know how and why to follow the emergency action principles. You know the signals that indicate a medical emergency and what to do to help. You can give rescue breathing and CPR, first aid for choking, and care for many emergency situations including bleeding, fractures, and burns. You understand how the body systems work together. You also know something about preventing injury and illness such as cardiovascular disease.

Now you can build on this knowledge to develop a healthier lifestyle. To do this, you may have to modify some existing behavior. This may be difficult to accomplish, since behavior change often requires that you change your attitudes and beliefs. Remembering that your present and future health and well-being depend on preventing illness and injury will help you modify your attitudes and beliefs toward health practices. These changes will ultimately result in changes in behavior.

Maybe, despite all the warnings, you are still smoking. Perhaps you work out regularly but still weigh more than you would like. This chapter will give you information to help you build a healthier lifestyle at home, work, and play.

If you have not already done so, fill out the Healthy Lifestyles Awareness Inventory in Appendix D. Doing so will help you learn the areas in which you need to change or modify behaviors to make your lifestyle healthier.

◆ Caring for Your Body

If you care for your body now, you will reap great dividends in the future. How you treat your body in ordinary daily activities—eating, exercising, relaxing, working, and sleeping—can work for or against you.

Nutrition

One of the most important things you can do to care for your body is to eat a healthy diet. A healthy diet is made up of balanced meals that provide nutrients essential to body maintenance, growth, development, and repair. Many of us eat foods that tend to be too high in salt, fats, and refined sugar and too low in fiber and fluids.

Changing your eating habits need not be difficult. For a start, read the labels on the foods you buy. Try to buy products that are low in salt, saturated fat, and cholesterol. Realize that information is given per serving size and look for the number of servings per package. As you read labels, look for the trade-offs. For example, many diet products, including some diet soft drinks, trade a few calories for a lot of salt. Many products that are low-fat, low-cholesterol, and low-calorie are also high in salt.

Eating less of foods that are high in salt, fat, and cholesterol can actually help prevent some diseases. To reduce salt intake, take the salt shaker off your table. To limit fat intake, eat or drink only low-fat dairy foods and use unsaturated oils and fats for cooking and eating.

Reducing your intake of these foods is only part of healthy eating. You must also increase your consumption of foods that are good for your body. Include more fiber in your diet by eating more fruits, vegetables, and grains. Eat wisely when eating at restaurants and fast-food places.

So, what should you eat? A healthy, balanced diet includes the following every day from the four basic food groups—carbohydrates, dairy products, protein, and fruit and vegetables (see Figure 18-1 on the next page):

• At least four servings of enriched, whole-grain breads or cereals. (One serving is one slice of bread or one-half cup of starch such as rice, potatoes, or cereals.)
• Two 8-ounce servings of low-fat dairy foods such as low-fat yogurt or low-fat or skim milk.

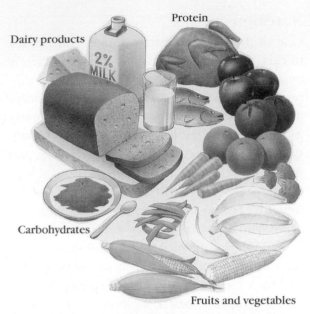

Dairy products

Protein

Carbohydrates

Fruits and vegetables

Figure 18-1 A well-balanced meal plan includes daily servings from the four basic food groups.

- Two to three servings of lean protein foods. (One serving is 2 ounces of chicken, fish, or turkey.)
- Four to five servings of fruits and vegetables. Include at least one serving of fruit high in vitamin C and one serving of a dark green, yellow, or orange vegetable every other day for vitamin A.

Drinking fluids is also crucial to your health. You should drink at least eight glasses of water each day. Try reaching for a tall glass of water sometimes instead of a soft drink.

Weight

Many adults are overweight. Some are overweight to the point of obesity. Obesity, defined as weighing 20 percent more than desirable body weight, contributes to diseases such as heart disease, high blood pressure, diabetes, and gallbladder disease. However, body weight is not the main problem. It is the presence of too much body fat that contributes to these diseases. See your physician or health care specialist for help if you want a measure of your body fat.

Losing weight, especially fat, is no easy task. Weight loss and gain depend on the balance of caloric intake and energy output. If you take in more calories than you use, you gain weight. If you use more calories than you take in, you lose weight. There are several guides to weight control. Table 18-1 provides guidelines for weight-loss strategies.

Day-to-day fluctuations in weight reflect changes in the level of fluids in your body. So, if you are watching your weight, pick one day and time per week as weigh-in time. Track your weight loss based on this weekly amount, not on day-to-day differences.

Weight loss or gain should always be combined with regular exercise—another part of a healthy lifestyle. Any activity—walking to the bus, climbing the stairs, cleaning house—uses calories. The more active you are, the more calories you use. Activity allows you to eat a few more calories and still maintain body weight.

Your eating habits should change as you grow older. A person who eats the same number of calories between the ages of 20 to 40 and maintains the same level of activity during this time will be considerably heavier at 40 than at 20. It is more important as you grow older to eat foods that provide your body with essential nutrients but are not high in calories.

Exercise

Most of us wish we had more time for exercise. Exercise is good for the heart, lungs, and blood vessels and increases muscular endurance, strength, and flexibility. If you have time for limited exercise only, it is best to build up cardiovascular fitness, the foundation for whole-body fitness.

Cardiovascular fitness can help you—

- Cope with stress.
- Deal with daily activities with more enjoyment.

Table 18-1   Weight-loss Strategies

Use some of the following strategies to help you lose weight—
* Keep a log of the times, settings, reasons, and feelings associated with your eating.
* Set realistic, long-term goals (for example, losing one pound per week instead of five pounds per week).
* Occasionally reward yourself with small amounts of food you enjoy.
* Eat slowly, and take time to enjoy the taste of the food.
* Be more physically active (take stairs instead of elevators, or park in the distant part of the parking lot).
* Reward yourself when you reach your goals (for example, with new clothes, sporting equipment).
* Share your commitment to losing weight with your family and friends who will support you.
* Keep a record of the food you eat each day.
* Weigh once a week at the same time and record your weight.
* Be prepared to deal with occasional plateaus as you lose weight.

Adapted from Payne, W.A., and Hahn, D.B: *Understanding Your Health,* ed. 2. St. Louis: Mosby—Year Book, Inc., 1989, p. 152.

* Control weight.
* Ward off infections.
* Improve self-esteem.
* Sleep better.
* Accomplish your personal fitness goals.

To achieve cardiovascular fitness, you must exercise your heart. To do this, you should exercise at least three times a week for 20 to 30 minutes and at your appropriate target heart rate (THR). Your target heart rate is 65 to 80 percent of your maximum heart rate. To find your target heart rate, subtract your age from 220, then multiply that figure by 0.65 to 0.80. For example, for a 20-year-old wanting to exercise at 65 percent of his or her maximum heart rate, the THR would be $(220 - 20) \times 0.65 = 130$ beats per minute (bpm). This means that you should get your pulse up to 130 bpm and keep it there for 20 to 30 minutes. As you exercise, take your pulse periodically at the wrist or neck (Fig. 18-2). Your exercise must be continuous and vigorous to maintain this rate. As you build cardiovascular fitness, you will eventually be able to exercise for longer periods of time and at a higher THR.

The "no pain, no gain" theory is not a good approach to exercise. In fact, experiencing pain usually means you are exercising improperly. Be sure to warm up before vigorous ex-

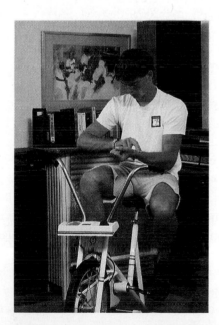

Figure 18-2   As you exercise, take your pulse periodically to see if you have reached your appropriate target heart rate.

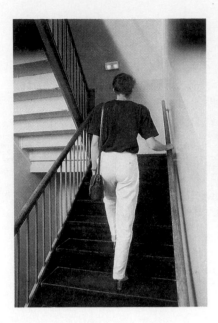
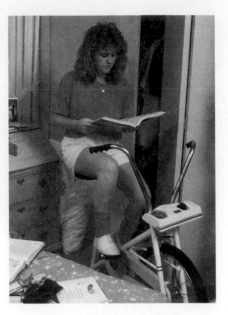

Figure 18-3 Build exercise into your daily activities.

ercise and cool down afterwards. Turn your daily activities into exercise (Fig. 18-3). Walk briskly instead of driving, whenever possible. Take the stairs instead of the elevator or the escalator. Pedal an exercise bike while watching TV, listening to music, or reading.

If you have been sedentary or have health problems, see your doctor before starting an exercise program.

Stress Control

Everyone will experience some stress throughout life. Dealing constructively with stress will help you achieve a healthy lifestyle. Reaching an immediate goal does not get rid of stress for very long. More stressful situations soon come along. After you leave school, for example, you start looking for a job. You may move and have to reorganize your life. You may get married and make many life changes. It is important to learn to manage stress early in life. People who do not learn to manage stress often develop negative habits such as smoking and overeating. Eventually, you can become dependent on habits such as these that can lead to poor health.

One of the best ways to handle stress is to develop hobbies that allow you to divert your attention to other things. For some people, this involves physical exercise. Another way is to avoid foods containing stimulants such as caffeine, found in coffee, tea, some soft drinks, chocolate, and some pain relievers. Caffeine may increase stress or make it more difficult to control. How much caffeine do you take in every day? If you decide to decrease your intake, do so gradually to avoid the headaches that can occur with withdrawal. Reducing stress by changing your lifestyle requires you to set attainable goals. If your goals are not realistic, you may never achieve them and, consequently, your level of stress may become worse.

Relaxation exercises are a form of focused meditation that help reduce stress by helping the body relax. You can do these exercises by sitting or lying quietly in a comfortable position with your eyes closed. Begin breathing in deeply through your nose and exhaling through your mouth. Focus on your breathing. Do this for about 10 minutes.

Breaking Unhealthy Habits
Smoking

During the past few decades, many people in the United States have become aware of the

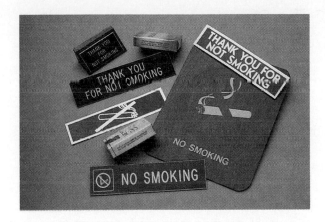

Figure 18-4 Because of the dangers of smoking, the government and many private groups have taken steps to discourage or ban smoking.

does, the agencies listed in Table 18-2 may be able to help you.

Alcohol

Alcohol is the most popular drug in Western society. About 100 million Americans drink beer, wine, or distilled spirits.

In addition to the hazardous relationship between drinking alcohol and driving, consuming alcohol in large amounts has other unhealthy effects on the body, as you read in Chapter 15.

Most people do not think social drinking is wrong. But a blood alcohol level of 0.05 per-

dangers of smoking. Smoking has been banned or restricted in many work sites around the nation, as well as on many airlines and in other public places (Fig. 18-4). Next time you are tempted to light up, consider that cigarette smoking is the single most preventable cause of heart and lung disease. There is no doubt that cigarette smoking causes most cases of lung cancer. Your risk of lung cancer starts to go down as soon as you stop. After ten years, your risk of lung cancer becomes the same as the risk for any nonsmoker.

Increased cancer rates are not the only dangers of smoking. Smoking is also a major cause of heart disease. The cigarette smoker has an increased risk of heart attack and sudden cardiac arrest over the nonsmoker. A pregnant woman who smokes harms herself and her unborn baby, chiefly because of the carbon monoxide and nicotine in cigarettes.

Users of smokeless tobacco also face serious risks. Chewing tobacco and snuff cause cancer of the mouth and tongue, so these products should also be avoided.

To stop smoking and stop using tobacco is difficult, but most ex-smokers and former users say they feel better physically and emotionally. Many programs designed to help the smoker break the habit are available. If you want to quit smoking or know someone who

---

Table 18-2 Sources of Help to Quit Smoking

American Heart Association
73720 Greenville Avenue
Dallas, TX 75231
(800) 527-6941
(214) 750-5300
Contact your local heart association

American Lung Association
GPO Box 596
New York, NY 10001
Contact your local lung association

American Cancer Society
1599 Clifton Road NE
Atlanta, GA 30329
(800) ACS-2345
(404) 320-3333

National Cancer Institute
Cancer Information Service
(800) 4-CANCER

Lungline
National Jewish Center
for Immunology
and Respiratory Medicine
1400 Jackson Street
Denver, CO 80206
(800) 222-LUNG
(303) 355-LUNG (Denver)

cent or higher impairs judgment and reflexes and makes activities like driving unsafe. How much drinking causes such a blood alcohol level? On an empty stomach, an average 160-pound person can reach this level after just two ordinary-size drinks in an hour or less—2 bottles of beer, 10 ounces of wine, or 2 drinks with 1¼ ounces of alcohol in each. Because of the time it takes for the body to process the alcohol, you should always limit yourself to one drink per hour.

Only time can make a person sober after having too much to drink. Black coffee and a cold shower may make a person feel more alert, but the body must process the alcohol over time for the impairment of judgment and coordination to pass. Therefore, any group driving to a party, for example, should always have a designated, nondrinking driver for the return trip.

Whether hosting a party or participating in one, you can act responsibly by keeping alcohol consumption under control. To do this, remember these general principles:

- Drink no more than one drink per hour.
- Have nonalcoholic beverages available.
- Do not drink before a party.
- Avoid drinking when angry or depressed.
- Eat plenty of food before and while drinking.
- Avoid salty foods—they may make you thirsty and cause you to drink more.
- Do not play drinking games.

Refer to Chapter 15 for a list of organizations that provide help and support for substance abuse problems.

Medical and Dental Care

Everyone should have regular medical, dental, and eye checkups. Preventing disease is far more effective than treating disease after it develops. With the growing costs of health care in the United States, prevention and early detection have increasingly become an important aspect of medical care. People need different types of medical examinations, depending on age, personal and family medical his-

Warning: Habits Can Be Hazardous

Sure, you need to stop smoking, or stop drinking, or stop eating, but how? Bad habits die hard. But you learned them at some point in your life, and you can unlearn them. It is never too late to try. Try these tips.

1. **Break the chain.** Be aware of how you link a negative habit to other behaviors. If you eat every time you sit down in front of the television set, separate those two behaviors. Do not eat when you watch television.
2. **Control the stimulus.** It's easier to stop drinking if you don't have a six-pack of beer in the fridge.
3. **Restructure your thinking.** Stop thinking of your morning break as a cigarette break. Try other stress reducers like taking a walk or drinking fruit juice. Have a plan of attack for times when you know you will be

tempted. For example, take gum or candy with you to work if that is where you smoke the most.

4. **Self-monitor.** Keep close track of your habit. By watching your eating, drinking, and smoking habits, you can fight temptation. As you begin to recognize when and where you are having the most difficulty breaking your habit, you will find ways to circumvent the problems yourself. For example, if you order a glass of water before lunch, your stomach will feel less empty, and you will begin to eat less.
5. **Join a self-help group.** There is safety in numbers. Sharing with a friend can help you make it past the rough spots. Self-help groups, such as Overeaters Anonymous and Weight Watchers, have proven successful for countless people.

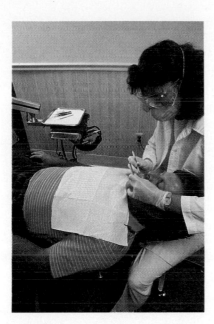

Figure 18-5 Visit your dentist twice a year for a cleaning and checkup.

tory, and other factors. Ask your physician what tests you may need and how often to have them.

See your dentist twice a year for a professional teeth cleaning and checkup (Fig. 18-5). Change your toothbrush often. Brush and floss each day to prevent periodontal (gum) disease, which destroys the soft tissue and bone that surround the teeth. This disease can strike anyone, but it becomes more serious as you age.

If you wear glasses, your eye doctor probably reminds you to get regular checkups. If you do not wear glasses, you should know that your eyesight can change anytime—making periodic checkups very important (Fig. 18-6). Glaucoma, a serious disease that can lead to blindness, can cause major damage even before you realize there is anything wrong. If you wear contact lenses, always follow the instructions for use and disinfection. Pay attention to the expiration date of your contact lens solutions, and discard them when recommended.

Protect your hearing. Beware of noise pol-

lution. Loud noise and music can contribute to hearing loss, increase your stress levels, and reduce your concentration. If others indicate that they can hear the music of your headset, it is at a level dangerous to your hearing. You should turn down the volume (see Figure 18-7 on the next page).

◆ Preventing Injuries

As you read in the introduction to the Injuries section, injuries are a major cause of death and disability in the United States. You can prevent injuries by using good safety practices. The following sections describe principles of safety for your home and motor vehicle and at work and recreation.

Fire Safety

In 1988, smoking caused 123,000 fires in the United States. Those fires killed 970 people, injured 5,800 people, and caused property loss in the United States of more than $300 million. In the United States, smokers are blamed for about 5 percent of all fires.

Fires are also caused by heating equipment, appliances, electrical wiring, cooking, and in many other ways. Regardless of the cause of fires, everyone needs to be aware of the danger fire presents and act accordingly.

Plan a fire escape route with your family.

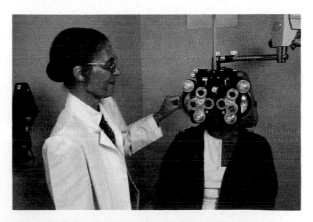

Figure 18-6 Whether you wear glasses or not, regular eye examinations are important.

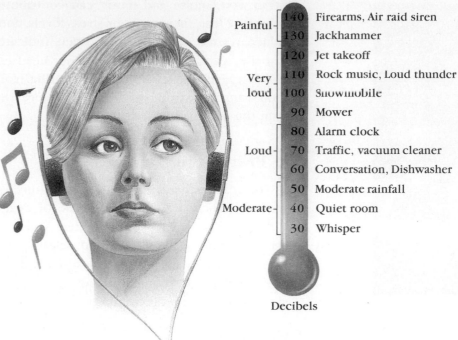

Painful	140	Firearms, Air raid siren
	130	Jackhammer
	120	Jet takeoff
Very loud	110	Rock music, Loud thunder
	100	Snowmobile
	90	Mower
	80	Alarm clock
Loud	70	Traffic, vacuum cleaner
	60	Conversation, Dishwasher
	50	Moderate rainfall
Moderate	40	Quiet room
	30	Whisper

Decibels

Figure 18-7 Beware of noise pollution; it can contribute to hearing loss.

The National Fire Protection Association urges that everyone plan and practice a fire escape plan (Fig. 18-8):

• Gather all family members and/or roommates at a convenient time. Sketch a floor plan of all rooms, including doors, windows, and hallways. Include each floor of the home.

• Plan and draw the escape plan with arrows showing two ways, if possible, to get out of each room. Sleeping areas are most important, since most fires happen at night. Plan to use stairs only, never an elevator.

• Plan where everyone will meet after leaving the building.

• Designate who should call the fire department and from which phone. Plan to leave the burning building first and then call from a phone nearby. Many, but not all, locations in the United States use 9-1-1 for the emergency number. When you travel, take a moment to find out the local emergency number.

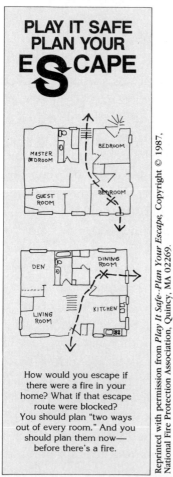

PLAY IT SAFE PLAN YOUR E S CAPE

How would you escape if there were a fire in your home? What if that escape route were blocked? You should plan "two ways out of every room." And you should plan them now—before there's a fire.

Figure 18-8 Plan a fire escape route for your home.

Practice the following guidelines for escape from fire:

- If there is smoke, crawl low to escape. Since smoke rises in a fire, breathable air is often close to the floor.
- Make sure children can open windows, go down a ladder, or lower themselves to the ground. Practice with them. Always lower children to the ground first before you go out a window.
- Get out quickly and do not, under any circumstances, return to a burning building.
- If you cannot escape, stay in the room and stuff door cracks and vents with towels, rags, or clothing. If a phone is available, call

the fire department—even if rescuers are already outside—and tell the dispatcher your location.

Contact your local fire department for additional safety guidelines. Install a smoke detector on every floor of your home. Eighty percent of homes in the United States have smoke detectors, but half do not work because of old or missing batteries, according to the International Association of Fire Chiefs. A handy way to remember the batteries is to change them twice a year when you reset your clocks for daylight saving time.

Knowing how to exit from a hotel in a fire could save your life. Locate the fire exits and extinguishers on your floor. If you hear an

---

Table 18-3 Fire Safety Tips

1. Never play with matches or lighters.
2. Keep matches and lighters away from heat sources and out of the reach of children.
3. Make sure matches and other smoking materials are completely out before throwing them away.
4. Never smoke in bed.
5. Keep basement, closets, and attic clear of rags, papers, and other materials that could catch fire.
6. Place portable heaters well away from any materials that could catch fire.
7. Turn off portable heaters when you go to bed.
8. Be sure every fireplace has a sturdy metal fire screen.
9. Leave a responsible person with your children when you go out, even for a little while.
10. Instruct babysitters on what to do in case of a fire.
11. Never leave children alone in a room with a portable heater or wood stove.
12. Have a fire escape plan with at least two ways out of every room, if possible.
13. Practice your escape plan by holding fire drills.
14. Have a battery-operated smoke detector on every level of your home.
15. Test smoke detectors regularly to ensure that they are in proper working order.
16. Have a working fire extinguisher easily accessible in your home.
17. Never leave paper, fabrics, paints, wood, or anything that could catch fire near a fireplace.
18. Never use a liquid that burns easily to start any fire, indoors or outdoors.
19. Never store gasoline or other highly flammable liquids indoors.
20. Keep handles of pots and pans on the stove turned in.
21. Remove knobs on gas stoves if there are toddlers in the house so that they cannot turn on the gas.
22. Never use appliances in wet areas.
23. If you have young children, cover electrical outlets with safety caps.
24. Do not spray aerosol cans near an open flame.
25. Do not put water on a grease fire.
26. Do not wear loose clothing when working around an open flame.

alarm while in your room, feel the door first and do not open it if it is hot (Fig. 18-9). Do not use the elevator. If the hall is relatively smoke free, use the stairs to exit. If the hall is filled with smoke, crawl to the exit. If you cannot get to the exit, return to your room. Turn off the ventilation system, stuff door cracks and vents with wet towels, and telephone the front desk or the fire department to report the fire and your location.

Safety at Home

Over 24 million injuries occur in homes each year. Removing hazards and practicing good safety habits will make your home safer (Fig. 18-10). Complete the Home Safety section of the Healthy Lifestyles Awareness Inventory to increase your awareness of home safety and help identify areas for improvements. Then

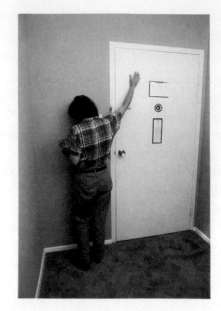

Figure 18-9   In a fire, do not open a door if it feels hot.

PREVENT ACCIDENTS AT HOME

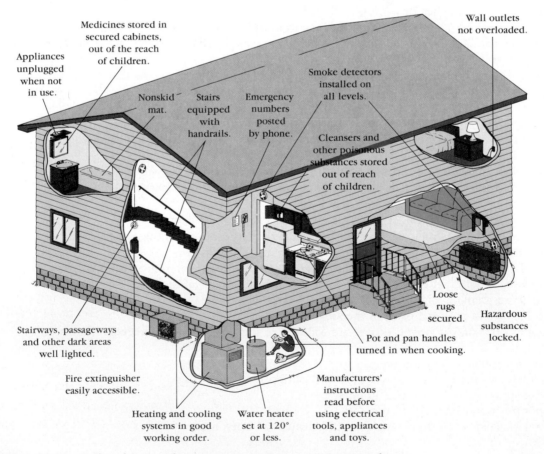

Medicines stored in secured cabinets, out of the reach of children.

Appliances unplugged when not in use.

Nonskid mat.

Stairs equipped with handrails.

Emergency numbers posted by phone.

Smoke detectors installed on all levels.

Cleansers and other poisonous substances stored out of reach of children.

Wall outlets not overloaded.

Loose rugs secured.

Hazardous substances locked.

Stairways, passageways and other dark areas well lighted.

Fire extinguisher easily accessible.

Heating and cooling systems in good working order.

Water heater set at 120° or less.

Pot and pan handles turned in when cooking.

Manufacturers' instructions read before using electrical tools, appliances and toys.

Figure 18-10   Follow home safety practices to prevent injuries at home.

make a list of needed improvements. Safety at home is relatively simple and relies largely on common sense. Taking the following steps will help to make your home a safer place:

◆ Post emergency numbers as well as other important numbers near the phone.
◆ Make sure that stairways and hallways are well-lighted.
◆ Equip stairways with handrails. If elderly people live in your home, you may need to put grab rails by the toilet and in the bathtub or showers. If small children live in your home, you need gates at the head and foot of the stairways.
◆ Keep medicines and poisonous substances separate from each other and from food. They should be out of reach of children and in secured cabinets, if possible.
◆ Keep your heating and cooling systems and all appliances in good working order. Check heating and cooling systems annually before use.
◆ Read and follow manufacturers' instructions for electrical tools, appliances, and toys.
◆ Turn off the oven and other appliances when not using them. Unplug certain appliances, such as an iron, curling iron, or portable heater, after use.
◆ Make sure your home has a working, easily accessible fire extinguisher.
◆ Keep any firearms in a locked place, out of the reach of children, and separate from ammunition.
◆ Have an emergency fire escape plan and practice it.

This list does not include all the safety measures you need to take in your home. If young children or elderly individuals live with you, you will need to take additional steps. See the *American Red Cross CPR: Infant and Child* workbook for more information on making your home safe for infants and small children. Practicing good safety habits at home lays the groundwork for establishing safety as an integral part of your life.

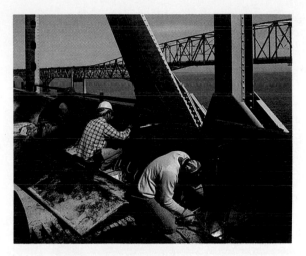

Figure 18-11 Safety clothing and/or equipment are required for some jobs.

Safety at Work

Most people spend approximately one third of their day at work. To improve safety at work, you should be aware of the following:

◆ Fire evacuation procedures
◆ Location of the nearest fire extinguisher and first aid kit

If you work in an environment where hazards exist, wear recommended safety equipment and follow safety procedures (Fig. 18-11). Both employers and employees must follow safety rules issued by the Occupational Safety and Health Administration (OSHA).

Motor Vehicle Safety

Buckle up—always. Wearing a seat belt is the easiest and best way to prevent injury in a motor vehicle collision. Infants and children should always ride in approved safety seats. All 50 states and the District of Columbia require the use of child safety seats.

Safety at Play

Make sports and other recreational activities safe by always following accepted guidelines for the activity (see Figure 18-12 on the next page).

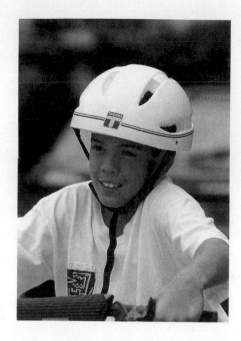

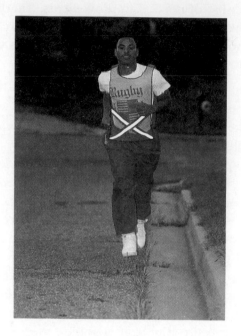

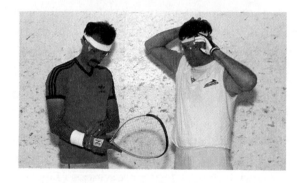

Figure 18-12 Wear proper safety equipment during recreational activities.

When bicycling, always wear an approved helmet. Children should, too, even if they are still going along the sidewalk on training wheels. Most bike mishaps happen within a mile of home. The head or neck is the most seriously injured part of the body in most fatally injured bicyclists. Look for a helmet approved by the Snell Memorial Foundation or the American National Standards Institute (ANSI). Keep off roads that are busy or have no shoulder. Wear reflective clothing and have reflectors on your bike wheels if you bicycle at night.

With any activity in which eyes could be injured, such as racquetball, wear protective goggles. Appropriate footwear is also impor-

tant in preventing injuries. For activities involving physical contact, wear properly fitted protective equipment to avoid serious injury. Above all, know and follow the rules of the sport.

If you do not know how to swim, learn how or always wear an appropriate flotation device if you are going to be in or around the water. Dangerous undercurrents can catch you even in shallow water. Be careful when walking beside rivers, lakes, and other bodies of water. Two thirds of all drownings happen to people who never intended to be in the water at all.

If you run, jog, or walk, plan your route carefully. Exercise only in well-lighted, well-populated areas. Keep off busy roads. If you must exercise outdoors at night, wear reflective clothing and move facing traffic.

Whenever you start an activity unfamiliar to you, such as boating, skiing, motorcycle riding, or any sport, take lessons to learn how to do the sport safely. Many mishaps result from inexperience. Make sure your equipment is in good working order. Ski bindings, for instance, should be professionally inspected, adjusted, and lubricated before each season. Costly, yes, but so are serious injuries.

◆ Good Health for Special Groups

Expectant Mothers

Good prenatal care begins even before your baby is conceived. Get your body in shape for pregnancy by getting down or up to your ideal weight, getting plenty of rest, and making sure you have been immunized against diseases such as rubella (German measles). Rubella can cause devastating birth defects.

Before becoming pregnant, you should stop smoking, stop drinking alcohol, and take no medications unless advised by your physician.

Did You Know. . .

. . .that the highest motor vehicle death rate is among males ages 20 to 24?

. . .that more motor vehicle deaths occur between 3:00 p.m. and midnight than during other hours?

. . .that more motor vehicle deaths occur on Saturday than on any other day?

. . .that more motor vehicle crashes occur in urban rather than rural areas but that more motor vehicle deaths occur on rural rather than urban roads?

. . .that even at a blood alcohol concentration (BAC) level as low as 0.02 percent, alcohol affects driving and crash likelihood?

. . .that the probability of a crash begins to increase significantly at 0.05 percent BAC?

. . .that crashes involving men are much more likely to be alcohol-related than those involving women?

. . .that alcohol involvement is highest in nighttime (9:00 p.m. to 6:00 a.m.) single-vehicle crashes?

. . .that, among passenger vehicle drivers fatally injured between 9:00 p.m. and 6:00 a.m., 62 percent have BACs at or above 0.10 percent?

. . .that drivers under 30 account for more than half of all drinking drivers who are fatally injured in crashes?

. . .that, per licensed driver, fatal crash rates for both males and females begin to increase at age 65?

. . .that 42 percent of all fatally injured motorcycle drivers either do not have a valid license to operate a cycle or the license has been suspended or revoked?

. . .that 57 percent of all motorcycle drivers 16 and older who are killed in single-vehicle crashes have very high BACs (0.10 or more)?

. . .that 22 percent of all motor vehicle deaths of people 65 and over involve pedestrians?

. . .that 74 percent of all motor vehicle deaths involve passenger vehicle occupants?

. . .that most serious pedestrian injuries result from striking the hood, windshield, or top of a vehicle—not from subsequent impact with the road or being run over?

. . .that 26 percent of deaths in roadside hazard crashes involve striking a tree, the most frequently struck fixed object?

. . .that 46 percent of people killed in roadside hazard crashes are 20 to 34 years old?

. . .that 82 percent of teenager motor vehicle deaths are passenger vehicle occupants?

Data from *Facts,* 1990 edition, published by the Insurance Institute for Highway Safety.

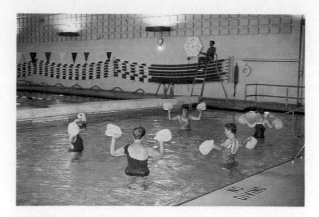

Figure 18-13 Older adults can benefit from regular physical activity.

You may be four to six weeks' pregnant by the time you know it, and these substances can be very harmful to the developing fetus.

If you learn about infant care in advance, you'll be better prepared for parenthood. Physicians, hospitals, and community organizations, such as the Red Cross, offer a variety of parenthood education classes. When you become pregnant, follow your obstetrician's or midwife's advice about nutrition, exercise, and other good health habits.

Older Adults

In the next 20 years, the United States population over age 65 will continue to increase. By the year 2040, it is estimated that older adults will comprise from 20 to 24 percent of the total population. Many of us will be assisting our parents to maintain their health.

For older adults, an active social life is a part of good health. Regular physical activity, such as daily walks, can provide both physical and psychological well-being (Fig. 18-13) Some older people have special dietary needs. Because appetite often dwindles with age, meals must be planned carefully for good nutrition.

Adults over 40 need medical checkups at least once a year. Taking too many medications can be a problem, so patients or their family members should often ask the doctor to review medications. Adults over 65 should also receive annual flu and tetanus immunizations.

Falls are the leading cause of injuries among older adults. Safety measures, such as good lighting, sturdy railings on staircases, and non-slip floors and rugs, can help ensure footing.

♦ Summary

Throughout this course, you have learned information and skills to cope with emergencies and save lives. In this chapter, you learned why and how to adopt a healthier lifestyle. Changing risky behaviors now can help prevent illness and injury later. Changing habits or acquiring new, healthier habits now will help you live a better, longer life. Kicking unhealthy habits does not happen overnight, but becoming aware of them is an important first step.

Study Questions

1. Describe two things you can do to improve your diet.

2. List three healthy ways to handle stress.

3. List two health dangers caused by the use of tobacco.

4. List three ways a person can keep alcohol consumption under control.

5. List three elements of a fire escape plan.

6. List two things you should know to help ensure your safety at work.

7. List four ways to prevent injuries during sports and recreational activities.

8. List four ways you can turn daily activities into exercise.

9. Calculate your target heart rate.

10. Identify the most important action you can take to avoid injury in a motor vehicle crash.

11. List activities you can do to improve cardiovascular fitness.

In questions 12 and 13, circle the letter of the correct answer.

12. Cardiovascular fitness increases muscular endurance, strength, and flexibility. It may also help you—

    a. Sleep better.
    b. Ward off infections.
    c. Cope with stress.
    d. a and c
    e. a, b, and c

13. Which of the following helps a person sober up after having too much to drink?

    a. Hot coffee
    b. A cold shower
    c. Time
    d. a and b
    e. a, b, and c

14. List four things you can do to improve safety in your home.

15. Write a healthy meal plan for one day. Include breakfast, lunch, and dinner. Use actual foods, for example, "one slice of wheat toast," and use foods you like to eat.

Answers are in Appendix A.

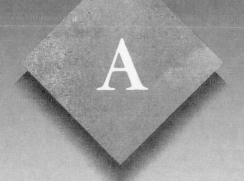

APPENDIX

A

Study Question Answers

CHAPTER 1

1. b, c, f, d, a
2. (1) Citizen responder (2) EMS dispatcher (3) First Responder (4) EMT-paramedic (5) Hospital care providers (6) Definitive care
3. Recognize that an emergency exists; decide to act; call EMS professionals; provide first aid
4. **Unusual noises**—breaking glass; screeching tires; moaning; calling for help; screaming; abrupt or loud unidentifiable noises; **unusual odors**—strong smell of gasoline, chlorine, smoke, unidentifiable fumes; **unusual appearance or behavior**—collapsed person; confused behavior; breathing difficulty; slurred, hesitant, confused speech; uncharacteristic skin color; sweating for no apparent reason; **unusual sights**—stalled vehicle; overturned pot; spilled medicine container; downed electrical wires
5. Presence of bystanders; uncertainty about the victim; nature of the injury or illness; fear of disease transmission; fear of doing something wrong
6. Call for an ambulance; watch for and meet ambulance; keep area free of unnecessary traffic; get blankets or other supplies; provide information about incident or victim; help comfort victim and others

7. Keep important information about yourself and your family in a handy place. Find out and post local emergency numbers in a handy place. Keep medical and insurance records up to date. Keep a first aid kit stocked and easily accessible in your home, work, and recreation areas. Learn and stay practiced in first aid skills. Make sure your house or apartment number is easy to read. Develop a plan of action for emergencies that may occur, such as a fire, flood, and tornado. Wear a medical alert tag if you have a potentially serious medical condition.
8. g, h, a, b, c, e, f, d
9. Screech of tires, crash of metal; car smashed into pole; pole at odd angle; wires hanging from pole; vehicle stalled in middle of the street
10. The EMS dispatcher may not have received the call until later because no one decided to act by calling 9-1-1 or the local emergency number, or because no one could get out of the traffic to call. The EMS dispatcher may have had a number of calls all coming in at the same time and been unable to dispatch the appropriate help. The EMS dispatcher may not have been given the correct location of the emergency. The ambulance may have become stuck in traffic on the way to the

crash because onlookers abandoned their vehicles. Once on the scene, emergency medical technicians may have evaluated a need for advanced medical help. Victims may have been trapped in vehicles, requiring extensive work to pry apart the wreckage.

CHAPTER 2

1. (a) respiratory (b) airway, lungs (c) circulatory (d) transports oxygen and other nutrients to cells and removes waste (e) skin, hair, nails (f) helps keep fluid in, prevents infection, sweat glands and pores in skin help regulate temperature, helps make vitamin D, stores minerals (g) bones, ligaments, muscles, tendons (h) supports body, allows movement, protects internal organs and structures, produces blood cells, stores minerals, produces heat (i) nervous (j) brain, spinal cord, nerves

2. o, d, l, m, g, c, k, i, a, e, h , f, j, b, n

3. d　　　　4. a　　　　5. b　　　　6. d

7. Any damage to the spinal cord or a nerve could interrupt or completely cut off the conduction of impulses to an area of the body. No nerve impulses would reach the area—it would be paralyzed.

CHAPTER 3

1. b, a, d, b, d, d, c, a, b, a, b, a

2. Survey the scene. Do a primary survey and care for life-threatening conditions. Call EMS personnel for help. Do a secondary survey, when appropriate, and care for other injuries or conditions that may need care.

3. (1) Is the scene safe? (2) What happened? (3) How many victims are there? (4) Are there bystanders who can help?

4. Tell him or her who you are; your level of training; what it is you would like to do.

5. Your exact location; telephone number from which the call is being made; caller's name; what happened; number of people involved; condition of victim(s); help that is being given

6. Unconsciousness, altered level of consciousness; breathing problems; persistent chest or abdominal pain or pressure; no pulse; severe bleeding; vomiting blood or passing blood; poisoning; seizures; severe headache or slurred speech; injuries to head, neck, and back; possible broken bones

7. Have someone else come with you. Be sure you know the quickest route to the hospital. Closely monitor the victim's condition.

8. Unconsciousness; open airway; loss of breathing; loss of heartbeat (no pulse); severe bleeding

9. Do a secondary survey only when no life-threatening conditions exist. In a secondary survey, you look for other injuries or conditions that may need care.

10. (a) 4, (b) 5, (c) 1, (d) 6, (e) 2, (f) 3

11. d　　　　12. c　　　　13. b　　　　14. c

15. b　　　　16. a　　　　17. d

18. Because a motor vehicle is involved, ask if anyone has called EMS personnel. If not, ask someone to do so. Then follow the emergency action principles. Survey the scene. Traffic may be dangerous to you or others. Ask questions. Find out details such as what happened and how many people were involved. If you determine that it is safe to approach, do so. Once at the victim's side, begin a primary survey. Find out if the victim is conscious, breathing, has a pulse, or is bleeding severely. While you begin appropriate care, instruct other bystanders to redirect traffic, watch for the ambulance, keep onlookers from crowding in, get any materials you need, and help you provide care, if necessary.

CHAPTER 4

1. b, f, a, g, h, e, d, c

2. Gasping for air; shortness of breath; breathing faster or slower than normal; making unusual noises such as wheezing, crowing, or gurgling; unusually deep or shallow breathing; unusually moist skin; flushed, pale, or bluish skin; dizziness or lightheadedness; pain in the chest; tingling in the hands or feet; apprehensiveness or fear

3. Trying to swallow large pieces of poorly chewed food; drinking alcohol before or during meals; wearing dentures; eating while talking excitedly or laughing, or eating too fast; walking, playing, or running with food or objects in the mouth

4. c, a, b

5. e　　　　6. a　　　　7. d　　　　8. d

9. c　　　　10. b　　　　11. e　　　　12. a

13. a　　　　14. b　　　　15. b　　　　16. c

17. 2, 3, 1, 4

18. 4, 2, 3, 1, 5

CHAPTER 5

1. e, c, g, i, d, b, h, a, f

2. There is no pulse.

3. Another trained rescuer arrives and takes over. EMS personnel arrive and take over. You are too exhausted to continue. The scene suddenly becomes unsafe.

4. Smoking; diets high in fat; high blood pressure; obesity; lack of routine exercise

5. c   **6.** d   **7.** d   **8.** b
9. e   **10.** b   **11.** c   **12.** b
13. Persistent chest pain associated with shoulder pain; perspiring heavily; breathing fast; looking ill
14. 2, 3, 1, 4, 5
15. d

CHAPTER 6

1. c, g, a, f, e, h, d, b, i
2. Transports oxygen, nutrients, and wastes; protects against disease by producing antibodies and defending against germs; maintains constant body temperature by circulating throughout the body
3. Blood spurting from a wound; blood that fails to clot after all measures have been taken to control bleeding
4. Apply direct pressure using your hand. If a sterile gauze pad or other clean material is available, place it between the wound and your hand. Elevate the injured area if possible. Maintain pressure by applying a pressure bandage. If these measures fail to stop the bleeding, apply pressure to a pressure point to slow the flow of blood to the area.
5. Discoloration of the skin in the injured area; soft tissues, such as those in the abdomen, that are tender, swollen, or hard; anxiety or restlessness; rapid, weak pulse; rapid breathing; cool, moist skin or pale or bluish skin; nausea and vomiting; excessive thirst; declining level of consciousness
6. Apply ice or a cold pack to the injured area. Be sure to place a cloth or another barrier between the source of cold and the skin to prevent damage to the skin.
7. b, d, c, a
8. 3, 1, 4, 2
9. A person who is close by could call EMS personnel, find materials for bandaging, reassure your father, watch for the ambulance, and get other materials, such as a blanket, that you might need to help maintain your father's body temperature.
10. a
11. Place an effective barrier between yourself and the victim's blood. Wash your hands thoroughly with soap and water after providing care. Avoid eating, drinking, and touching your mouth, nose, or eyes while providing care or before washing your hands.

CHAPTER 7

1. b, c, a
2. Restlessness; fast breathing; drowsiness; pale, cold, moist skin; rapid, weak pulse; unconsciousness; irregular breathing

3. Medical emergencies: sudden illnesses and severe injuries
4. Monitor ABCs. Care for any life-threatening problems. Help the victim rest comfortably. Help the victim maintain normal body temperature. Reassure the victim. Provide care for specific conditions.
5. c   **6.** b   **7.** d   **8.** e
9. b
10. Shock is life-threatening because the circulatory system fails to circulate oxygen-rich blood to all parts of the body, causing vital organs to fail to function properly.
11. Elevating the legs helps to maintain blood flow to the vital organs.

CHAPTER 8

1. b, f, a, e, c, d
2. b, d, a, c
3. a, c, d, b
4. Swelling or reddening around the wound; area around the wound may feel warm or throb with pain; wound may have a pus discharge; victim may develop a fever and feel ill; red streaks may develop that progress from the wound in the direction of the heart
5. Hold dressings in place. Apply pressure to control bleeding. Protect a wound from dirt and infection. Provide support to the injured part.
6. **Abrasion**—a rubbing or scraping away of the skin such as occurs when you skin your knee; **laceration**—usually a cut from a sharp object, such as when you cut yourself with a knife, but can result from a blunt force splitting the skin such as the chin striking the ground; **avulsion**—a complete or partial tearing away of a portion of the skin and sometimes other soft tissues or of an entire body part; **puncture**—piercing of the skin by a pointed object or a bullet
7. Heat, chemicals, electricity, and radiation
8. Superficial, partial-thickness, full-thickness
9. e   **10.** d   **11.** e   **12.** d
13. d   **14.** d   **15.** b   **16.** b
17. c   **18.** a   **19.** e   **20.** b
21. c   **22.** e   **23.** c

CHAPTER 9

1. h, b, f, c, a, i, k, d, j, g, e
2. Swelling; pain; discoloration of the skin; deformity; inability to use affected part normally
3. Splint only if you can do it without causing more pain and discomfort to the victim. Splint an injury in the position you find it. Splint the injured area and the joint above and below the injury site.

Check for proper circulation before and after splinting.

4. Anatomic, soft, rigid

5. d   6. d   7. b   8. e

CHAPTER 10

1. b, a, c, e, d

2. A fall from a height greater than the victim's height; any diving mishap; a person found unconscious for unknown reasons; any injury involving severe blunt force to the head or trunk; any injury that penetrates the head or trunk; a motor vehicle crash involving a driver or passengers not wearing safety belts; any person thrown from a motor vehicle; any injury in which a victim's helmet is broken; lightning strike

3. Changes in the level of consciousness; severe pain or pressure in the head, neck, or back; tingling or loss of sensation in the extremities; partial or complete loss of movement of any body part; unusual bumps or depressions on the head or spine; blood or other fluids in the ears or nose; profuse external bleeding of the head, neck, or back; seizures; impaired breathing or vision as a result of injury; nausea or vomiting; persistent headache; loss of balance; bruising of the head, especially around the eyes and behind the ears

4. Wearing seat belts including shoulder restraints; wearing approved helmets, eyewear, faceguards, and mouthguards, when appropriate; preventing falls; obeying rules in sports and recreational activities; avoiding inappropriate use of drugs; inspecting work and recreational equipment; thinking and talking about safety

5. Place the victim on his or her back. Do not attempt to remove any object impaled in the eye. Place a sterile dressing around the object. Stabilize any impaled object in place as best you can. You can use a paper cup to support the object. Close and cover the unaffected eye to keep blood, fluid, or dirt from entering it.

6. b   7. e   8. d   9. a

10. a   11. b   12. d   13. e

14. Do not put direct pressure on the wound. Apply direct pressure around the area of the wound to help control bleeding. Call EMS personnel if you have not already done so.

15. You know the victim is breathing and has a pulse. If you are able to check consciousness, check for severe bleeding, and find no life-threatening conditions, leave the victim as he is. Send someone to call EMS personnel or call yourself. With the victim still lying on his side, stabilize his head

and neck using in-line stabilization. If the victim's head is severely angled to one side, he complains of pain, pressure, or muscle spasms on initial movement of the head, or you feel resistance when trying to align the head, support the head in the position in which you found it. Maintain an open airway. Monitor the ABCs, control any external bleeding. Maintain normal body temperature.

CHAPTER 11

1. c, a, b, e, d

2. Call EMS personnel. Monitor ABCs. Control bleeding. Minimize shock. Limit movement.

3. Difficulty breathing; severe pain at the injury site; flushed, pale, or bluish discoloration of the skin; obvious deformity; coughing up blood

4. Shallow breathing; pain in the injured area; holding the injured area

5. A sucking sound coming from the wound with each breath

6. Severe pain, bruising; external bleeding; nausea; vomiting (sometimes vomit containing blood); weakness; thirst; pain, tenderness, or a tight feeling in the abdomen; organs possibly protruding from the abdomen; with a pelvic injury, possible loss of sensation in legs or inability to move them

7. e

8. Difficulty breathing; sucking sound when victim breathes

9. Help him rest in a comfortable position. Minimize shock. Cover the wound with a dressing that does not allow air to pass through, such as plastic wrap. Call EMS personnel. Monitor ABCs.

CHAPTER 12

1. c, e, b, d, a

2. Falling on the hand of an outstretched arm

3. Pain; tenderness; swelling; discoloration; deformity; inability to use the limb; severe external bleeding

4. Injured leg appears noticeably shorter than the other leg; injured leg is turned outward; severe pain; inability to move the leg

5. Control bleeding, rest, apply ice, elevate the injured part. If you suspect a serious injury, immobilize the injured area and minimize shock. Call EMS personnel if necessary.

6. d   7. e   8. e

9. Control bleeding. Have someone call EMS personnel. Immobilize the leg, using the ground for a splint if this is possible. Monitor ABCs. Minimize shock. Apply ice or a cold pack.

CHAPTER 13

1. f, c, h, g, e, a, d, b
2. Changes in levels of consciousness; nausea; vomiting; dizziness, lightheadedness, and weakness; changes in breathing, pulse, and skin color
3. Do no further harm. Monitor ABCs. Notify EMS personnel when necessary. Help the victim rest comfortably. Minimize shock by maintaining normal body temperature. Provide reassurance. Provide any specific care needed.
4. When the seizure lasts more than a few minutes; when the victim has repeated seizures; when the victim appears to be injured; when you are uncertain about the cause of the seizure; when the victim is pregnant; when the victim is a known diabetic; when the victim is an infant or child; when the seizure takes place in water; when the victim fails to regain consciousness after the seizure
5. High blood pressure; cigarette smoking; diets high in saturated fats and cholesterol; lack of regular exercise
6. e   7. a   8. c   9. a
10. b   11. e   12. d
13. Do a secondary survey to see if the person was injured during the seizure. Provide any care necessary. Reassure and comfort the victim. Ask bystanders to move away and give the victim room. Stay with the victim until he or she is fully conscious and aware of the surroundings.

CHAPTER 14

1. f, e, b, g, c, a, h, d
2. Nausea; vomiting; diarrhea; chest or abdominal pain; breathing difficulty; sweating; loss of consciousness; seizures
3. The type of substance; the amount of substance; how it entered the body; the victim's size, weight, and age
4. Grasp the tick with fine-tipped tweezers, as close to the skin as possible and pull slowly, steadily, and firmly. Once the tick is removed, wash the area immediately with soap and water. Apply an antiseptic or antibiotic ointment. Look for signals of infection. If the tick or its mouthparts stay in your skin, obtain medical care. If a rash or flu-like symptoms develop, seek medical help.
5. Wear long-sleeved shirts and long pants. Tuck pant legs into socks or boots; tuck shirt into pants. Wear light-colored clothing. Use a rubber band or tape the area where pants and socks meet so nothing can get under clothing. Stay in the middle of trails and avoid underbrush and tall grass. Wear hiking boots. Avoid areas populated with snakes. If you see a snake, look for others. Walk back on the same path. Inspect carefully for insects or ticks after being outdoors. If you are outdoors for a long time, check yourself several times during the day, especially in hairy areas of the body. Spray pets that go outdoors with repellent and check them for ticks often. Use a repellent if you are in a grassy or wooded area or if the area is infested with insects or ticks.
6. Keep all repellents out of the reach of children. Never spray permethrin on your skin or a child's skin. Never use repellents on children's hands. Use repellents sparingly. Wash repellent-treated skin after coming indoors. If you suspect you are having a reaction to a repellent, wash treated skin immediately and call your physician.
7. (1) Wash the wound. (2) Immobilize the affected part. (3) Keep the affected area lower than the heart if possible. (4) Call EMS professionals. (5) If possible, carry a victim who must be transported, or have him or her walk slowly. (6) If the victim cannot get professional medical care within 30 minutes, consider suctioning the wound using a snakebite kit.
8. For contact with a poisonous plant, wash the area thoroughly with soap and water. If a rash or weeping lesion has begun to develop, apply a solution of baking soda and water to the area several times a day. Use lotions to soothe the area. If the condition worsens, seek medical care. For a spilled chemical on the skin, flush the affected area continuously with large amounts of water. Call the EMS system immediately. Continue to flush the area until EMS personnel arrive.
9. Keep medications and household products out of the reach of children and in secured cabinets. Use childproof safety caps on containers of medications and other poisonous products. Keep products in original containers with labels in place. Use poison symbols to identify poisonous products. Dispose of outdated products. Use potentially dangerous chemicals only in well-ventilated areas. Wear proper clothing for work or recreation that may put you in contact with a poisonous substance.
10. c   11. c   12. e   13. d
14. c   15. d   16. a
17. The area around the sting site becomes red or swollen. Your friend feels nauseated, dizzy, or weak; or vomits; or experiences breathing difficulty.

CHAPTER 15

1. f, c, d, e, a, h, b, g

2. Difficulty breathing; chest pain; altered level of consciousness; moist or flushed skin; mood changes; nausea; vomiting; sweating, chills, fever; headache; dizziness; rapid pulse; rapid breathing; restlessness; excitement; irritability; talkativeness; hallucinations; confusion; slurred speech; poor coordination; trembling

3. Alcohol; nicotine; caffeine; aspirin; laxatives; sleeping pills; diet pills

4. Use common sense. Keep prescriptions in their appropriate containers. Clearly label all medications including when, how, and how often they should be taken. Throw out leftover prescriptions. Never take another person's prescription or even one prescribed for you at a previous time.

5. Survey the scene to be sure it is safe. Do a primary survey and care for any life-threatening conditions. Call the local Poison Control Center or your local emergency number. Question the victim or bystanders. Find out what substance was taken, how much was taken, and when it was taken. Help maintain normal body temperature. Withdraw if the victim suddenly becomes violent or threatening. If you suspect someone has used a designer drug, tell EMS personnel.

6. b, c, a, d

7. c   **8.** e

9. Containers; drug paraphernalia; signals of other medical problems

CHAPTER 16

1. c, e, d, a, b

2. Air temperature; humidity; wind; clothing; how often you take breaks from activity; how much and how often you drink fluids; intensity of activity; health status

3. Heat cramps; heat exhaustion; heat stroke

4. Changes in body temperature; changes in skin temperature, color, and moisture; headache; nausea; dizziness and weakness; exhaustion; progressive loss of consciousness; rapid, weak pulse; rapid, shallow breathing

5. Refusing water; vomiting; changes in level of consciousness

6. Move the victim away from the heat source. Have the victim rest in a cool place and drink cool water slowly. Loosen tight clothing. Remove clothing soaked with perspiration. Apply wet towels or sheets to the victim's body. Fan the victim. Apply ice and cold packs to the wrists, ankles, armpits, neck, and groin.

7. Frostbite; hypothermia

8. Avoid being outdoors in the hottest or coldest part of the day. Change your activity level according to the temperature. Take frequent breaks. Dress appropriately. Drink large amount of fluids

9. d   **10.** e

11. Pale; sweating heavily; feeling weak, nauseated, dizzy

12. You could have worn lightweight clothing that allowed the air to pass through and a hat; have taken frequent breaks; and have drunk water often.

13. She could have you rest comfortably and give you cool water to drink slowly.

14. White, waxy, cold fingers that lack feeling

15. Handle the affected areas gently. *Do not rub.* Warm the areas gently by soaking them in water no warmer than 100° to 105° F. Test the water. If it is uncomfortable to the touch, it is too warm. *Do not* let the affected areas touch the bottom or sides of the container. When the affected areas look red and feel warm, bandage them with a dry, sterile dressing, and seek professional medical attention.

16. Decreased level of consciousness; glassy eyes; possible numbness in the arm

17. Call the local emergency number. Then look for additional blankets, hot water bottles, and heating pads, and place any available source of heat on the victim after checking for any wet clothing or blankets.

CHAPTER 17

1. Move a victim only if there is immediate danger such as a fire, lack of oxygen, risk of drowning, risk of explosion, collapsing structure, or uncontrollable traffic hazards.

2. Dangerous conditions at the scene; size of the victim; your physical ability; whether others can help you; the victim's condition

3. Only attempt to move a person you are sure you can comfortably handle. Bend at the knees and hips. Lift with your legs not your back. Walk carefully using short steps. When possible, move forward rather than backward. Always look where you are going. Support the victim's head and spine. Avoid bending or twisting a victim with possible head or spine injury.

4. Walking assist; fireman's carry; two-person seat carry; clothes drag

5. Reaching assist; throwing assist; wading assist

6. Be aware of possible dangers. Watch children at

all times. Wear a Coast Guard-approved personal flotation device (PFD). Keep PFDs within reach, or stay with as least one other person whenever you are around water. Never swim alone. Wear nonslip rubber shoes or boots on a boat or when around slippery rocks. Do not use alcohol or other substances that impair judgment or physical ability.

7. c **8.** e **9.** c **10.** e
11. b
12. With a downed electrical wire hanging over the car, you should not attempt a rescue of any sort. Explain to bystanders that the wire may have an electric current running through it and not to get near the car or the wire. Tell the occupants of the car to stay in it. Call your local emergency number and explain the situation. They will send the proper authorities.

CHAPTER 18

1. Buy and eat products that are low in saturated fat and cholesterol. Use unsaturated oils and fats for cooking and eating. Eat less salt by removing the salt shaker from the table and adding less salt when cooking. Include more fiber in your diet by eating more fruits, vegetables, and grains.

2. Exercise regularly. Develop hobbies. Avoid foods containing stimulants such as caffeine. Do relaxation exercises. Set realistic, attainable goals.

3. Lung cancer and cardiovascular (heart) disease

4. Limit your drinks to one per hour. Have nonalcoholic beverages available. Do not drink before a party. Avoid drinking when angry or depressed.

Eat plenty of food before and while drinking. Avoid salty foods. Do not play drinking games.

5. Develop and draw an escape plan with two exits from each room if possible. Plan where everyone will meet after leaving the building. Designate who should call the fire department and from which phone outside the burning building.

6. Know the fire evacuation procedure and the location of the nearest fire extinguisher and first aid kit. Wear recommended safety gear and follow safety procedures.

7. Know and follow rules recommended for the activity. Wear appropriate protective gear. Wear reflective clothing, when appropriate. Make sure your equipment is in good working order. Take lessons and learn how to participate safely in a new activity. Compete at a skill level appropriate for your skills and physical condition.

8. Walk or bike instead of driving. Take the stairs instead of elevators or escalators. Pedal an exercise bike while watching TV, listening to music, or reading.

9. Subtract your age from 220. Multiply the answer by 0.65 to 0.80. The answer is your target heart rate.

10. Wear a seat belt.

11. For example, walk; jog; run; bike; swim; hike; cross-country ski

12. e **13.** c

14. Refer to the list on page 377 and to the Home Safety section in the Healthy Lifestyles Awareness Inventory.

B

First Aid and Disease Transmission

◆ Introduction

A disease that can be passed, or transmitted, from one person to another is called a communicable, or infectious, disease. Many diseases can be passed from one person to another, some more easily than others. It is natural to have concerns about disease transmission if you have to provide care in an emergency situation. As you read in Chapter 1, those concerns have increased over the past few years as a result of the high level of public awareness of AIDS. This appendix presents basic information about how infections occur and the potential for disease transmission during first aid care. It also explains how you can

protect yourself and others against disease transmission while giving first aid care.

◆ How Infections Occur

Infection is a condition caused by disease-producing microorganisms. When the body is invaded by these microorganisms, the disease process begins. Most infections are caused by bacteria and viruses.

Bacteria are one-celled microorganisms present throughout our environment. Bacteria do not depend on another organism for life and can live outside the body. Relatively few bacteria infect humans, but those that do can cause serious disease, such as tetanus. It is difficult for the body to fight a bacterial infection. Physicians may prescribe antibiotics that either kill the bacteria or weaken them enough that the body can overcome their effects.

Unlike bacteria, viruses are dependent on another organism to live. Once in the body, they are difficult to eliminate because few medications are effective in fighting viral infections. The body's immune system is the primary defense against them. Viruses cause many diseases, including the common cold.

◆ How Diseases Can be Transmitted During First Aid Care

Your body has a natural defense system that protects it against disease—the skin and the immune system. However, in situations that require first aid care, communicable diseases can be transmitted by—

- Contact (touching).
- Breathing.
- Bites.

Contact

Contact transmission occurs when one touches an infected person or a contaminated object. Microorganisms in a person's blood and other body fluids can enter another person's body through breaks or cuts in his or her skin or through the membranes of the eyes or mouth, causing infection. Direct contact with blood or other body fluids carries the greatest risk of infection. Infections transmitted by blood are referred to as blood-borne infections.

Infection can also be transmitted by contact with objects that have been contaminated with the blood or other body fluids of an infected person. Even though your intact skin protects you from diseases transmitted by contact, sharp objects handled carelessly can pierce your skin and transmit infection to you.

Therefore, be extremely careful when handling potentially contaminated objects and avoid touching blood with your bare hand unless absolutely necessary.

Breathing

Infections transmitted through air are called airborne infections. You can become infected if you breathe in droplets that become airborne when someone who has an infection, such a cold or flu, sneezes. You are at no greater risk of such an infection when giving first aid than when associating with family, friends, or colleagues, or when in public places.

Bites

An animal, such as a dog or raccoon, or an insect, such as a tick, can transmit disease through a bite. Rabies and Lyme disease are transmitted in this way. A human bite can also transmit disease. Providing first aid care rarely involves danger of being bitten by an animal or a person. Therefore, in an emergency situation, contracting a disease through a bite is equally rare.

◆ Specific Communicable Diseases

Some communicable diseases, such as the common cold, are more easily transmitted than others. Although it does cause minor discomfort for the sufferer, the common cold is short-lived and rarely has serious consequences. Other diseases, such as hepatitis B and HIV infection, are far more dangerous. Hepatitis B is a serious liver disease that can last for months. A person infected with HIV (human immunodeficiency virus), who eventually develops AIDS (acquired immune deficiency syndrome), can become a victim of many infections that have fatal consequences.

However, these serious diseases are not easily transmitted. They are not spread through casual contact. For instance, the principal ways people become infected with HIV include sexual contact—through semen or vaginal fluid; blood-to-blood contact—through sharing needles or syringes with an infected person; and mother-to-child contact—before, during, or just after birth, or, rarely, through breast milk. The virus does not live in a dry environment for more than a few hours and is killed by alcohol, chlorine bleach, and other common disinfectants. Once it is killed, you cannot reactivate the virus by adding water.

The risk of infection by HIV through any other means is extremely low. In a first aid situation in which the rescuer comes into contact with a person's blood, he or she would be at higher risk of infection with other diseases, such as hepatitis, than with HIV.

You may be concerned about disease transmission via saliva if you have to give rescue breathing. Saliva is not known to transmit HIV. There is only a theoretical risk of infection with HIV from saliva.

If you are in a situation in which you might frequently be called upon to give first aid that might require rescue breathing, you should consider taking a more advanced CPR course that will train you in the use of a resuscitation mask. Using a resuscitation mask allows you to give rescue breathing without making mouth-to-mouth contact.

◆ How to Reduce the Risk of Infection

Remember that you are most likely to give first aid to yourself or someone you know, such as a family member, whose health status you are probably aware of. One of the easiest steps you can take to prevent infection while giving first aid is to maintain good personal hygiene practices such as handwashing before and immediately after giving care.

In addition, since germs can enter the body through breaks in the skin, you should always try to take precautions to prevent direct contact with a person's body fluids when giving first aid.

To reduce the risk of infection while you are giving care, you should do the following:

◆ Avoid touching or being splashed by body fluids when possible.

◆ Place an effective barrier between you and the victim's body fluids. For example, if you have to control bleeding, ask the victim to help you by applying direct pressure, or place a dressing or other clean, dry cloth between your hand and the wound. Examples of other barriers are a piece of plastic wrap or disposable gloves.

◆ Cover any cuts, scrapes, or skin conditions you may have by wearing protective clothing such as disposable gloves.

◆ Wash your hands thoroughly with soap and water immediately after providing care, even if you wore gloves. Use a utility or rest room sink, not one in a food preparation area.

◆ Avoid eating; drinking; and touching your mouth, nose, or eyes while providing care or before washing your hands.

◆ Avoid touching objects that may be contaminated with blood or other body fluids.

◆ Avoid handling any personal items, such as pens and combs, while providing care or before washing your hands.

◆ Be prepared with an adequately stocked first aid kit that includes waterless antiseptic hand cleaners and disposable gloves.

The precautions listed above are part of widely accepted practices. If you take appropriate safety measures, risk of infection is minimal. Always give first aid care in ways that protect you and the victim from disease transmission. Use protective barriers that are appropriate to the emergency, and wash thoroughly as soon as possible after giving care.

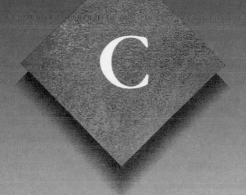

Good Samaritan Laws

◆ What Every Citizen Should Know About the Good Samaritan Laws

Helping at the scene of an emergency often raises questions about one's personal liability. So that people are not discouraged from responding to emergencies, most states and the District of Columbia have enacted laws to protect those who respond. These laws are popularly known as Good Samaritan laws, based on the parable of the man who, during a journey, aided a stranger on the side of the road. This appendix provides essential information about Good Samaritan laws. As someone who is prepared to assist injured or ill victims, you should understand how your state laws protect you when you provide emergency care.

What Are Good Samaritan laws?

Good Samaritan laws are state laws enacted to give legal protection to citizens and medical professionals who act in good faith to provide emergency assistance to ill or injured persons at the scene of an emergency.

What Do These Laws Mean?

Each state's laws are worded differently. However, in general, the protection of the Good Samaritan laws applies to situations in which an individual provides care although under no legal obligation or duty to do so. When citizens like you respond to an emergency and act as a reasonable and prudent rescuer would under the same or similar conditions, Good Samaritan immunity generally prevails. This legal immunity protects you, as a rescuer, from being sued and found financially responsible for the victim's injury. For instance, a reasonable and prudent rescuer would—

- Move a victim only if the victim's life was endangered.
- Check the victim's airway, breathing, and circulation before providing further care.
- Summon professional help to the scene by calling the local emergency number or the operator.
- Continue to care for any life-threatening conditions until EMS personnel arrive.
- Ask a conscious victim for permission before giving care.

Good Samaritan laws were enacted to encourage people to help victims whose lives may be endangered. They require only that the "Good Samaritan" use common sense and a reasonable level of skill, not to exceed the scope of the individual's training, in emergency situations. The "Good Samaritan" is not expected to perform miracles or endanger his or her own life in order to provide care. Good Samaritan immunity is not in any way dependent on the outcome—whether the victim lives or dies. It is expected that each person would do his or her best under the circumstances to save a life or prevent further injury or harm.

Citizens are rarely sued for assisting at an emergency scene. However, the existence of Good Samaritan laws does not mean that you cannot be sued. These laws do not provide blanket protection from liability. In rare instances, courts have ruled that these laws do not apply in cases when an individual rescuer's response was grossly or willfully negligent or reckless, or in which the rescuer abandoned the victim after initiating care.

How Can You Find Out About Your State Laws?

If you are concerned about protection under your state's laws, find out what your state's laws say. Consult a legal professional, or ask a librarian to help you in finding the laws and appropriate material referencing them at your library.

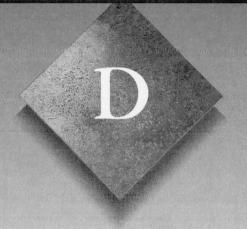

Healthy Lifestyles Awareness Inventory

A healthy lifestyle is a combination of positive beliefs and practices. How healthy is your lifestyle? What do your habits say about the life you lead? Complete the following inventory and see how your habits add up. Mark the response that best describes your behavior. Total your points after each survey. Add these subtotals and check your score with the corresponding feedback at the end of each section. The feedback provides a broad interpretation of how your behavior relates to a healthy lifestyle. Record your subtotals and totals on the scorecard on page 407.

◆ Caring for Your Body

	Always (3)	Often (2)	Rarely (1)	Never (−1)	N/A (0)
Part I: Nutrition					
1. I eat a balanced diet.	☐	☐	☒	☐	☐
2. I limit my intake of saturated fats and cholesterol.	☐	☒	☒	☐	☐
3. I limit my intake of salt.	☒	☐	☐	☐	☐
4. I bake, broil, or grill foods rather than frying them.	☐	☒	☐	☐	☐
5. I eat fruits, vegetables, and low-fat yogurts when snacking rather than "junk" food.	☒	☒	☐	☐	☐
6. I read labels for information about the nutritional quality of food.	☐	☒	☐	☐	☐
7. I maintain an appropriate weight.	☐	☐	☐	☐	☒
8. If I need to lose weight, I avoid fad, starvation, or miracle diets that are harmful to my health.	☒	☐	☐	☐	☐

Part I Subtotal: 14

	Always (3)	Often (2)	Rarely (1)	Never (−1)	N/A (0)
Part II: Exercise					
9. I participate in continuous, vigorous physical activity for 20 to 30 minutes or more at least three times per week.	☐	☐	☒	☐	☐
10. I follow an exercise program appropriate for my level of fitness.	☐	☒	☒	☐	☐
11. I warm up properly before vigorous activity and cool down afterwards.	☐	☒	☐	☐	☐
12. I use exercise equipment properly and safely.	☒	☐	☐	☐	☐
13. I swim only when others are present.	☐	☐	☒	☐	☐

	Always (3)	Often (2)	Rarely (1)	Never (−1)	N/A (0)
14. I wear highly visible clothing when exercising outdoors such as walking, running, or biking.	☐	☒	☒	☐	☐

Part II Subtotal: 9

Part III: Managing Stress

	Always (3)	Often (2)	Rarely (1)	Never (−1)	N/A (0)
15. I schedule my day to allow time for leisure activity.	☐	☐	☒	☐	☐
16. I get an adequate amount of sleep.	☐	☐	☒	☐	☐
17. I express feelings of anger or worry openly and constructively.	☒	☐	☐	☐	☐
18. I say "no" without feeling guilty.	☐	☒	☐	☐	☐
19. I make decisions with a minimum of stress and worry.	☐	☒	☐	☐	☐
20. I set realistic goals for myself.	☐	☒	☐	☐	☐
21. I accept responsibility for my actions.	☒	☐	☐	☐	☐
22. I seek professional help when stress becomes too difficult to manage.	☐	☐	☐	☐	☒
23. I allow myself to cry.	☒	☐	☐	☐	☐
24. I manage stress so that it does not affect my physical well-being.	☐	☒	☐	☐	☐
25. I discuss problems with friends or relatives.	☒	☐	☐	☐	☐

Part III Subtotal: 22

Part IV: Work

	Always (3)	Often (2)	Rarely (1)	Never (−1)	N/A (0)
26. Work is a place I like to go.	☐	☒	☐	☐	☐
27. I like my supervisors and working companions.	☐	☒	☐	☐	☐
28. I take advantage of learning opportunities at work.	☒	☐	☐	☐	☐

	Always (3)	Often (2)	Rarely (1)	Never (−1)	N/A (0)
29. I take advantage of opportunities for advancement at work.	☒	☐	☐	☐	☐
30. I am satisfied with my balance of work and leisure time.	☐	☐	☒	☒	☐
31. I take all my annual vacation in a given year.	☒	☐	☐	☐	☒

Part IV Subtotal: [11]

Part V: Tobacco, Alcohol, and Other Substances

	Always (3)	Often (2)	Rarely (1)	Never (−1)	N/A (0)
32. I avoid smoking cigarettes, cigars, pipes, or using other forms of tobacco, such as chewing tobacco or snuff.	☐	☒	☐	☐	☐
33. I try to avoid inhaling the smoke of others.	☐	☒	☐	☐	☐
34. I avoid using illegal substances, such as marijuana, uppers, and crack.	☒	☐	☐	☐	☐
35. I drink fewer than five alcoholic beverages per week.	☒	☒	☐	☐	☐
36. I avoid driving a car or other motor vehicle or operating a boat while under the influence of alcohol or other substances that impair judgment or reactions.	☒	☐	☐	☐	☐
37. I avoid riding in cars, in other motor vehicles, or in boats with people under the influence of alcohol or other substances that impair judgment or reactions.	☒	☐	☐	☐	☐
38. If necessary, I avoid using alcoholic beverages or other substances while taking prescription or over-the-counter medications.	☒	☐	☐	☐	☐
39. I keep all doctors informed of medications I am taking to avoid harmfully combining medications.	☒	☐	☐	☐	☐

	Always (3)	Often (2)	Rarely (1)	Never (−1)	N/A (0)
40. When taking prescription medication, I follow my doctor's instructions.	☐	☒	☐	☐	☐
41. When taking over-the-counter medications, I follow the instructions on the label.	☒	☐	☐	☐	☐

Part V Subtotal: ☐ 26 ☐

Part VI: Medical Care

	Always (3)	Often (2)	Rarely (1)	Never (−1)	N/A (0)
42. I seek appropriate care or cut back on activities, as necessary, when I feel unwell or tired.	☐	☐	☒	☐	☐
43. I maintain an accurate, written, current personal health history.	☐	☐	☒	☐	☐
44. I brush my teeth at least twice a day.	☒	☒	☐	☐	☐
45. I floss my teeth at least once a day.	☐	☐	☒	☐	☐
46. I ask questions of health care providers.	☒	☐	☐	☐	☐
47. I use a sunscreen with ultraviolet (UV) protection when spending time in the sun.	☐	☒	☐	☐	☐
48. I wear sunglasses with UV protection when out in the sun.	☐	☒	☐	☐	☐
49. I use adequate measures to protect myself and my partner(s) from sexually transmitted diseases.	☒	☐	☐	☐	☐
50. I practice good personal hygiene by bathing daily and washing my hands frequently	☒	☐	☐	☐	☐
51. I have regular medical checkups.	☒	☐	☐	☐	☐
52. I have regular dental checkups.	☒	☐	☐	☐	☐

	Always (3)	Often (2)	Rarely (1)	Never (−1)	N/A (0)
53. I have regular eye examinations.	☒	☐	☐	☐	☐
54. I routinely examine my testicles/breasts for the presence of masses or other unusual signals.	☐	☒	☐	☐	☐
55. I maintain adequate health insurance coverage.	☒	☐	☐	☐	☐

Part VI Subtotal: [33]

Add subtotals I to VI
to determine your total score.

Total: **CARING FOR YOUR BODY**   [   ]

Caring for Your Body: Feedback

>110 = At the top! You are taking *great* care of your body! Keep up the good work. Take note of the behaviors for which you scored 1 or less and make them regular habits in your life.

92 to 110 = On your way! You are taking adequate care of your body but need some improvement. Check your answers and note the behaviors with a score of 2 or less. To perform at your maximum potential and minimize the risks of illnesses that may develop later in life, make these behaviors a more frequent part of your life.

55 to 91 = On the edge! You are at risk. Although you may be taking moderate care of your body, it needs attention now! To learn to take proper care of your body, refer to Chapter 18. Any behaviors for which you scored 2 or less need improvement. Incorporating them into your daily life will enable you to perform at your maximum potential and minimize the risks of illnesses that may develop later in life.

<55 = You are at risk! Sooner or later, your body will begin to show and feel signs of neglect. Perhaps you are unaware of how to care for your body. Chapter 18 details how you can change your habits and take better care of yourself. If you are unsure about how to get started, consult a professional health care provider. To perform at your maximum potential and minimize the risks of illnesses that may develop later in life, you must start caring for your body now. Your goal is to change habits in order to improve the quality of your daily life.

If you scored low in this section, remember that there are many ways to change how you care for your body. Each of the areas addressed in this part of the inventory has an impact on your health. Changes you make in one area frequently will be beneficial in another area. See Chapter 18 for more information on improving your lifestyle.

Proper nutrition combined with exercise and adequate rest and relaxation will help keep your body in peak form. This will enable your body to respond and react most efficiently to demands placed on it. Eating a balanced diet also helps prevent disease.

Exercise helps you relieve stress, increases your cardiovascular efficiency, and helps you maintain your desired weight. All of these benefits serve to lower your risks of cardiovascular disease, high blood pressure, and stroke. Consult your physician if you have any questions or concerns about nutrition or exercise. You may also refer to Chapters 5 and 18 for help.

Do not forget relaxation! It is an important part of a healthy lifestyle. Try to manage stress. Prioritizing daily activities, making time for yourself each day, and exercising are three ways to help do so.

If you scored low in the Work section, remember that every job has its ups and downs. It may be necessary to evaluate your situation. Make a list of problems and possible solutions. By taking advantage of opportunities at work, you may be able to move into a job role that is more satisfying. This is important, since most adults spend at least eight hours a day at work. Career counselors are one source of help available to you.

If you scored low in the tobacco, alcohol, and other substances section, you need to think seriously about the consequences of your actions. For example, when you choose to drink and drive, your actions affect other people. The same is true of smoking or using other substances. Give serious consideration to the outcomes of these behaviors. Not only are these actions detrimental to your health, they are potentially dangerous for others also. For more information, refer to Chapters 15 and 18. Chapter 15 includes a list of sources you can turn to for help. Other sources are listed in the telephone directory.

If you scored low in the Medical Care section, remember that preventing disease is much more effective and less expensive in the long run than treating it. Look at the items scored 2 or less and make a commitment to correct them. Taking care of yourself now is the first step toward preventing disease in the future. See Chapter 18 for more information.

◆ Occupant and Recreational Safety

	Always (3)	Often (2)	Rarely (1)	Never (−1)	N/A (0)
Part VII: Occupant Safety					
56. I wear a safety belt when driving or riding in a motor vehicle.	☐	☒	☐	☐	☐
57. I obey traffic laws.	☒	☐	☐	☐	☐
58. I honor pedestrian cross-walks.	☒	☐	☐	☐	☐

	Always (3)	Often (2)	Rarely (1)	Never (−1)	N/A (0)
59. I drive anticipating the errors of others.	☒	☐	☐	☐	☐
60. I wear a helmet when I operate or ride on an open motor vehicle such as a motorcycle or all-terrain vehicle (ATV).	☐	☐	☐	☐	☒
61. When going out, if I anticipate alcohol will be consumed, I make sure there is a designated driver.	☒	☐	☐	☐	☐
62. I ride only with a driver who is not under the influence of alcohol or other substances that impair judgment or reactions.	☒	☐	☐	☐	☐
63. I use turn indicators when turning or changing lanes.	☐	☒	☐	☐	☐
64. When driving, I try to leave adequate room between my car and the car in front of me.	☒	☐	☐	☐	☐
65. I obey traffic laws when cycling.	☐	☒	☐	☐	☐
66. I keep my vehicle in good working order and have it inspected regularly.	☐	☒	☐	☐	☐

18   9

Part VII Subtotal: 26

Part VIII: Recreational Safety

	Always (3)	Often (2)	Rarely (1)	Never (−1)	N/A (0)
67. I keep recreational equipment in good working condition.	☐	☐	☐	☐	☒
68. I wear a helmet when cycling or skateboarding.	☐	☐	☐	☒	☒
69. I wear protective equipment to prevent injury when participating in certain recreational activities.	☒	☐	☐	☐	☐
70. I wear goggles when participating in sports such as racquetball, squash, or handball.	☒	☐	☐	☐	☐

	Always (3)	Often (2)	Rarely (1)	Never (−1)	N/A (0)
71. I wear a lifejacket (Personal Flotation Device—PFD) when participating in water activities such as boating, fishing, and waterskiing.	☐	☐	☑	☐	☐
72. I know and follow the rules that govern my recreational activity.	☑	☑	☐	☐	☐
73. I participate in recreational activities at a level appropriate to my skills.	☑	☑	☐	☐	☐
74. I avoid swimming or diving after consuming alcoholic beverages or other substances that impair judgment or reactions.	☑	☐	☐	☐	☐
75. I enter the water "feet first first time" to check unknown water depths and conditions before diving.	☑	☐	☐	☐	☐
76. I make sure lifejackets (PFDs) are worn by everyone on the boat.	☐	☐	☐	☐	☑
	12	4	1	−1	

Part VIII Subtotal: 16

Add subtotals VII and VIII to determine your total score.

Total: OCCUPANT AND RECREATIONAL SAFETY 42

Occupant and Recreational Safety: Feedback

>**42** = Good job! You are actively tuned in to dangers on the road and at play. Pay attention to those behaviors for which you scored 2 or less. Turn these behaviors into healthy habits.

35 to 42 = Close, but no prize! You can benefit by paying more attention to safety on the road and at play. Focus on those behaviors for which you scored 2 or less. Decrease your chances of injury by making these behaviors a part of your healthy lifestyle.

21 to 34 = Who needs trouble? While you do pay attention to a few safety aspects on the road and at play, your current habits invite trouble. Safety procedures were designed to protect you. Improve any behaviors for which you scored 2 or less.

<21 = You are an accident waiting to happen! Pay attention to all behaviors with a score of 2 or less and read Chapter 18. It will help you incorporate these areas in your lifestyle. You are not invincible; act now.

If you scored low, you are putting yourself and those around you at unnecessary risk. Take measures now to correct those items scored 2 or less. Be sure to read the sidebar on page 379. Your local Department of Motor Vehicles or Public Safety and your insurance company should also be able to provide you with information about occupant safety.

If you scored low in the Recreational Safety section, remember that injury-prevention measures taken now can affect the rest of your life. In a split-second, an innocent mistake like not wearing the appropriate safety gear or not following the rules can result in an injury that causes a lifelong disability. See Chapters 10 and 18 for more information about injury prevention. Consult your activity's rulebook for rules to follow during participation. Ask a coach or reputable sporting goods dealer, or contact the organization that regulates your activity to find out about recommended protective gear, equipment, and conditioning exercises.

◆ Home and Work Safety

	True (2)	False (−1)	N/A (0)
Part IX: Home Safety			
77. I post the local emergency number(s) near my telephone(s).	☒	☐	☐
78. I routinely maintain battery-operated smoke detectors where I live.	☒	☐	☐
79. The stairs where I live are equipped with handrails.	☐	☐	☒
80. All passageways where I live, including staircases, are adequately lighted.	☒	☐	☐
81. I keep all medicines safely and securely stored out of the reach of children.	☒	☐	☐
82. I make sure that all medicines are secured with childproof packaging and caps securely in place.	☒	☐	☐
83. I keep cleansers and other poisonous material safely and securely stored, out of the reach of children, and separate from medicines and foods.	☒	☐	☐
84. The heating and cooling systems where I live are kept in good working order.	☒	☐	☐
85. I read the manufacturer's instructions for tools and electrically operated appliances before operating.	☒	☐	☐

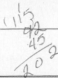

	True (2)	False (−1)	N/A (0)
86. I follow the manufacturer's instructions for safe operation of space heaters.	☐	☐	☑
87. When pots and pans are on the stove, I keep their handles turned in.	☑	☐	☐
88. I turn off the oven and other appliances after use.	☑	☐	☐
89. I keep irons and other heating appliances unplugged when I am not using them.	☑	☐	☐
90. I keep a working fire extinguisher where I live.	☑	☐	☐
91. I have an emergency plan in the event of injury, sudden illness, or natural disaster such as fire, flood, tornado, hurricane, and earthquake.	☑	☐	☐
92. I practice these plans with my family/roommates.	☑	☐	☐
93. I store firearms unloaded, in a locked place, out of the reach of children.	☐	☐	☑
94. I store firearms in a separate place from ammunition.	☐	☐	☑
95. When lifting objects, I use proper lifting techniques.	☑	☐	☐
96. To obtain high, out-of-reach objects, I use a sturdy stool or stepladder.	☑	☐	☐

Part IX Subtotal: ☐ 32

Part X: Work Safety

	True (2)	False (−1)	N/A (0)
97. I follow safety procedures at work.	☑	☐	☐
98. I know fire evacuation procedures at work.	☑	☐	☐
99. I know the location of the nearest fire extinguisher at work.	☑	☐	☐
100. I can quickly obtain first aid supplies at work if necessary.	☑	☑	☐
101. I know the location of the nurse's office or the emergency response team at work.	☐	☐	☑
102. I am aware of safety hazards that exist at work.	☑	☐	☐
103. I wear recommended safety equipment at work, such as protective shoes, hard hats, gloves, and goggles.	☑	☐	☐
104. When lifting objects, I use proper lifting techniques.	☑	☐	☐

	True (2)	False (−1)	N/A (0)
105. To obtain high, out-of-reach objects, I use a sturdy stool or stepladder.	☑	☐	☐

Part X Subtotal: ⟨13⟩

In parts IX and X, if you marked more than three responses N/A, give yourself 1 point for each N/A.

Add subtotals IX and X to determine your total score.

Total: HOME AND WORK SAFETY ⟨45⟩

Home and Work Safety: Feedback

>**28** = Two thumbs up! By following recommended safety practices, it looks as if you have made your home and work safe places to be. A safe home environment can prevent many mishaps. However, do not be lax. Change any behaviors with a score of less than 2 and try to anticipate the unexpected.

13 to 28 = It is a beginning! You have taken your first steps toward making your home and work environments a safe place. Give behaviors for which you scored less than 2 serious consideration. Then make changes! See Chapter 18 for details.

<**13** = You may be playing with fire, literally! Get started! Safety practices at home and work are important to your well-being. Read Chapter 18 and see how you can make your home and workplace safer. Then make changes to correct any behaviors with a score of less than 2. Your life and the lives of others may depend on it!

If you scored low in the Home Safety section, you have already identified areas for improvement. Refer to Chapter 18 for more tips on making your home a safe place. Practicing home safety is injury prevention at home. If you have questions about making your home safer, ask your instructor for a list of reliable sources of information and help.

If you scored low in the Work Safety section, you need to learn how to make work a safer place. See Chapter 18 for more information. Your supervisor may also be able to provide helpful information. Most important, if your company has recommended safety practices—follow them!

SCORE CARD I

Healthy Lifestyles Awareness Inventory

CARING FOR YOUR BODY

Part I: Nutrition

Part II: Exercise

Part III: Managing Stress

Part IV: Work

Part V: Alcohol, Tobacco, and Other Drugs

Part VI: Medical Care

Subtotal:

OCCUPANT AND RECREATIONAL SAFETY

Part VII: Occupant Safety

Part VIII: Recreational Safety

Subtotal:

HOME AND WORK SAFETY

Part IX: Home Safety

Part X: Work Safety

Subtotal:

TOTAL SCORE:

SCORE CARD II

Healthy Lifestyles Awareness Inventory

CARING FOR YOUR BODY

Part I: Nutrition ☐

Part II: Exercise ☐

Part III: Managing Stress ☐

Part IV: Work ☐

Part V: Alcohol, Tobacco, and Other Drugs ☐

Part VI: Medical Care ☐

Subtotal: ▨

OCCUPANT AND RECREATIONAL SAFETY

Part VII: Occupant Safety ☐

Part VIII: Recreational Safety ☐

Subtotal: ▨

HOME AND WORK SAFETY

Part IX: Home Safety ☐

Part X: Work Safety ☐

Subtotal: ▨

TOTAL SCORE: ▨

Glossary

Pronunciation Guide

The accented syllable in a word is shown in capital letters.

river=RIV er

An unmarked vowel that ends a syllable or comprises a syllable has a long sound.

silent=SI lent

A long vowel in a syllable ending in a consonant is marked ‾ .

snowflake=SNO flāk

An unmarked vowel in a syllable that ends with a consonant has a short sound.

sister=SIS ter

A short vowel that comprises a syllable is marked ˘ .

decimal=DES ĭ mal

The sound of the letter **a** *in an unaccented syllable is spelled* **ah**.

ahead=ah HED

Abdomen The middle part of the trunk, containing organs such as the stomach, liver, and spleen.

Abrasion (ah BRA zhun) A wound characterized by skin that has been scraped or rubbed away.

Absorbed poison A poison that enters the body through the skin.

Addiction The compulsive need to use a substance; stopping use would cause the user to suffer mental, physical, and emotional distress.

Airway The pathway for air from the mouth and nose to the lungs.

Airway obstruction A blockage of the airway that prevents air from reaching a person's lungs.

Allergy An abnormally sensitive reaction to a substance.

Alveoli (al VE o li) Tiny air sacs in the lungs where gases and waste are exchanged between the lungs and the blood.

Amnesia (am NE zhe ah) A loss of memory often caused by a concussion or other head injury.

Anaphylaxis (an ah fī LAX sis) A severe allergic reaction; also called anaphylactic shock.

Angina (an JI nah) **pectoris** (pek TO ris) Chest pain that comes and goes at different times;

commonly associated with cardiovascular disease.

Angulated (ANG gu la ted) - Sharply bent.

Antibiotic (an tǐ bi OT ik) A substance used to block the growth of certain microorganisms or kill them.

Antibody (AN tǐ bod e) A disease-fighting protein that helps protect the body against specific infections.

Antidote A remedy for counteracting the effects of a poison.

Antiseptic A substance that blocks or slows the growth of certain microorganisms but does not kill them.

Antivenin A material used to counteract the poisonous effects of snake or insect venom.

Arm The entire upper extremity from the shoulder to the hand.

Arteries (AR ter ez) The large blood vessels that carry oxygen-rich blood from the heart to all parts of the body.

Arthritis (ar THRI tis) An inflamed condition of the joints, causing pain and swelling and sometimes limiting motion.

Aspiration (as pǐ RA shun) Taking blood, vomit, saliva, or other foreign material into the lungs.

Asthma (AZ mah) A condition that narrows the air passages and makes breathing difficult.

Atherosclerosis (ath er o sklě RO sis) A form of cardiovascular disease marked by a narrowing of the arteries in the heart and other parts of the body.

Aura An unusual sensation or feeling a victim may experience before an epileptic seizure; may be a visual hallucination; a strange sound, taste, or smell; an urgent need to get to safety.

Automatic external defibrilator (de FIB rǐ la tor) **(AED)** A device used to monitor heart rhythms and administer an electric shock to cardiac arrest victims in an attempt to restore proper heart rhythm.

Avulsion (ah VUL shun) A wound in which a portion of the skin and sometimes other soft tissue is partially or completely torn away.

Bacteria (bak TE re ah) Microorganisms capable of causing infection.

Bandage Material used to wrap or cover a part of the body; commonly used to hold a dressing or splint in place.

Bile A yellow-green secretion of the liver that is stored in the gallbladder and released to help the body digest and absorb fat.

Bladder An organ in the pelvis in which urine is stored until released.

Blood clot A coagulated mass formed by the clotting of blood.

Blood pressure The pressure of the blood on the artery walls.

Blood volume The total amount of blood circulating within the body.

Bone A dense, hard tissue that forms the skeleton.

Booster shot A smaller dose of a vaccine given to help maintain the antibodies produced as a result of an initial immunization.

Brain The center of the nervous system that controls all body functions.

Breathing emergency An emergency in which breathing is so impaired that life is threatened.

Bronchi (BRONG ke) Air passages that lead from the trachea to the lungs.

Burn An injury to the skin or other body tissues caused by heat, chemicals, electricity, or radiation.

Capillaries (KAP ǐ ler ēz) Tiny blood vessels between the arteries and veins that transfer oxygen and other nutrients to all body cells.

Carbon dioxide A colorless, odorless gas that is a waste product of respiration.

Cardiac (KAR de ak) **arrest** A condition in which the heart has stopped or beats too weakly or too irregularly to pump blood effectively.

Cardiopulmonary (kar de o PUL mo ner e) **resuscitation** (re sus ǐ TA shun) (CPR) The technique that combines rescue breathing and chest compressions for a victim whose breathing and heart have stopped.

Cardiovascular (kar de o VAS ku lar) **disease** A disease of the heart and blood vessels; commonly known as heart disease.

Carotid (kah ROT id) **arteries** The major blood vessels that supply blood to the head and neck.

Cells The basic units of all living tissue.

Chest The upper part of the trunk, containing the heart, major blood vessels, and lungs.

Choking Blockage of the airway by food, fluids, or other foreign objects.

Cholesterol (ko LES ter ol) A fatty substance made by the body and found in certain foods. Too much cholesterol in the blood can cause fatty deposits on artery walls that may restrict or block blood flow.

Circulatory (SER ku lah tor e) Relating to the movement of blood through the heart and blood vessels.

Citizen responder A layperson who recognizes an emergency and decides to help.

Clavicle (KLAV i kl) See collarbone.

Closed wound A wound in which soft tissue damage occurs beneath the skin's surface and the skin is not broken.

Clotting A process by which blood thickens at a wound site to seal an opening in a blood vessel to stop blood loss.

Collarbone A horizontal bone that connects with the sternum and the shoulder; also called the clavicle.

Concussion (kon KUSH un) A temporary impairment of brain function, usually without permanent damage to the brain.

Consent Permission to provide care, given by the victim to the rescuer.

Contusion (kon TOO zhun) A closed wound caused by force to the body; also called a bruise.

Coronary (KOR o ner e) arteries The blood vessels that supply the heart muscle with oxygen-rich blood.

Corrosive Having the power or tendency to destroy or eat away, sometimes through chemical action.

Cravat A triangular bandage folded to form a long, narrow strip.

Critical burn Any burn that is potentially life-threatening, disabling, or disfiguring; a burn requiring medical attention.

Cyanosis (si ah NO sis) A blue discoloration of the skin and membranes of the mouth and eyes, resulting from a lack of oxygen in the blood.

Deformity A change in shape from the normal.

Dependency The desire to continually use a substance.

Depressants Substances that depress the central nervous system to slow down physical and mental activity.

Dermis (DER mis) The deeper of the two layers of skin.

Designer drug A potent and illegal street drug formed from a medicinal substance whose chemical composition has been modified ("designed").

Diabetes (di ah BE tez) A condition in which the body does not produce enough insulin.

Diabetic (di ah BET ik) A person with the condition diabetes mellitus.

Diabetic emergency A condition in which a person becomes ill because of an imbalance of insulin.

Diaphragm (DI a fram) A dome-shaped muscle that aids breathing and separates the chest from the abdomen.

Direct pressure The pressure applied by one's hand on a wound to control bleeding.

Disease An abnormal condition of the body that impairs normal function of cells, tissues, or body systems.

Disease transmission The transfer of disease.

Dislocation The displacement of a bone from its normal position at a joint.

Dressing A pad placed directly over a wound to absorb blood and prevent infection.

Drowning Death by suffocation when submerged in water.

Drug Any substance other than food intended to affect the functions of the body.

Emergency A situation requiring immediate action.

Emergency action principles (EAPs) Four steps to guide a person's actions in any emergency.

Emergency medical services (EMS) professionals Trained and equipped community-based personnel dispatched through a local emergency number to provide emergency care for ill or injured people; commonly, ambulance personnel.

Emergency medical services (EMS) system A network of community resources and medical personnel that provides emergency care to victims of injury or sudden illness.

Emergency medical technician (EMT) Someone who has successfully completed a state-approved Emergency Medical Technician training program. There are several different levels of EMT's, including paramedics at the highest level.

Epidermis (ep ĭ DER mis) The outer layer of skin.

Epiglottis (ep ĭ GLOT is) The flap of tissue that covers the trachea to keep food and liquid out of the lungs.

Epilepsy (EP ĭ lep se) A chronic condition characterized by seizures that vary in type and duration; can usually be controlled by medication.

Esophagus (e SOF ah gus) The tube leading from the mouth to the stomach.

Exhale To breathe air out of the lungs.

External bleeding Visible bleeding.

Extremities (ex TREM ĭ tez) The arms and legs, hands and feet.

Fainting A loss of consciousness resulting from a temporary reduction of blood to the brain.

Femoral (FEM or al) **arteries** The large arteries that supply the legs with oxygen-rich blood.

Femur (FE mur) The thighbone.

Finger sweep A technique used to remove foreign material from a victim's upper airway.

First aid Immediate care given to a victim of injury or sudden illness until more advanced care can be obtained.

First Responder A person trained in emergency care who may be called upon to provide such care as a routine part of his or her job.

Forearm The upper extremity from the elbow to the wrist.

Fracture A break or disruption in bone tissue.

Frostbite A serious condition in which body tissues freeze, more commonly in the fingers, toes, ears, and nose.

Full-thickness burn A burn injury involving the layers of skin and the underlying tissues.

Genitals The external reproductive organs.

Germs Disease-producing microorganisms.

Good Samaritan laws Laws that protect citizens giving first aid in an emergency.

Hallucinogens (hah lu SĬ no jenz) Substances that affect mood, sensation, thought, emotion, and self-awaremess; alter peceptions of time; and space and produce delusions.

Head-tilt/chin-lift A technique for opening the airway.

Heart A fist-size muscular organ that pumps blood throughout the body.

Heart attack A sudden illness involving the death of heart muscle tissue when it does not receive enough oxygen-rich blood.

Heart disease Cardiovascular disease.

Heat cramps Painful spasms of skeletal muscles following exercise or work in warm or moderate temperatures; usually involve the calf and abdominal muscles

Heat exhaustion A form of shock, often resulting from strenuous work or exercise in a hot environment.

Heat stroke A life-threatening condition that develops when the body's cooling mechanisms are overwhelmed and body systems begin to fail.

Hemorrhage (HEM or ij) A loss of a large amount of blood in a short period of time from arteries, veins, or capillaries.

Hormone A substance that circulates in body fluids and has a specific effect on cell activity.

Humerus (HU mer us) The bone of the upper arm.

Hyperglycemia (hi per gli SE me ah) A condition in which too much sugar is in the bloodstream.

Hyperventilation (hi per ven tĭ LA shun) Abnormally increased breathing rate.

Hypoglycemia (hi po gli SE me ah) A condition in which too little sugar is in the bloodstream.

Hypothermia A life-threatening condition in which the body's warming mechanisms fail to maintain normal body temperature and the entire body cools.

Immobilization (im mo bi li ZA shun) The use of a splint or other method to keep an injured body part from moving.

Immune (ĭ MŪN) **system** The body system that protects against infection.

Immunization (im u nĭ ZA shun) The introduction of a specific substance into the body that builds resistance to an infection.

Impaled object An object that remains embedded in a wound.

Infection A condition caused by disease-producing microorganisms in the body.

Ingested poison A poison that is swallowed.

Inhalants (in HA lants) Substances inhaled to produce an intoxicating effect.

Inhale To breathe in.

Inhaled poison A poison breathed into the lungs.

Injection The placing of a substance into the body through a bite, a sting, or a hypodermic needle.

Injected poison A poison that enters the body through a bite, a sting, or a hypodermic needle.

Injury A condition that occurs when the body is subjected to an external force, such as a blow, a fall, or a collision.

In-line stabilization A technique used to minimize movement of the victim's head and neck while providing care.

Insulin (IN su lin) A hormone that enables the body to use sugar for energy; frequently used to treat diabetes.

Insulin-dependent diabetes A type of diabetes that occurs when the body produces little or no insulin.

Integumentary (in teg u MEN tar e) Relating to the body system that includes the skin, nails, and hair.

Internal bleeding Bleeding inside the body.

Involuntary Without conscious control or direction.

Joint A structure where two or more bones are joined.

Laceration (las e RA shun) A cut, usually from a sharp object; may have jagged or smooth edges.

Leg The entire lower extremity from the pelvis to the foot.

Ligament (LIG ah ment) A fibrous band that holds bones together at a joint.

Liver A large abdominal organ that has many functions; when injured, it can bleed severely.

Lower leg The lower extremity between the knee and the ankle.

Lungs A pair of organs in the chest that provides the mechanism for taking oxygen in and removing carbon dioxide during breathing.

Lyme disease An illness transmitted by a certain kind of infected tick.

Medical emergency A sudden illness requiring immediate medical attention.

Medication A drug given to prevent or correct a disease or condition or otherwise enhance mental or physical welfare.

Membrane (MEM bran) A thin sheet of tissue that covers a structure or lines a cavity such as the mouth or nose.

Microorganism (mi kro OR gah nizm) A bacteria, virus, or other microscopic organism that may enter the body. Those that cause an infection or disease are called germs.

Muscle Tissue that lengthens and shortens to create movement.

Musculoskeletal (mus ku lo SKEL e tal) Relating to the muscles and the skeleton.

Narcotics (nar KOT iks) Powerful depressant substances used to relieve anxiety and pain.

Near-drowning A situation in which a person who has been submerged in water survives.

Nerve A part of the nervous system that sends impulses to and from the brain and all body parts.

Noninsulin-dependent diabetes A type of diabetes that occurs when the body produces insufficient quantities of insulin.

Nutrients Substances that provide nourishment.

Open wound A wound resulting in a break in the skin surface.

Organ A group of specialized cells and tissues that work together to do a specific job.

Overdose A situation in which a person takes enough of a substance that it has toxic (poisonous) or fatal effects.

Oxygen A tasteless, colorless, odorless gas, essential in order to maintain life.

Pancreas (PAN kre as) An organ in the abdomen that makes insulin for the body.

Paramedic Someone certified after successfully completing a state-approved paramedic training program. Paramedics represent the highest level of EMTs.

Paraphernalia Equipment.

Partial-thickness burn A burn injury involving both layers of skin, characterized by wet, red skin and blisters.

Pelvis (PEL vis) The lower part of the trunk, containing the intestines, bladder, and reproductive organs; a group of bones that surrounds the pelvic area.

Personal flotation device (PFD) A buoyant device such as a cushion or lifejacket; designed to be held or worn to keep a person afloat.

Pharynx (FAR ingks) A part of the airway formed by the back of the nose and throat.

Plasma (PLAZ mah) The liquid part of blood.

Platelets Structures in the blood made up of cell fragments; essential for blood clotting.

Poison Any substance that causes injury, illness, or death when introduced into the body.

Pores Tiny openings in the skin that help regulate body temperature.

Poison Control Center (PCC) A special health center that provides information in cases of poisoning or suspected poisoning emergencies.

Pressure bandage A bandage applied snugly to create pressure on a wound or injury; used to help control bleeding.

Pressure points Sites on the body where pressure can be applied to major arteries to slow the flow of blood to a body part.

Primary survey A check for conditions that are an immediate threat to a victim's life.

Profuse bleeding Rapid and heavy bleeding.

Pulse The beat felt in arteries with each contraction of the heart.

Puncture A wound that results when the skin is pierced with a pointed object such as a nail.

Rabies A disease caused by a virus transmitted through the saliva of an infected animal.

Radial (RA de al) artery The artery that supplies the hand and fingers with blood.

Red blood cells The solid component of blood that transports oxygen and carbon dioxide.

Reproductive organs Male and female organs with reproductive functions, including internal organs and the genitals.

Rescue breathing The technique of breathing for a nonbreathing victim.

Respiration The breathing process of the body that takes in oxygen and eliminates carbon dioxide.

Respiratory (re SPI rah to re *or* RES pah rah tor e) Relating to the breathing process.

Respiratory arrest The condition in which breathing has stopped.

Respiratory distress The condition in which breathing is difficult.

Rib cage The cage of bones formed by the 12 pairs of ribs, the sternum, and the spine.

Risk factors Conditions or behaviors that increase the chance that a person will develop a disease.

Rupture A tear or break in an organ or body tissue; to tear or break.

Scapula (SKAP u lah) See shoulder blade.

Secondary survey A check for injuries or conditions that could become life-threatening problems if not cared for.

Seizure (SE zhur) A disorder in the brain's electrical activity, marked by loss of consciousness and uncontrollable muscle movement.

Shock The failure of the circulatory system to provide adequate oxygen-rich blood to all parts of the body.

Shoulder blade A large, flat, triangular bone at the back of the shoulder in the upper part of the back; also called the scapula.

Shoulder separation Dislocation of the shoulder in which the shoulder blade is separated from the collarbone.

Skeletal muscles Muscles that attach to bones.

Skin A tough, supple membrane that covers the entire surface of the body.

Skull The bony structure of the head.

Sling A bandage used to hold and support an injured part of the body, often an arm.

Soft tissue Body structures that include the layers of skin, fat, and muscles.

Spinal column The column of bones (vertebrae) extending from the base of the skull to the tip of the tailbone (coccyx).

Spinal cord A bundle of nerves extending from the brain at the base of the skull to the lower back; protected by the spinal column.

Spine A series of bones (vertebrae) that surrounds and protects the spinal cord; also called the backbone.

Spleen An organ in the abdomen; one of its functions is to store blood.

Splint A device used to immobilize body parts.

Sprain The stretching and tearing of ligaments and other soft tissue structures at a joint.

Sterile Free from living microorganisms.

Sternum (STER num) The long, flat bone in the middle of the front of the rib cage; also called the breastbone.

Stimulants Substances that affect the central nervous system to speed up physical and mental activity.

Stomach One of the main organs of digestion, located in the abdomen.

Strain The stretching and tearing of muscles and tendons.

Stroke A disruption of blood flow to a part of the brain that causes permanent damage; also called a cerebrovascular accident (CVA).

Substance abuse The deliberate, persistent, excessive use of a substance without regard to health concerns or accepted medical practices.

Substance misuse The use of a substance for unintended purposes or for intended purposes but in improper amounts or doses.

Sucking chest wound An injury in which the chest cavity is punctured allowing air to pass freely in and out of the chest cavity.

Superficial burn A burn injury involving only the top layer of skin; characterized by red, dry skin.

Survival floating A facedown floating technique that enables a victim in warm water to conserve energy while waiting for rescue.

Tendon (TEN don) A fibrous band that attaches muscle to bone.

Tetanus (TET ah nus) An acute infectious disease.

Thigh The lower extremity between the pelvis and the knee.

Tissue A collection of similar cells that act together to perform specific body functions.

Tolerance A condition that occurs when a substance user has to increase the dose and frequency of use to obtain the desired effect.

Trachea (TRA ke ah) A tube leading from the upper airway to the lungs; also called the windpipe.

Traction (TRAK shun) splint A mechanical device that reduces the deformity of a leg fracture by stretching the muscles to prevent the leg from shortening.

Transient (TRANZ e ent) **ischemic** (is KE mik) **attack (TIA)** A stroke-like episode that does not cause permanent damage.

Trauma A wound or injury caused by violent force; the force or mechanism, such as a fall, pressure, or shock, that causes such an injury.

Trunk The part of the body containing the chest, abdomen, and pelvis.

Upper Arm The upper extremity from the shoulder to the elbow.

Veins Blood vessels that carry oxygen-poor blood from all parts of the body to the heart.

Venom Poison, usually transmitted by bites or stings.

Ventricular (ven TRIK u lar) **fibrillation** (fi bri la shun) An abnormal heart rhythm occurring when no organized electrical impulse controls heart contractions, causing the heart to fail to pump blood.

Vertebrae (VER te bra) The 33 bones of the spinal column.

Virus A disease-producing microorganism.

Vital organs Organs whose functions are essential to life, including the brain, heart, and lungs.

Vital signs Important information about the victim's condition, obtained by checking breathing, pulse, and skin characteristics.

Voluntary With conscious control or direction.

Withdrawal A condition produced when a person stops using or abusing a substance to which he or she is addicted.

Wound An injury to the soft tissues.

Sources

Baker, S.P.; O'Neill, B.; and Karpf, R.S. *The Injury Fact Book*. Lexington, Massachusetts: Lexington Books, D.C. Heath and Co., 1984.

Buchanan, J.F., and Brown, C.R. "Designer Drugs: A Problem in Clinical Toxicology." *Medical Toxicology,* 3:(1988):1-17.

Climko, R.P.; Roehrich, H.; Sweeney, D.R.; and El-Razi, J. "Ecstasy—a review of MDMA and MDA." *International Journal of Psychiatry in Medicine,* 16:(4) (1987):359-371.

Committee on Trauma Research; Commission on Life Sciences; National Research Council; and the Institute of Medicine. *Injury in America*. Washington, D.C.: National Academy Press, 1985.

Consumer Guide with Chasnoff, I.J.; Ellis, J.W.; and Fainman, Z.S. *The New Illustrated Family Medical & Health Guide*. Lincolnwood, Illinois: Publications International, Ltd., 1988.

Getchell, B.; Pippin, R.; and Varnes, J. *Health*. Boston: Houghton Mifflin Co., 1989.

Hamilton, E.M.N., and Whitney, E.N. *Nutrition, Concepts and Controversies*. ed. 2, rev. Eleanor Noss Whitney. St. Paul: West Publishing Co., 1982.

Lamar, J.V., Jr. "Crack." *Time*, June 2, 1986.

Lierman, T.L., editor. *Building a Healthy America: Conquering Disease and Disability*. New York: Mary Ann Liebert, Inc., Publishers, 1987.

Litovitz, T.L.; Schmitz, B.S.; and Holm, K.C. "1988 Annual Report of the American Association of Poison Control Centers National Data Collection System." *American Journal of Emergency Medicine,* 7(5)(September 1989):496.

Marion Laboratories. *Osteoporosis: Is it in your future?* Kansas City: Marion Laboratories, 1984.

National Capital Poison Center, Georgetown University Hospital, 3800 Reservoir Rd., N.W., Washington, D.C. 20007, 202-625-3333

National Committee for Injury Prevention and Control. *Injury Prevention: Meeting the Challenge*. New York: Oxford University Press as a supplement to the American Journal of Preventive Medicine, Volume 5, Number, 3, 1989.

National Safety Council. *Accident Facts, 1989 Edition*. Chicago: National Safety Council, 1989.

National Safety Council; and Thygerson, A.L., editors. *First Aid Essentials*. Boston: Jones and Bartlett Publishers, 1989.

Payne, W.A., and Hahn, D.B. *Understanding Your Health*. St. Louis: Mosby—Year Book, Inc., 1989.

Rice, D.P.; MacKenzie, E.J.; and Associates. *Cost of Injury in the United States: a Report to Congress 1989*. San Francisco, California: Institute for Health and Aging, University of California, and Injury Prevention Center, The Johns Hopkins University, 1989.

Strauss, Richard H., editor. *Sports Medicine*. Philadelphia: W.B. Saunders Co., 1984.

The White House. *National Drug Control Strategy*. September 1989.

U.S. Department of Health and Human Services; Public Health Service; Alcohol, Drug Abuse, and Mental Health Administration; and National Institute on Alcohol Abuse and Alcoholism. *Seventh Special Report to the U.S. Congress on Alcohol and Health*. Alexandria, Virginia: Editorial Experts, Inc., January 1990.

Wardlaw, G.M., and Insel, P.M. *Perspectives in Nutrition*. St. Louis: Mosby—Yearbook, Inc., 1990.

Index